Polka-Dot Bath

Marklyn Beck

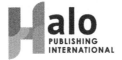
Halo
PUBLISHING
INTERNATIONAL

ISBN: 978-1-61244-916-6
LCCN: 202091934

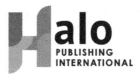

Halo Publishing International, LLC
8000 W Interstate 10, Suite 600
San Antonio, Texas 78230
www.halopublishing.com

Printed and bound in the United States

Contents

Preface

Inquiring minds want to know - just call me Marlene.

I've been known to say and wholly mean, "Life's a trip, a trip for which you can't even pack, as—regardless of all your plans, thoughts, considerations, and preparations—you never really know where life is going to take you until you get there. As often as not, it's not exactly where you were headed; sometimes it's a far cry from there. But *there* you are."

That's what this book is all about. I'm going to tell you what to expect when you get *there* and where *there* is. My guess is that it's a far cry from where you think you're headed. But you're headed *there*, just as sure as the sky changes colors and the clock changes time. In fact, if you're over fifty, you're headed *there* just as fast and furious as springtime changes the weather! You might want to speed read; buy yourself some time to promote change before you do get *there*.

No guessing to it; this is fact. Without some serious systems overhaul, you aren't going to like it when you do get *there*. And on this particular subject I readily self-profess expertise.

I've been a nurse for twenty-eight years, an LVN for one, and an RN for twenty-seven. I've worked with geriatrics, more commonly referred to as "old people," for twenty-seven of those twenty-eight years. I have *seen* our societies' throwaways. Like that charming little thrift shop downtown, nursing homes are chock-full of treasures that are tossed out like junk.

While my daughter was growing up, I maintained an eight-to-five schedule, but I always planned to make a change to long-term care once she was grown, out on her own. Like everyone else, I had heard the horror stories about nursing homes. I wanted to see if the horror stories were true; I wanted to try to make a difference if they were. So I've been employed in long-term care facilities, aka nursing homes, for a total of thirteen years. I've worked in seven different facilities, for six different corporations, in five different cities. And I've held every position from

Administrator, to Director of Nursing, to Assistant Director to charge nurse, aka floor nurse. I'm thinking that puts me in the position for a fair assessment, and I'm here to tell you that throughout the system the patterns may vary somewhat in color or light, but they are consistent.

The good news is that I haven't *personally* seen a single sign of the horror stories I'd heard about. The bad news is that I've seen a gazillion different versions of horror stories I'd never heard about or even imagined possible. You see, that's what makes it so bad. The things that do commonly happen—the things that happen day after day in facility after facility—are wrongful things about which no one dares to speak. Things so infinitely *wrong* that they are fast tucked away with hopes of being forever concealed by the settling dust. Things about which no one could possibly know, except those who dare not speak. But you, you *need* to know, so someone must speak. I happen to have just the right combination of love, courage, and stupidity to do the job.

So now you know what this book is about; you know who I am and what makes me an expert on the subject. But why am I writing it? It's simple. I am determined to flip the light switch that reveals the realities of long-term care, the current realities of our elderly, and the future realities for you, me, our friends, families, our children and our children's children... These things have been quietly, but no doubt intentionally, tucked away in the dark for way too long. I'm hoping that once the light is on, allowing us to see, we might clean out our societal closet.

One last thought, and I tend to shoot pretty straight, so duck if you offend easily.

Truth is, I was ranting to God one morning about where life has taken our elderly, when the seed for this book was planted. I ranted on about the heartbreaking, anger-inducing wrongs I'd seen at work the day before. This having drudged up a mental ambush of *things* that will forever haunt the halls of my heart. I pretty much wanted to know what He was going to do about it.

God interrupted and said, "I created you."

If I don't do something, knowing all that I know, having seen all that I've seen, and having heard all that I've heard, I will deserve exactly *where* life is taking me. I don't want to go *there*, and I sure as heck don't want to deserve it. So I pretty much need to know what *I'm* going to do about it.

So I'm telling you.

Similarly, if you don't do something, knowing all that you will know after reading this book, you will deserve precisely *where* life is taking you. Trust the expert; you do not want to go *there*, and you most certainly do not want to deserve it. So you pretty much need to know what *you* are going to do about it.

Before I go any further, please allow me a moment:

Nurses, though many of you appear to think of nursing as a Girl Scout or Boy Scout badge, thank you. Regardless of your true heart and/or professionalism, you have my respect for doing what you do and continuing to keep steppin' day after day despite the *all* of it.

However, put on your big-boy and big-girl pants and read this with an open heart and mind. It makes a tremendous difference in perspective.

Although nursing is no doubt a chosen career for you, it is an unchosen need for those in your care. The undeniable and overwhelming problems in the nursing profession are not your patients' or residents' fault. What time you get off or who chews you out about overtime, how exhausted or stressed you may be... these things, though no doubt significant, are not nearly as significant as the care your patients receive ...or don't receive.

If you recognize yourself in any aspect of these pages, please, stop and think, do not take offense; seek change. Lastly, wait for the sequel. What matters here, today, is the people within these pages and the multitudes of similar souls in similar circumstances, along with those of us (*you* and me) who are headed *there*.

Now then, with that said...

This book, this is the how; how things really are *there*. We'll get to the why.

Introduction

I wanted to take my daughter, Ava Kate, for a ride in a hot air balloon, something she, too, has always wanted to do. I checked into the details, and it turns out that they serve champagne and a fruit and cheese tray that can be savored as you drift across the sky, floating through the clouds. It struck me suddenly; I could almost hear an angelic choir as the thought hit me. I told Ava I planned to get her tipsy, grab her ankles, and dangle her over the edge of the basket until she agreed to sign a legal document ensuring I would never be placed in a nursing home. Ava loved that, she laughed hard, but, by dang, she hasn't let me schedule that ride! I'm thinking I maybe shouldn't have told her my plan...

The good, the bad, and the ugly. I'm gonna tell it. It's way past time that somebody did. You need to know. That said, I'm just going to tell you like it is, just as I've seen it. I'm completely unable at this point—probably ever—to sugarcoat the reality of it all. I'm about to open the closet.

All the "stuff" human beings have so diligently, sometimes laboriously, tucked away in the dark is about to tumble down off the shelves as I tell you nothing short of the absolute truth. Some of it, to some people, won't sound as bad as it is; some of it, to some people, will sound worse than it is. Regardless, it all *is*. That's what you need to remember. It *is*. It *is* your future. It *is* your loved ones' present. This *is* where life is taking you, although this is almost certainly not where you think *you* are headed.

Before I dig in, allow me to point out that I am not suggesting perfection. You have people serving people, human beings serving human beings. When human beings are involved, perfection is not even in the realm of possibility. However, I am suggesting better. Much better, in fact. Better is always possible; better is a must. The key word here is "human." As you read, remember that you are reading about human beings. Our elderly are simply us, you and me, with more miles under their feet; miles resulting in wrinkles on the outside. Inside, however, elderly people are just as wrinkle free as you and me. They still dream, still wish, still hope, and still have feelings, a sense of humor, and opinions. Folks, they are not dead. They are not old, empty shells waiting to be buried in the sand. Don't bury them alive.Our elderly are every bit as alive today as they were the day they were born. And sadly, the vast majority are just as vulnerable. Unfortunately, they are not nearly as cute and cuddly. So, as a society, we throw them away and forget about them. Before we human beings twisted this world inside out, the elderly were respected, revered, literally sought out for their experience and wisdom. The elderly knew they were considered extremely valuable. Now we idolize our young and naïve; we toss out our old and wise. Our elderly know they are considered extremely useless.

I went to a job interview once, having received an employment proposition from a recruiter, via email. It offered yet another angle on the lives and care of our elderly. Thus, I wanted very much to check it out.

The interviewer was a corporate nurse who, while sloppily munching his way through three bags of barbecue Fritos, informed me that he was the interim administrator while the company sought a replacement for the administrator they had "canned". He then sat back in his big leather chair, stuffed his hand back into a Frito bag, and blurted, "So you're in long-term care. WHY?!" His lip curled in disgust as he leaned his chair dramatically backward.

Resisting the urge to hand him a napkin, I replied, "Well, to be honest, sir, I had long heard the horror stories about nursing homes. I wanted to see how much truth was in them, and I wanted to see if I could make a difference."

Flinging himself forward, a look of disbelief on his face, he slapped his Frito bag down on his desk and dusted his hands as he proclaimed, "How naïve! You can't make a difference. You're kidding yourself. Nursing homes are just a place to stick people when you've got nothing else to do with them."

Shifting in my seat to maintain professional composure, I quietly responded, "Well, in essence, sir, that is precisely the perspective—reality, if you will—that I desire to change. Further, though I am fully cognitive, wearily so, that I alone cannot make a difference for all individuals in nursing homes, I do feel I have made, I do make, a difference for those in my care."

Shaking his head with a vengeance, he declared arrogantly, "I have just added another RN position to this facility." Scooping his Frito bag from his desk, he leaned back in his chair once more and smugly finished, saying, "Now *that's* making a difference. Nurses are overloaded, and the nurses here deal with crazy, old, hopeless people all day, every day. I lightened their miserable load."

I stood, smiled, thanked him for his time, and exited before my thoughts became words.

This guy—this Frito-devouring, smugly arrogant dude—is a corporate nurse for a corporation that provides psychiatric services specifically to our geriatric population, aka old people. Many of their patients, if not most, are admitted due to depression, some with suicidal thoughts and/or attempts; these receiving treatment to help them find reason, desire, and motivation to continue breathing. A vast number of the geriatric patients they serve are coming from and returning to nursing homes. You know, "the place we stick people when there just isn't anything else to do with them." Frito dude is overall responsible for ensuring the implementation and maintenance of a program designed to provide effective treatment for emotional disorders, to inspire and instill hope and a desire to live in these "crazy, old, hopeless people" that make up his nurses' "miserable load."

One undeniable fact is that if God doesn't grant you and me an early departure, if we don't have a ton of money to hire private caregivers to provide for us at home, and/or if we don't literally luck out in being one of those very rare souls who maintains good health, functional ability, mental clarity, and financial security until the day we die … we're up next folks! No doubt about it.

I've heard my father say many times, "Once you hit fifty, it's a downhill slide." Well, if I've got to downhill slide into the reality of a nursing home as I now know them to be, I'm going to be kicking and screaming the whole way down!

Speaking of kicking and screaming, meet Mabel:

Mabel's real name was Marybell. However, her younger brother never mastered the mouthful; all he could manage was May-bil, so over time Mabel stuck.

Mabel was a quiet, soft-spoken, genteel southern lady. She seldom spoke at all, saying only what needed to be said. Otherwise, provided Mabel had her snuff, a spit cup, "proper clothes," and a "proper hat," she sat content-edly in her rocker recliner for hours on end, leaving it only at mealtimes and bedtime.

One evening I noticed Mabel hadn't yet been taken to the dining room for dinner, so I went in her room to get her.

"I need to go to the bathroom first, please, ma'am," Mabel said softly.

So, I helped Mabel transfer from her recliner to her wheelchair, then wheeled her into the bathroom. After toileting, I turned Mabel to the sink. "Let me help you wash your hands."

Mabel smiled so big I thought her dentures might fall out. "I never get to wash my hands!" she sang softly. "Are you sure you have time to help me with that, too?"

"Well, of course."

"Why, thank you, ma'am," Mabel delighted in her ever-hushed tone.

Helping Mabel stand at the sink, I kept her chair right behind her, touching the backs of her knees, just in case she tired too quickly.

"Oh shit!" Mabel squawked suddenly. "Who the hell is *that?*"

I was stunned to absolute silence, never having heard such language or anything near such volume from Mabel! If I hadn't heard it with my own ears, I would not have believed it. It worked out okay, as Mabel wasn't waiting for a response. Immediately, oblivious to my presence, Mabel stood gaping into the mirror with wide eyes, knuckles white as she gripped the sink with both hands, completely absorbed in the moment.

I watched as Mabel's face changed from surprise to outright suspicion. Her brow creased, and she slowly moved her head, first one way, then the other, while staring into the mirror. Still not convinced, Mabel raised her bent finger and touched the tip of her nose. Her eyes popped back open as wide as saucers, and her chin dropped nearly to the floor as she stood gaping into that mirror.

"Oh my," she whispered. "Ooooh my, oh my." She slowly shook her head.

So there we were, staring. I was staring at Mabel; Mabel was staring into the mirror. Both of us were as silent as snow. I literally jumped when Mabel suddenly pierced the silence with an explosion of laughter, laughing so hard she lost her balance! Instinctively, I reached out, guiding her hips down into the seat of her wheelchair as I, too, burst out laughing right along with her, having no clue as to what either of us was laughing about. Mabel slapped her thighs, rocking so hard with laughter that her hat plopped from her head onto her lap as tears streamed down the creases in her cheeks, then dripped off her chin. Finally, gasping for air, Mabel shrieked, "By damn, I think that ugly old thing is *me!*" She roared ever louder.

Laughing even harder, I leaned against the wall, then slunk to the floor next to Mabel's chair to keep from falling myself.

Staff members popped up in the doorway to see what on earth was causing the commotion, but Mabel and I were unable to stop laughing to explain. Mabel's contagious laughter spread like a delightful virus, and within moments the hallway outside Mabel's doorway was jammed with staff and residents, all laughing hysterically, not a single one of them having any clue what was so funny.

Ultimately, all quietened down. Catching their breath and wiping tears from their eyes, everybody wandered off to their prospective locations, no longer able to await an explanation or simply too revived by the joyful laughter to care.

Mabel composed herself, wiping her face with her hands. Then, picking up her hat from where it had fallen onto her lap, she replaced it on her head and straightened it just right.

"Well, I guess we best be getting along now, please, ma'am," she said softly, a mischievous smirk lingering at the corners of her mouth.

Mabel squared her shoulders as I wheeled her to the dining room. Placing her at her table, I bent to lock the brakes on her wheelchair. Mabel leaned forward and whispered into my ear, "I still *feel* like me." She shrugged. "But I sho don't look like me no more!" She snickered. "I hadn't seen my own face in years! I've sat quietly in that chair and got old. If I'd known, I'd have been up kicking and screaming!" Mable slapped a wrinkled hand over her mouth, stifling another outburst of laughter. Then she cleared her throat and placed that same cool, wrinkled old hand over mine, "My apologies for my ugly language in the bathroom. It just slipped out. I do beg your pardon. Can that just be our little secret, please, ma'am?"

"What language? I didn't hear a thing."

Mabel squeezed my hand, then settled back in her chair, lifted her chin, and winked. "Thank you, ma'am." Her black eyes were as shiny as new marbles.

"My pleasure, ma'am."

Basics are Big

Allow me to introduce you to a few more treasures:

John:

A quiet, soft-spoken loner. A long recovering alcoholic who never married nor had children. A quick-witted soul with a mischievous sparkle in his ever-observant pale blue eyes and a sarcastic edge to his few words, John went with the flow, never created wrinkles. He seldom said much, but when he did, he spoke volumes in his slow country drawl.

State was in the building, conducting their annual survey. This notorious staff-cutting corporate office was paying staff overtime, which they usually stood so firmly against, to either come in or stay over and help management catch up on the facility's nearly *five hundred* belated, mandatory patient care needs assessments, hopefully before the end of survey.

So there I sat at the nurses' station, working diligently on assessments due long before I ever walked back in the front door, when I peered over the counter to see John shuffling out of the dining room with one hand gripping his walker, the other gripping a cup of coffee, and nothing on his feet but socks. They were regular socks, not the grip socks facilities provide to help prevent falls. Bear in mind now that the lobby was carpeted, but the dining room floor was slip-ready laminate.

"Mr. John? Where on earth are your shoes?" I laughed.

He stopped mid-step and gazed briefly and blankly over my head as he took a deep breath, as if it took every ounce of his strength to explain the obvious to the ignorant.

"Weeell, when they moved me to this room from my old room"—he shrugged, brows raised—"I didn't have shoes no more."

Oh, simple as that, I thought to myself. Knowing said room change took place months earlier, coinciding with yet another corporate mandated staff cut, I replied as I stood, "Oh, come on now, let's go find your shoes."

"Okay." He shrugged, then shuffled my way.

So, off we went together, down the hall to John's room. I flipped the light switch, and John sat on the side of his bed as I opened his small, free-standing double closet, which was jam-packed on both sides with John's belongings, as he currently had no roommate. Right away I noticed the bulging white trash bags tied up at the bottom of the closet. John watched without expression, sipping his coffee as I pulled the bags out into the room. His eyes popped open, and a grin spread ear to ear when I dug deep, then pulled out a pair of black sneakers.

"Well, look at that. I do have shoes," he drawled with genuine wonder, his pale blue eyes big and round as he scratched his balding head.

John spoke more in that half hour than he had the entire time I'd known him, watching as I pulled one thing after another out of those bags. Sadly, many items had long been replaced at his expense, including his electric razor, personal items like antiperspirant and a toothbrush, and his clock. John liked to know the correct time. He pointed proudly at his new clock, which had been purchased for him months prior, with his meager funds of course, to replace the "lost" clock.

"I like this new one with the big numbers. I can see it real good," he commented casually. "I don't need that one no more. You can give it to somebody who needs it."

Then I pulled out a brand-new pair of white sneakers, and John's face turned red as he chuckled heartily. "Well, I'll be! I got more!" he said almost loudly, his mouth gaping. "Kinda feels like Christmas," he added to himself.

I set the white sneakers on the laminate floor next to the black ones and continued to empty the bags, throwing the mixed-in trash away and finding a place to put items as I went. Then I pulled out a small metal box holding three pencils.

John gasped, stared, then drawled just loud enough to be heard, "I been looking for them pencils for a long, long time."

By "looking," I feel certain John meant he had been pondering where they might be.

John took that pencil box like I was handing him lost treasure. Slowly, almost reverently, he took the three pencils from the box and clutched them in his old fist as he lay back on his bed, tears welling in the corners of his eyes.

"My buddy gave me these before he died," he mumbled softly to the ceiling.

I stopped. "That guy that used to pick you up twice a week and take you to the AA meetings?"

"Yeah." He looked at me, surprised. "You remember him?"

"Well, yes, I do. You were always happiest on those days. He was a good friend. Nice guy."

"Yeah. He was. Best friend a man could have." He smiled, chuckled softly, and shifted his gaze toward the sunlight streaming in through the window.

Bending over, I pulled a drawing pad from the bottom of one of the bags. John looked over and began shifting his body to sit up. I waited, then handed him the pad as he stared at it in awed silence.

"I didn't know you liked to draw!" I exclaimed.

"Oh yeah. I'm purty good at it. Been drawin' my whole life."

"Well, you've got your pencils and your pad. I want a picture!"

John's eyes sparkled. "Okay." He chuckled.

Wadding the trash bag, I rolled my eyes. "I want my picture, Mr. John. I'm no dummy. I can tell when I'm being blown off."

"Aww, now, nobody can blow *you* off." He chuckled. "It ain't *even* possible."

After tossing the empty bags into the trash can, I was starting for the door when Mr. John stopped me.

"I'd like to put the black ones on now, if you don't mind," he requested, almost as if he were embarrassed.

Realizing John did not want to let go of his pencils to put his shoes on, I readily turned back to help him. Moments later I left Mr. John lying back on his bed with his black sneakers on, ankles crossed, still clutching those pencils in his right fist as he gazed out the window.

"Turn that light out as you leave, please. And thank you for everything," he mumbled quietly.

On the bright side, I never saw Mr. John out of bed without his shoes on again. On the not-so-bright side, me being me, I was furious. I looked in John's records. He had been moved to his new room two years, three months, three weeks, and four days before that day. Thus, he'd been *that* long without shoes. Knowing of two recent falls he'd had in his room, I looked. Each time he'd fallen, it was documented that he'd been reminded to wear shoes or grip socks when out of bed. Yet he had neither available to him. To top it all off, out of the whopping sixty dollars a month/fifteen dollars a week he was allotted from his check, they'd replaced, at his expense, all the personal items that had been stuffed in a trash bag in his closet the entire time. Well, they'd replaced everything but shoes.

On a happy note, I still have the picture of the sneakers John drew for me. He *is*; he's "purty" good!

Anna, aka Ms. D:

Ms. D had the most beautifully intense blue eyes I had ever seen. She was a true lady: gentle, kind, soft-spoken, and proper.

I was getting report one afternoon from Lynn, the nurse I was relieving. Lynn was extremely hyperactive. Did I say extreme? Because I meant *extreme*! Lynn was anxiety-ridden, and anxiety-inducing, though she had a good heart and was truly a conscientious nurse. But Lynn was no doubt one of those people whose hands, head, and body are as involved in speaking as their mouth is. She had innumerable nervous habits, twitches, and truly strange, almost unnerving expressions. At times I wanted to swear her eyes went in two different directions. And though irrelevant in the big scheme of things, Lynn seldom washed her hair. Thus, I found it distracting that the top of her hair clung to her head as the bottom swung with her endless motion. I say this simply to emphasize the difficulty of just getting report from her. A tiring process.

Anyway, there I stood, struggling to hide my frustration and maintain polite composure while getting report from a human explosion, when I noticed a soft, monotone "water" in the background, over and over and over again, every few seconds.

Strangely, as I glanced around, it appeared no one else heard this incessant repetition. As the explosion continued, I gazed around the entire area and noticed Ms. D sitting in her wheelchair, facing the TV (that day's activity was 'movie time'). Her head was down, and her long gray hair, which we knew she preferred up in a tidy bun, hung limp and unkempt. She sat unmoving, except for her lips, which repeated "water" incessantly. I noticed a therapist standing just behind her, watching the movie over the top of her head. I glanced at the Activity Director, who was sitting at a nearby table, painting some of the ladies' fingernails. I watched a member of the kitchen staff roll the cart of evening snacks, along with jugs of juice and Kool-Aid, past the back of Ms. D's chair. 'Kitchen' spoke to the therapist, who had obviously lost interest in the movie, as he turned and walked away, disappearing around the corner and down the hall. Then 'Kitchen' rolled the snack cart into the lobby, parked it in its designated place, walked back past Ms. D and then on through the dining room back to the kitchen. Ms. D repeating "water" all the while.

"I'm sorry," I blurted to Lynn, the human explosion. "I can't stand it any longer! She's thirsty; she's not asking for the moon!"

Hurrying out of the nurses' station, I grabbed a plastic cup from the nearest medication cart, filled it with water from the pitcher, stuck a straw in it, and scurried over to Ms. D.

That precious woman took that cup and started sucking on the straw as if her very life depended upon it, which, I guess it did at that. Suddenly, she stopped, panting as she pulled the straw from the cup and placed it on her lap. Then turning the cup upside down, she drained it without stopping, handed it back to me and said, "water." Over halfway through the third cup, Ms. D stopped drinking, sighed heavily, handed me the cup with a wet-lipped smile, and said, "Thank you."

I walked away as Ms. D resumed her usual repetition of "help me." Her dementia had progressed to the extent that she repeated "help me" incessantly, except when she was sleeping deeply. Ms. D repeated "help me" while being helped. A very dignified woman who had raised several successful children and then buried her husband of sixty years, Ms. D had been cared for in her son's home until her dementia progressed to the point that she began the incessant "help me," which, in all fairness, would have driven even Mother Teresa up the proverbial wall if she'd had to hear it twenty-four-seven.

That evening, while feeding Ms. D at dinner, I noticed that she was much more interested in the fluids than the food. I also noticed that she reeked of ammonia. Once her thirst was satisfied, she started repeating "bathroom." So I requested her aide take her to her room to use the restroom.

Her aid replied, "She just say that. She never go once we get her in there. She just say things. She don't know what she sayin'."

I then requested that the aid take her to her room, check to see if she was soiled, and, if so, clean her up and change her brief.

"She dry. She always dry. I only has to change her at bedtime, and sometime she dry then, but I changes her anyway cuz her brief be all worn out by then. I takes care of my residents."

"Why would her brief be all worn out by then?" I heard myself ask out loud.

"Cuz she usually done had it on all day. We don't change 'em unlessen they wet or shitty," the aid replied indignantly, as if speaking to sheer stupidity itself.

I attempted to educate the aid on the fact that if a resident isn't voiding or wetting the brief, it is most likely due to lack of fluid intake.

The aid rolled her eyes. "She drinkin' fluids *now*, I see." She spouted sarcastically, as I assisted Ms. D with a drink.

Though she wasn't on my unit, I suggested to her nurse that they might want to check for a urinary tract infection. This based on what the aid had said, as well as the ammonia odor. I also began checking Ms. D's water jug, which was kept at her bedside. I found it empty the first time, so I filled it with ice water and, of course, assisted her with a drink. The next day the jug wasn't empty. More importantly, it appeared to be sitting precisely where I'd left it. I washed her jug out, filled it with ice water, assisted her with a drink, and then took my Chapstick out of my pocket and drew a circle around the base of the cup on the overbed table, knowing no one ever wiped the overbed tables. After trashing my Chapstick, I taped a note next to the jug, saying, "I require assistance with fluids. Please offer me a drink when you are providing any care for me. Thank you!" I drew a smiley face on the note, hoping to soften any possible, but likely, resulting attitude.

My note disappeared, but the jug never moved, the water level never changed, and my circle never vanished. Long story short, despite my efforts, Ms. D ended up in the hospital for four days with severe dehydration, urinary tract infection, and sepsis.

I was long gone—that's another story—by the time Ms. D got to leave this messed up world to go to her heavenly home. However, my sad but educated guess is that she went thirsty, with cracked lips and likely a raging urinary tract infection, repeating "water" as she drew her last dry breath.

Folks, even a *dog* deserves water.

Ms. D was a lovely lady who sang with her grandchildren every Thanksgiving. I know this because I'm tiny, and during a respite stay, long before her dementia progressed to severe and she returned to stay for good, Ms. D mistook me for one of her grandchildren. I was chattering with her about Thanksgiving while providing care one afternoon when she suddenly reached out and hugged me tight exclaiming, "Oh, honey, I have missed you! Don't tell the others, but you are my favorite grandchild! Let's start our Thanksgiving singing early, just the two of us!"

So I sat on the side of her bed and joined in on the tune. Then I cracked up laughing when Ms. D grinned big, slapped her wrinkled hand over her mouth like a kid, and said with eyes wide, "Oh my, you've lost your singing voice!"

One last thing. Ms. D was the beloved mother of our medical director. If she didn't—couldn't—get water, is your dad going to? And if one can't get *water*, what else is one doing without?

Hoppy:

Hoppy got his nickname as a small boy, and he did not want to be called anything else. A little dude with creamy brown skin, enormous copper-brown eyes, and eyelashes so long you could see them from the door, Hoppy knew he was handsome. I commented one evening on his eyes and his eyelashes. Hoppy replied quite seriously, "I know. I've always been handsome." Then he grinned mischievously and added, "But you might be the prettiest lady that ever told me so."

Hoppy was well loved. Family visited nearly every day. He was apparently a busy man once upon a time, as he had framed newspaper clippings all over his walls with pictures of him and articles about his efforts in the community. His granddaughter told me he had once been asked to run for mayor, but Hoppy had grinned and replied, "Oh no. I can't get all wrapped up in politics. I like to get things done!"

Hoppy had suffered a stroke many years before I met him. His legs were contracted, and he had a G-tube, which is a tube that is inserted into the stomach as a way of administering medications and nutrition. Hoppy had difficulty swallowing, which put him at risk of aspiration: breathing things he swallowed into his lungs. He could still eat pureed foods and drink thickened liquids, but not enough to sustain adequate nutrition, so Hoppy received medications, water, and nutritional formula via his stomach tube.

One evening, while administering Hoppy's bedtime medication, he asked for a pain pill. Hoppy was so debilitated and contracted that he cried out in pain when he had to be repositioned for the provision of care or to prevent pressure sores. I administered the pain pill via his stomach tube. But before I left his bedside, Hoppy asked for a drink. I looked, but he had no thickened water at his bedside. He usually had a glass on his table that was left over from dinner. I went up the hall to get him something to drink, but we had no thickened liquids anywhere, and Hoppy would aspirate for sure if his liquids weren't thickened. No thickener was to be found either.

I called the on-call management staff to report the circumstances. I was told, "He'll be okay until morning. He won't dehydrate overnight." I was appalled. I could not go tell this thirsty man—whom I'd just given a pain pill that would only increase his thirst—that I had nothing for him to drink. Disregarding the on-call staff, I called the Assistant Director of Nursing. She was nicer about it, but told me the same thing: "Nobody is going to come unlock the kitchen tonight. He'll be okay. Just wet the inside of his mouth with a moist Toothette (which is a sponge on a stick)."

I hurried back down the hall to do just that, despite the guilt I felt. When I sailed back into his room, toothette in hand, Hoppy exclaimed, "Oh good, you're back. I'm so *thirsty*!" His mouth sounded sticky and dry. Suddenly, I realized that I had no way of knowing how much fluid he'd had by mouth all day, *if* he'd had any at all. Then, after further thought, I realized the fluid I had administered with his four o'clock medications may well been all he had received via his tube that day. Knowing "the real world", I hurried back up the hall and called another facility in town. Ultimately, I drove over and borrowed three individual containers of thickened water and juice. Hoppy had tears in his eyes by the time I made it back to his room.

"Hey, hey, my friend! It's all good! It's okay!"

"Ma'am, I didn't think you were coming back. They told me to stop turning my light on, so I was trying to go to sleep so I could forget how thirsty I am."

"Oh, Hoppy, you should know I'm coming back. I'm never going to leave you thirsty. And you turn your light on anytime you need to. Don't worry about what they say. *They* aren't thirsty."

Hoppy was busy quenching his thirst. But when he finished, he flashed me the most beautiful, drippy-lipped smile I've ever seen! I'd have told him so, but knowing Hoppy, he'd have just said, "I know."

Georgie:

I first met Georgie in her tiny, sunbathed kitchen as her home health nurse. Her screen door banged noisily closed behind me just as I spotted her standing at her open kitchen window, "smelling the garden" drifting in on the ever-so-slight summer breeze. Georgie was a stout, dignified, delightful little woman with a crop of sandy white hair; sun-stained, leathered skin; and an undying spirit. Long before determined legally blind and deaf, her eyes and ears having abandoned her almost completely, Georgie still had crystal-clear recall of her love for books and music. Keeping herself busy tidying her little house, doing her laundry, and "traveling memory lane", Georgie still prepared her own breakfast of cereal, toast, and orange juice. Her son, who lived next door, brought her lunch and dinner. Georgie was about to celebrate her one hundredth birthday, and her family was throwing her a big party, which Georgie thought was purely "silly". "But I'm a goin'." She shrugged and chuckled, "I wouldn't hurt nobody's feelins for nothin'."

I had the honor of being present the day some ladies from her church showed up to present Georgie with an award: Fearless and Faithful Warrior for Christ; Woman after God's own heart. I cried. Georgie cried. The ladies cried. We all laughed at one another for crying. We sang "Amazing Grace" together, like kids around a campfire. It was a good day. Before I left that day, Georgie asked quietly, "I know this is going to sound strange," she chuckled, "but, would you let me feel your face so that I can see you in my mind?"

I knelt down in front of her.

"Ahh, yes." She smiled radiantly. Clapped her old hands together. "Beautiful inside and out."

The next time I saw her, two full years had passed, and Georgie was being admitted to my unit in the nursing home. Georgie was struggling, but she maintained her faith. She was always uplifting to others, but in her heart, she was baffled as to why God hadn't yet called her home. Georgie told me she "aimed to figure it out."

Having grown up, and having raised her own family on a farm, Georgie liked country cooking and vegetables fresh from the garden. Her son and I noticed she'd lost a little weight, so I started setting her meal up for her, making certain that she heard where the food was located on her plate and that she was assisted as needed. Georgie told me she liked butter and sugar on her cornbread. The other staff reminded me daily, with horrified faces, that Georgie was a diabetic. However, considering Georgie was one hundred and two years old, deaf, blind; she had faith as strong as Billy Graham's; she was ready to go to Heaven, and was absolutely right with God, by *dang*, I put butter and sugar on her cornbread; therefore putting meat back on her bones and a smile on her honey-sweet face. Sue me!

One evening I noticed Georgie hadn't come to the dining room for a few days; the aid told me she was eating in her room. Recalling that Georgie had fallen in her room again just a few days earlier, I went to see her after dinner. She was already lying down, but she seemed okay. Not her perky self, but she said she was fine. Still, I made a mental note, and I mentioned it to her nurse, my co-worker.

When I arrived at work on Monday afternoon, I went down the hall to see Georgie first thing. I found my old friend lying in bed in a dark room, the blinds closed, and the curtains pulled. My mind flashed back to the little house her son had built for her. The house had been designed so that Georgie's bedroom, the bathroom, and the kitchen all lined up on one side of the house. It was built at an angle to the road so that the sun rose on the bedroom side of the house. Thus, the sunlight kissing her eyelids had served as Georgie's alarm clock.

"Good morning!" Georgie sang with an enormous smile as I slid the curtains back. "Goodness, I'm glad you're here. I believe that was the longest night I've ever lived through!" She chuckled. "Why, I was a startin' to think it was never gonna end. I guess I just wasn't sleepy."

I was opening the blinds when the nurse aid walked into the room. "Good morning, Ms. Georgie," she said as she headed in my direction. "Oh!" She jumped back, startled. "I didn't see you there!"

"I see you didn't!" I laughed. "And what's up with the good morning thing? It's already two in the afternoon!"

"Oh." She laughed. "Ms. Georgie started telling me good morning every day when I opened her curtains, so I started saying it, too." She shrugged as she started helping Georgie sit up to change her clothes.

"You find Georgie in bed like this every day?"

"Yeah, for the past few weeks anyway."

"What's up with that?"

"I don't know. I figure she's taking a nap."

"With a gown on, the curtains pulled, and the blinds closed tight?" I cried. "For a nap? Who among the aids is *that* considerate?"

"Did you say nap? Oh goodness, I hope not! I don't need a nap!" Georgie chuckled. "I'm about as rested as a body can stand!"

"You have a point," the aid mumbled, her brow furrowed.

"No, Ms. Georgie!" I laughed. "She's going to help you get out of that bed!" Glancing back to the aid, I said, "Yeah, I have a point all right, and I've got a feelin'."

"Oh, God bless you!" Georgie raised both hands in the air. "I'm ready! I thought morning would *never* come!"

Later, at dinner, Georgie was as chirpy as a bird. I put sugar on top of her buttered cornbread, and life rolled on as we knew it.

The next day I ran errands so that I could stop by and check on Georgie. I stopped by at about eleven a.m., slipped quietly into Georgie's room, and found her lying in bed in a dark room, lights off, blinds closed, curtains pulled. Yet she was wide awake. She didn't know I was there, so I sat in the rocking chair her son had provided for her. I waited. The nurse aid came in a short while later and set her lunch tray on the overbed table, then slid the table over her bed. The aid never said a single word, though Georgie asked who was there and if it was time to get up. The aid walked out, and Georgie just lay there.

"I guess it's not." Georgie sighed heavily.

I sat there for over an hour and a half altogether, knowing I was going to be late getting back to work. Eventually, the aid came back to get the lunch tray. I observed as she replaced the lid on Georgie's plate full of untouched food and picked up the tray. The plastic was still covering the tea, and the silverware was still rolled up. I observed as Georgie told the aid she needed to use the toilet. "I've been waiting, but it looks like it's another long night. I'm just not sleeping all night anymore," Georgie said, shrugging.

The aid told Georgie she'd be back, to help her to the bathroom, after getting the rest of the trays. Georgie never asked what trays she was talking about. I slipped over to the door while the aid was getting Georgie's tray, then flipped the light on as the aid turned to exit the room.

"She didn't eat. She didn't even know her food was there. And please tell me she isn't kept in the dark all day, every day," I begged.

"She all right. She don't eat much, no way. Sometimes nothin'. And if I keeps the room dark, she don't keep trying to get up all by herself all the time and fallin'. I'm keepin' her safe."

"This strong, dignified, precious woman is accustomed to being as independent as possible. She doesn't realize she can't get up safely by herself anymore. She needs our help, not deprivation of light, food, and socialization," I barked. "Help her to the bathroom before you do anything else, please," I finished as I took the tray and set it back down.

I told the director of nursing I wasn't going home to change for work until Georgie was eating warm food and that aid was out of the building.

Later that evening I told Georgie's son I fully understood his feelings. He said he didn't want to move her elsewhere; he wanted to keep her there so I could keep an eye on her. That was it; he didn't say another word. He just looked me in the eye, tears in his own, hugged me, and walked away, heading back home to care for his sick wife.

A couple of weeks later, an aid pushed an exhilarated Georgie into the dining room, and Georgie's eyes glowed as she called my name. "I figured it out! I know why the Lord hasn't called me home yet," she shouted. "I know what I'm supposed to do, and I'm about to do it!"

Georgie immediately proceeded to shout about Jesus, the love of Jesus, and salvation. She ended by inviting everyone to pray together. She began praying as many began grumbling about the noise, telling me to make her be quiet. I bowed my head and prayed with Georgie.

Georgie ate everything on her plate and asked for a second piece of "that sweet buttered cornbread," which I readily retrieved from the kitchen.

Georgie went home to heaven late that night, to eternal joy and everlasting light.

Marlene:

Marlene used to work at the bank and was highly active in the community. I was often told, "Marlene ran this little town back in her day."

Marlene still had a mind and memory as sharp as a tack. If one wanted to make certain one remembered something, one could tell Marlene. Similarly, if one wanted to know something, one could ask Marlene. Marlene knew everything because she was nosy! But, by golly, Marlene owned it. She readily admitted to being nosy, adding with a shrug, "Well, I like to know things." How fully accountable she was!

Marlene crept around quietly in her wheelchair, which she slowly propelled with her one good leg, propping her bad leg on top of her good foot. Marlene loved to listen in on conversations, loved repeating those conversations, and loved meddling. And—my kind of girl—Marlene loved snacks. Still trying to run things, Marlene called city representatives, the bank, or the mayor about random concerns, real or otherwise on a daily basis. Why? Marlene never quit.

"Bag lady" was what I used to call her affectionately, as she had bags hanging all over her wheelchair. Marlene took her room with her when she left it, and this always included at least two boxes of Kleenex, which served a variety of purposes. One could easily track Marlene down, as she left a trail of Kleenex behind her wherever she went. But most memorable about Marlene? She had sparkling brown eyes, a completely adorable smile, and a giggle that would melt the heart of Mr. Snow Miser himself. And Marlene loved bingo!

Because of Marlene's physical status, she tired easily and rather quickly. She became a high fall-risk when fatigued, as she tended to slide right out of her chair, no longer having the strength to sit up. Thus, a nap, or at least an afternoon rest, was crucial. However, getting Marlene in and out of bed required the use of a lift with a sling, and it took two people to utilize this lift safely. It was somewhat cumbersome, difficult to maneuver, and time-consuming.

One day I overheard the aid trying to persuade Marlene to lie down, but Marlene was shaking her head, adamantly refusing. She was quiet, though, as Marlene's condition prevented her from having sufficient muscle strength to speak above a loud mumble, except during bingo. In fact, when having difficulty hearing Marlene, we told her, "Use your bingo voice." Marlene would grin, breathe deep, and be heard! Anyway, on questioning, Marlene told me she wanted to play bingo at "bingo time." That was why she didn't want to lie down. That seemed simple enough to me.

"Okay, so lie down for a bit, and then they can get you up for bingo. You can eat dinner after bingo, then lie back down. Easy breezy," I said.

"They won't get me back up." She shook her head, pursing her lips.

"Sure they will. You have to be up for meals, anyway, because you choke easy and can't safely eat in bed."

"Yeah, but they won't get me up, and I won't get to play bingo," she continued, shaking her head. Marlene wasn't one bit concerned about the risk of choking, only the risk of missing bingo.

I went to find the aid, who told me with a huge, friendly smile, "Naw, Marlene tired. She don't need to get back up."

When I attempted to explain Marlene's desire to play bingo and to remind the aid of Marlene's risk of choking when eating in bed, the aid interrupted nicely. "Naw, it's too hard getting Marlene up and down. She need to lay down and stay there. She tired, anyway. She gone fall."

Another aid chimed in as she waddled by, "Hey, if she doesn't want to lay down, great. Just leave her up in her chair. That means only one round on Marlene today."

"What?!" I cried as they both scattered in the wind. "So, wait a minute, the folks up in their wheelchairs don't get their briefs changed?!"

No reply, as there was no one there.

I got the other nurse to help me lay Marlene down, and I changed her soggy brief. I later found the aid and had them get her up for bingo. I wrote them both up for not providing adequate and timely incontinent care to those in wheelchairs and for fully intending to have Marlene eat in bed, placing her at risk of aspiration.

Marlene won a puzzle book and giggled delightedly as she fumbled around, scattering Kleenex as she dug it out of one of her many bags to show it to me before having me pile it in the drawer with her other bingo prizes. Marlene would have preferred winning a snack, but with Marlene any prize is worth winning.

I reported to the director of nursing about what I'd heard regarding "only one round," and she agreed that it certainly *sounded* like the residents up in their wheelchairs didn't get changed. She was pleased that I'd written them up and said she was going to address the problem immediately with all aids and nurses. She agreed it was unacceptable.

To my knowledge, it was never "addressed" with anyone. I observed thereafter, and, folks, unless the individual is cognitive and requests to be changed, they don't get changed if they're up in their wheelchairs. And some of them who aren't cognitive enough to request to be changed are up in their chairs *all day long*, thus sitting in urine most of the day.

In Marlene's case? Fully cognitive enough to request a change, but afraid she wouldn't be gotten back up and would miss bingo. Afraid she wouldn't be able to eavesdrop. Afraid she would be stuck in bed "forever". Marlene would rather be wet and uncomfortable in her chair than cut off from what little life she had.

I started a scheduled changing for those in wheelchairs. Sadly, I had to literally supervise and check briefs for compliance. I noticed Betty (a resident who thought the picture of Strawberry Shortcake in her coloring book was a picture of her as a little girl) no longer peed puddles beneath her wheelchair in the lobby. It turned out Betty hadn't been "refusing" to have her brief changed, after all. Betty said it "feels good to be all nice and dry".

But I'm not there anymore. I wonder if there is a puddle of urine in the lobby beneath Betty's chair. I wonder if Marlene is in bed, missing bingo, choking on her dinner, or sitting up in a wet brief so she can eavesdrop instead of just exist. I wonder.

Stan:

Stan was a tall, obviously once handsome man with a northerner's blunt edge. Stan could be every *bit* as irritable as he could be charming, and he swung from one spectrum to the other as unpredictably as a tornado. With a wide, easy smile, which he flashed in an almost practiced manner, he brazenly exhibited his eye for the ladies. Unfortunately, Stan had a crush on me. Sauntering up to my medication cart one day, without realizing or caring that he was interrupting my care of others, Stan borrowed my pen, asked me for a piece of paper, and then wrote me a love note and signed it *Love, Stanny*.

Never one to give up on a lady, Stan tried to give me money one "check day" so I could get my hair done, adding, "That's what you women do, isn't it? Huh? Get your hair done?" with a hearty but sincere chuckle. Stan openly and readily professed, always with a chuckle, that "all" his wives had been prostitutes when he met them. "But I didn't care. They were beauties!" he said, shrugging and flashing that wide, easy smile.

"All. How many wives have you had, Stan?"

"Five"

I rolled my eyes, laughing.

"Law says I can have one more." He smiled and winked.

However, though the ladies were a priority, Stan's greatest concern in life was money. He routinely counted the days until his "next check," and he asked repeatedly, all day, every day, "What day is it today?"

I bought him a calendar, hung it in his room, and told him to make a habit of crossing the day off each night before he went to bed. That way, when he got up each morning, he'd know exactly what day it was and how many days it was until his next check. Stan was ecstatic! "Good idea! He said. Then, the next day he began to hunt staff down to find out what day it was so he could check his calendar and make sure he had remembered to mark the previous day off.

As much as he denied to himself his declining ... stamina, Stan fell asleep near every time he sat down. One afternoon while passing through the lobby, I noticed Stan sitting by the window, his teeth flopping around in his mouth, almost blowing through his lips with every snore.

"Stan." I tapped his shoulder. "You're about to blow your dentures out. Put some denture adhesive in." I laughed. "Adhesive? What's that?" He laughed, finding it comical for some reason I still don't understand. But this reminded Stan of something he'd forgotten that he didn't find comical.

"I need some of that stuff…those little round things that you put in the cup to clean your teeth at night." He grinned, raising his extra-large hand in the air and forming a circle with his thumb and fingers. "You know what I mean. The little round things. Yeah?"

"Denture cleanser."

"Yeah." He chuckled. "Okay, call it what you want. I just need some. And I probably need a cup, too, while you're at it."

"You want me to clean them while I'm at it, too?" I smirked.

"Well, if you want to come around at bedtime tonight, we can clean them together." He winked.

"Behave. I'll put some denture cleanser and a cup in your bathroom before dinner."

"Thanks." Stan clicked his tongue, indicating he was done with the whole thing.

Before dinner I went to the supply room, which I dreaded doing, as it was such a jumbled mess. But I went. I dug around for over half an hour, finding only a cup and no cleanser. But a cup was at least promising. Noticing we had a bin full of toothpaste and another full of toothbrushes, I went in search of Dee. Dee was responsible for stocking supplies and putting briefs out for the residents. Dee informed me disinterestedly, "We don't order denture cleanser."

"We have to! We can't *not* order denture cleanser!" I was baffled.

"Well, we don't. So, I guess we can."

"But that's a basic need."

"I been here for a year and a half, and I ain't never seen none. And I handle supplies," she emphasized.

"Well, why don't we order it?"

"Girl, I don't know! I guess she just don't order it."

I went to the director of nursing's office and knocked. She said to come in, so I opened the door. There she sat with the assistant director of nursing, the MDS coordinator, and the treatment nurse.

"Stan needs denture cleanser. I can't find any, and Dee tells me we don't order it. I can pick him some up at the Dollar Store on my break tonight, but he will need it ongoing."

The director, along with the others, looked at the assistant director, who replied, "I'll order some. We must just be out. Dee is supposed to inventory each week and tell me what we need. I don't know if she doesn't tell me."

One blaming the other, both refusing to own the fact that it simply never crossed their minds.

I thanked her, then later picked up some denture cleanser for Stan to use until the order came in. Now, I must admit I fell short here. I missed a big red flag. Several weeks later I was reorganizing the nutrition room. In it was a freestanding storage closet in which they kept personal care items readily available for the aids to provide to the residents. I noticed we had no denture cleanser in the closet, and it appeared there were about the same amount of toothpaste tubes as there had been when I started working there months before. (Bear in mind, all the personal items, except Kleenex, were only slightly larger than travel size.) It also appeared the lotion and mouthwash bins were unchanged from months prior. The only item that appeared to be used and restocked was the shaving cream. I decided to restock as I organized. During this process, I discovered that the tubes of toothpaste in the bin had expired a full two years before I ever started working there. Upon further inspection, I found that the mouthwash had expired just under a year before my employment. I threw all of it in the trash, stacked the bins, found a cart, and headed for the supply room. I filled all the bins with supplies and hurried for the door, already way behind. But as I reached for the doorknob, a thought struck me. I stopped and checked the expiration dates. Of the supplies I'd just taken from the supply room, only the lotion and mouthwash were current. All the toothpaste was expired, every single tube. And they had only ordered one box of denture cleanser.

I checked Stan's bathroom, and he still had half of the box I'd purchased. I then counted all the residents who had dentures, which ultimately amounted to seventy-eight percent of the residents. Not surprising considering the population we served.

Before I left that night, I checked every single resident's personal care items. I can say, without exaggeration or hesitation, that the only ones with toothpaste or denture cleanser were those who could and would ask (that being very few), and those with family members who struggled to see to it that their loved one's needs were met. Roughly two out of ten residents had oral care items. However, because of the location and condition of many of those items, I feel confident in saying one out of ten were actually performing, or receiving, oral care of any kind.

In fact, when I talked to Stan about gently brushing his gums and washing his mouth out with mouthwash, or at least water, after removing his dentures, he responded, "Are you serious?!" He grinned. "Nobody has ever told me that! I've *never* done that! Maybe that's why my mouth hurts on this side." He wiggled his tongue on the inside of his right cheek. "That's why I don't like to wear that stuff that sticks my teeth in my mouth. You know. That stuff you mentioned earlier? Makes my mouth hurt." Then, as an afterthought, Stan chuckled and asked, "What did you call it?"

"Denture adhesive."

"Yeah. Adhesive. You can remember the names of all that stuff. Pretty and smart." He flashed his cocky smile.

I rolled my eyes and shook my head. "You never quit, Stan. Let me take a look."

"What?" He laughed.

I pulled my flashlight out of my pocket, and Stan sat down in a chair. In short, Stan was scheduled with the dentist, who placed him on antibiotics for an abscess. Once it was healed, I never again saw Stan's teeth flopping when he snored. In fact, Stan flashed his smile and pointed out to me one day that he was "wearing that sticky stuff now."

Most facilities have a dentist who comes to the facility, and Peridex is commonly ordered for the residents he or she sees every time he or she comes. Peridex is a treatment for gum disease.

I remembered a little lady I helped get ready for bed who was shocked silly—she had literally gaped at me—when I said, "Okay, where's your toothbrush? Let's clean those pearly whites before you snuggle in."

"We don't brush my *teeth!*" she exclaimed, like I was suggesting we shave her head.

I remembered the man who drove us nuts calling every single night to remind us (the nurses) to remind the aid to "help Mother brush her top teeth, and be sure to put the bottom dentures in the cup with some cleanser. Her teeth have always been extremely important to her." I recalled the day I met that man. He had said, "I don't mean to be a problem. But I promised Mother years ago that I would make sure her teeth were brushed if she should ever be unable to brush them her-self." He laughed and added, "I know the nurses think I'm crazy, but my grandmother got an infection from a tooth, and it somehow went to her brain. She started having seizures and died a horrible death at home. It left a mark on my mother. I never really thought I'd have to follow through on that promise, but here I am."

I remembered the lady who was losing weight, she was bedbound, had dementia, and was physically unable to feed herself. I'd been told she was a picky eater. I started feeding her every day, hoping to resolve the unexplained weight loss. The first day I fed her, I noticed she had no teeth. When I asked her about it, she said, "Aww, I throwed them nasty thangs away a long time ago. Nobody ever cleaned 'em, and they had funky stuff all over 'em! I just spit 'em out on my tray, and they hauled 'em away!" She grinned victoriously, then shuddered. "I don't want no new ones, 'cause ain't nobody gone clean them, neither. I ain't puttin' no nasty teefs in my mouf never agin."

Again, I could go on forever. Oral care is pertinent to one's overall wellbeing: self-esteem, appetite, and comfort! But, overall, oral care is *not* happening in long-term care settings. It just isn't happening.

Stella:

Stella had big, almost black eyes, a charmingly crooked smile, and long, thick hair that was still as coal black as the day she was born. Her skin was as tough as leather because of the sun, as she had grown up on a farm, ridden horses, and baled hay with her daddy. "I was a daddy's girl to the max," she told me with a huge grin.

Stella married a boy who worked on her daddy's farm. Lewis was his name. When her daddy died, her stepmother sold the farm, and Lewis moved Stella into town. She hated living in town, but she never said so because "Lewis needed a job and he was doing the best he could". Stella planted a small garden in their backyard and bought a few chickens so she could have at least a small part of the farm life she so loved and missed. Stella confided that she had longed to have a family of her own. She thought children would help ease the heartache and fill the hole left in her heart when she lost her daddy and the farm. But for whatever reason, Stella never got pregnant, and she and Lewis "couldn't afford doctors and tests".

Stella had worked as a checker at a local grocery store. She owned an old Ford step-side, but any day the sun was shining, she left home early and walked the four miles to work, then caught a ride home or had Lewis pick her up. Stella hated being "cooped up". Laughing, she told me she occasionally got caught in a sudden, unexpected rainstorm, but it was worth the risk to feel the sun on her skin as long as she could before going indoors to work.

Lewis had been dead nine years, and Stella was barely into her sixties when she had a massive stroke, which left her totally dependent.

She couldn't speak, swallow, lift a finger, or wiggle a toe. After extensive therapy, she was able to swallow a pureed diet if she was fed small bites slowly, drank thickened liquids, and took two sips of liquid between each bite. We were working with her in the hopes of Stella regaining her ability to feed herself with special adaptive equipment. Therapists were also working with Stella on mobilizing her own wheelchair, giving her exercises to strengthen her arms and dexterity.

It had been seven years since Stella's stroke, and she had come a long way. However, the therapist told me it seemed Stella had given up a few years before. She'd made amazing progress, then suddenly stopped. Stella wouldn't try. She wouldn't talk to anyone. She sat with her eyes down and just took the bites and drinks as offered. She wouldn't respond to attempts to interact. More specifically, Stella would blatantly ignore the attempts.

One evening at dinner, Stella reached her max. In one surprisingly productive motion, she reached up, grabbed the edge of her dinner plate, and slung it against the wall as she yelled, "No more!" Tears were streaming down her face. She then reached over to her neighbor's plate and stole her neighbor's dinner roll, then swung it clumsily but quite successfully to her mouth and took an enormous bite.

As she reached over to her other neighbor's plate, I swiftly rolled her wheelchair back from the table. Stella started cursing a blue streak. Wheeling her through the lobby, I headed quickly for the door, going straight outside so that Stella could yell and curse all she wanted without disturbing or scaring anyone else. Strangely, Stella immediately grew silent. To keep her from feeling like a spectacle, I pushed her chair along the sidewalk. Stella reached her slender hand out to touch a bush in passing. I stopped. Stella began randomly touching leaves, feeling the surface of them. She was silent as she lifted her face to the sky, closing her eyes. A few minutes passed before she reopened them. When she did, she gazed all around her, staring at the small wooded area on our left, then raising her face to the sky once more, she suddenly squealed and pointed. "A bird! Look at the bird!" She giggled like a small child.

Saying nothing, I began slowly pushing her wheelchair along the winding path, a feeling growing in my gut. Stella stretched out her hand, touching everything within reach. Finally, I pushed her off the sidewalk into the grass so she could touch things off the path. Ultimately, I had to take Stella back inside. After pushing her to her room, I sat down on the side of her bed, facing her chair.

"Stella, I saw you. You had no problem grabbing that plate and flinging it against the wall. You had no difficulty grabbing that roll or biting it. Yet you don't feed yourself. You don't even try to do anything for yourself. What's up, my friend? What can we do to help you help yourself? You are very much alive. I'd like to see you live."

Stella stared at me. I stared at Stella. After several minutes I stood to go, leaned down and hugged Stella. As I released her, she grabbed me and held on tight, sobbing against my shoulder. I waited, stroking her hair. Stella released her grip after crying herself out.

"I'm so sorry I acted like that."

"Oh, no problem. I enjoy plates soaring past my head, getting cursed out and ignored, and having snot roll down my sleeve." I laughed. "Keeps me from getting bored."

Stella laughed hard as she rolled her wheelchair the few feet to her bedside table. Opening the drawer, she pulled out a stack of calendars.

"I see you can roll your chair, too, missy. You have all sorts of surprises today." I winked.

"I'm so sorry. I never meant to be a problem for you. I can see you really care. But..." Stella stopped.

"But what, Stella? Talk to me. We can't help if we don't know what the problem is."

"Thank you for taking me outside. Thank you so much!"

"No problem, Stella. You were scaring everybody. You needed somewhere you could scream and yell. But you didn't. You got quiet. Care to share?"

Stella handed me the calendars. I looked at her, confused.

Quietly, Stella began, "I marked the days off once I could use my hands again. The first few years aren't marked, but I keep a calendar for those years, too, so I know how many years, months, weeks, and days it's been." Tears again streaming down her face, Stella continued. "I mark them off every night when they put me to bed. I never imagined life could be like this. We take so much for granted."

"Stella, I'm pretty darned good at decoding, but you're challenging even my skills. What are you marking off?"

"The days I haven't felt the sun," she whispered.

"Oh my God. Stella, you stopped living because you hadn't felt the sun? Why didn't you tell someone? That's an easy fix! We can fix that!"

Stella started sobbing, then wiped her nose on her sleeve. I handed her the box of Kleenex and waited. "I asked. I asked everybody that helped me do anything. I asked them every day to please take me outside, just for a few minutes. Everybody said they would. At first, I believed them. I got excited and waited. I'd remind them, and then everyone started getting irritated with me. So I stopped asking. I don't want them mad at me. I'm not in a position to have anyone mad at me. Then I worked *really* hard, so I could push my chair myself. I was slow, but I could do it. But they *still* wouldn't let me go outside. Somebody had to go with me, they said. But nobody ever had time. I know it sounds childish—maybe it is childish—but if I can't ever go outside again, what's the point? I don't care if I can push my chair or eat that gruel with a spoon. So I quit. I'm so sorry."

"Don't apologize, Stella. We let *you* down. I'm so sorry. And thank you for sharing. We shall fix the problem. It may take me a day or two, but, Stella, you will go outside every day the weather is good. Okay? All I ask is that you never, ever give up on yourself again." I hung Stella's current calendar on her wall. "You can't cross today off, you know. You felt the sun. I saw you." I smiled.

"It felt so *good*!" Stella's eyes teared up again.

"Stop it! No more tears! You're going to have mascara running down my face, and I'll have to go home so I don't scare people!"

Stella laughed.

I spoke with administration, told them the whole story.

The administrator asked quietly, "How many calendars does Stella have?"

"Seven."

"Dear God, she hasn't been outside for seven years?" He gazed thoughtfully out his window.

"Nope. Thing is, if you think about it, unless they go to the doctor or have family that takes them out, most of them never breathe fresh air or feel the sunshine again. Stella just happens to be a sun lover who spoke up. Actually, she blew up."

We fixed up an area outside where Stella could sit in the sun or the shade while being out of traffic's way and easily visible to staff. We offered Stella a room that provided the warmth and light of the afternoon sun through a window which provided a view of her sitting spot. With Stella's guidance, I planted her a tiny garden outside her window, which she watered every day it didn't rain. I took her vegetables home when she harvested and cooked them *just* the way she told me to, though she might argue that point just a little, maybe a lot.

I advocated for outdoor time for all. I got nowhere quick. Oh, I got promises, but no action.

I've always enjoyed teasing visitors who ask, "What's the code to get out the front door?"

I reply with a chuckle, "Oh, there is no code. Once you come in, you don't go out."

They usually chuckle or laugh out loud as I give them the code. But the thing is, for the vast majority of individuals who live in nursing homes, it's the truth. They come in and seldom if ever see the outdoors again. Never.

On a happy note, before I left, Stella was still eating pureed "gruel" (With a lot of salt, pepper, and butter. Stella quoted me at every evening meal, saying, "Yeah, yeah, yeah, everything's better with butter." She'd wink.), but she was feeding herself with no problems, and she was moving her wheelchair like greased lightning! Farm life was paying off. Stella could even stand and pivot with assistance.

Stella shines with the sun. I hope she's still shining.

Penny:

Penny was fairly young in comparison to the average age in a nursing facility. Wheelchair-bound with a spitfire "*tude*", Penny was somewhat angry at the world. Adult Protective Services had placed Penny in the home due to unsafe living conditions, rightly so considering what Penny herself had shared with me; though she still wanted to go home. A beauty in her day, life and poor health had taken their toll, and Penny literally struggled with the fact that she wasn't a beauty in the eyes of the world anymore. She wore her mass of salt-and-pepper hair long and wild, framing her ghostly pale face and her long, pointed nose. But, now and then, she'd regain her old hope and tidy up. I wish I could show you the picture I took of her one day. She rolled slowly out into the hallway, and I reflexively raised an eyebrow and grinned, as she looked much like she'd been aggressively attacked by hair clips and a giant, glossy lipstick.

"What?" she asked, looking up at me with her head leaned to the side, appearing both surprised and a tad annoyed.

"Your hair, my friend. What on earth happened to your hair?" I squealed as a wad of clipped hair flopped from one side of her head to the other.

Penny grinned, peering up from amidst the wads. "I fixed it for dinner."

"Oh, okay."

"Well, does it look bad? You're supposed to be my friend. Don't let me go to dinner looking ridiculous," she snipped.

"Well then, umm, go take another look."

"I can't see in the mirror. It's too high. I'm using a small hand mirror. Take my picture with your phone. Let me see." So I did. "Oh! Good grief!" Penny laughed. "I can't go to dinner like this! My lipstick is even lopsided!"

"Come on, let me fix your hair. You fix your lipstick. Gorgeous color, by the way. But hurry. I have blood sugars to check."

So, I cleaned up the clippy battlefield, and Penny fixed her lipstick. While I was brushing Penny's hair, she asked softly, "You think you'll ever remarry? You've been single for a long time now."

"Hmm, I don't know." I shrugged thoughtfully. "Haven't really thought about it. Maybe not."

"You probably won't, you know. You are beautiful and strong, and those very things will probably get in your way." The hand mirror drooped in her hand. "I don't think I ever will, either. Not anymore. I wish I'd married Joe. But I guess I thought I had forever at the time. And he wasn't exciting enough for me. Stupid, huh?"

Placing the mirror on her cluttered bedside table, Penny rolled slowly out the door, propelling herself with swollen feet, their movement restricted by the enormity of her fluid-filled legs. "I need toilet paper again," she grumbled over her shoulder as I tidied up her mess. "They never give us more than one roll. Oh, and I'm out of clean pants again." Penny turned her head and glanced back at me as I followed her out into the hallway.

Our eyes rolling simultaneously, Penny wheeled slowly off towards the dining room. I stood gazing at the back of Penny's still wild, but much tamer, gray head; sighed heavily; scurried the other direction to laundry; and grabbed two rolls of TP to put in her bathroom. Finally, after searching through massive piles, bins, and dryers, I found a pair of clean pants with Penny's name on them.

After catching back up with myself to the greatest extent possible, I found housekeeping and once again requested extra toilet paper be placed in Penny's bathroom each day.

The housekeeper scowled and replied as always, "I'm only sposed to put one roll in each bathroom. One roll on the roller, iffen it ain't got one, and one roll on the back of the pot. That's it, and that's all I'm gone do."

"There are two to four ladies sharing that toilet and toilet paper. Furthermore, Penny takes two different fluid pills twice a day. She needs two rolls all by herself. If she doesn't have toilet paper, she starts refusing the fluid pill. If she refuses the fluid pill, she ends up in acute heart failure. Please, please put extra paper in the bathroom. I do not have time to get toilet paper every day, and she *needs* it. Thank you for understanding."

I walked away, hopeful. However, every single day, at some point, Penny called for me to get toilet paper. Ultimately, I went to the administrator, yes, for toilet paper. It got no better. You'd have thought Penny was asking for gold. So I started providing her toilet paper each day before I started my shift. Then one Friday, she asked me to give her six rolls so she would have some over the weekend. "No one will get me any, so I have to use paper towels, and they're kind of rough," she said.

I gave her six rolls every Friday. And, by dang, I bought her a full-length mirror and had maintenance hang it on the back of the door so she could see to fix her hair. I'd never realized it before, but all the mirrors throughout the facility were hung high above the bathroom sink, which is placed at standing level, as if the majority of the residents aren't in wheelchairs.

In fact, it touched my heart to the extent that I asked numerous residents at dinner. One hundred percent of them informed me, "I haven't seen my own face in years." Ninety-nine percent if you count Deason's son, who was having dinner with him and said he'd seen his own face that morning. Thank you, Jason.

Thing is, I don't work there anymore. I can't help but wonder sometimes if Penny has toilet paper. Is she taking her fluid pills? Is her heart still pumping? What, pray tell, does her hair look like today? That matters to Penny, so it matters to me. When it's my turn, I want a mirror I can easily see into. I want my hair fixed. By dang, I want my mirrored mauve lipstick. And Lord help me, I want toilet paper. And don't make me beg for it. Please and thank you!

Me:

I want shoes. I love my sneakers. Sneakers give me happy feet.

I may not like bingo, but if I do, please let me play. If I don't, please have something interesting, preferably fun, for me to do to make it worth getting out of bed each day. And if I choke when I eat in bed, please don't put me in bed before mealtime and leave me there.

I need toilet paper. Let's get real here. It's not as if I'm asking for a luxury item.

I want clean pants, and please don't gripe at me because I need you to find me some. After all, you won't let me go get them myself.

I want my hair fixed and my lipstick on. Please provide me a mirror I can see into, even if I look like a clown when I'm all dolled up. I feel better with my hair done and my face on. I just do.

I want clean teeth and fresh breath. If I can't do it myself, please help me.

I don't want to be thirsty. Please, oh please, don't make me be thirsty!

I need light and socialization. Even if I just sit quietly, let me be around other people and feel life. Please don't keep me in the dark or isolate me from others.

Dear goodness, I want sunshine! I need sunshine! *Please* let me feel the sunshine and breathe fresh air. It does a body good.

I may be old. I may be wrinkled. I may be slow. But I'm still me. Please *see me.*

Your shell is going to have cracks someday. It's going to lose its luster. Do you want to be discarded, unseen, and passed by as if the pearl that is you doesn't still live and breathe inside of that shell?

*Note:

These are just a few stories of just a few individuals regarding just a few basic needs. We have far more needs, and sadly, I could give you literally endless examples from each and every facility in which I have been employed, and on a vast array of needs. These are not isolated issues. In fact, I promise not to reference a single isolated care issue throughout the entirety of these pages. That would not serve my purpose here. My purpose is to enlighten you on the common threads and the definite realities of your loved one's present...of your future.

Candy for Clyde

Clyde, a school bus driver by choice, supplemented his income with handyman work so that he could provide for his family yet still be able to drive his bus. There was no horseplay or bullying on Clyde's bus. He just wasn't going to allow it. He always threatened to "set 'em straight right quick!"

One day he was telling me about it, saying "But them kids knew they had a true friend in ole Clyde. Kids need limits and rules. They need to know they matter enough for you to go to the trouble to make 'em, stick to 'em, and hold *them* to 'em." He finished, then randomly grabbed the blinds, struggling to tug them down from the window, no longer cognitively aware of my presence.

Clyde's dementia was severe, having progressed to the extent that he required assistance with every aspect of his life. Openly despising the very thought of getting out of bed, Clyde was an undeniable drama queen every time he was transferred from bed to chair or chair to bed. Yes, I said drama *queen*. The man could roar like a lion, but most often he squealed like a girl. Then, just as soon as his scrawny little butt hit the cushion on his wheelchair, he stopped.

"Well, come on, let's go," he'd say, cool as a pickle and gentle as a lamb, as if encouraging you to get with the program and stop the dilly-dallying.

Thus, we only got Clyde up for meals so he could go to the dining room, where staff could feed him. If left to eat alone in his room, Clyde didn't eat his food; he wore it—with a huge, oblivious, adorable grin, I might add. Clyde was dropping weight, so I started feeding him myself. He still wore a bit of his dinner, and thanks to his ever-busy hands, I wore a little myself. But I learned quickly that if I distracted Clyde by getting him to talk about whatever random thing that would capture his attention, he'd accept the food and swallow. Clyde and I had some interesting conversations, one of which revealed his desire for a red airplane. I just happened to glimpse the Christmas tree while grasping for our next topic, so I asked Clyde what he wanted for Christmas.

"A plane," he replied, void of tone or expression.

"What color?"

Without hesitation he exclaimed almost reverently, "Red! I want a *red* one!" He grinned, raising his big, recently clouded, gray eyes skyward as he opened his mouth, robotically accepting the spoon.

In addition to feeding him myself, I added a high caloric bedtime snack to Clyde's diet in attempt to facilitate prevention of further weight loss. I soon discovered ole Clyde had a sweet tooth, and I didn't have to talk at all to get my friend to eat chocolate pudding! One evening I bought him a Three Musketeers bar from the vending machine and took it in as a special treat. I had it in my pocket when I walked into his room with his bedtime medication. Clyde narrowed his eyes, scrunching his fuzzy brows, and stared at me as I approached his bed.

"What you got in your pocket there?" he asked quietly.

"My pocket?"

"Yeah, your pocket. I see something kinda shiny in your pocket."

"Here, buddy, take your bedtime medicine." I rolled my eyes, trying not to smile, then raised the tiny spoonful of crushed meds in pudding to his lips while he continued staring at me as if he were a detective, hot on the trail.

"If I take that medicine, you gonna show me what's in that pocket?"

"Fair enough. It's a deal." I could not resist a chuckle.

Clyde locked his narrowed eyes on mine, slowly opening his mouth for the medicine. He swallowed, grimaced, smacked his lips. "Now let's see what's in that pocket." He peered over the side of his bed at my jacket pocket.

Slowly, I slipped my hand into my pocket, relishing the changes in Clyde's expression as it went from suspicion to anticipation to sheer, unadulterated delight as I pulled that candy bar from my pocket.

Clyde threw his stubby little head back against his pillow and shouted, "Candy! Candy for Clyde!" as he clapped his hands.

I walked out of his room with a full heart and a huge smile as Clyde devoured his candy bar, chocolate already smearing his chin and the tip of his nose, me and my pocket no longer in the blissful mix.

Ultimately, Clyde owned me. Every time I passed his doorway, he'd holler out, "Hey, where you been? I been looking fer you."

"I been looking for you, too," I'd reply while passing.

"Well, you ain't been lookin' very hard. I been right here," I would hear him mumble predictably as seeing me pass slipped from his memory altogether.

Without fail, I delighted in the sight of Clyde's little head raised up off his pillow as he ogled the doorway to see who was passing, and the sound of his voice as he expressed his sincere, uncensored thoughts and feelings.

One night I was feeding Clyde his bedtime snack when he suddenly looked at me, fully cognitive of my presence, and said, "I'ma tell you somethin'. File it away somewhere so's you can pull it out and refresh yersef from time to time. You're a beauty, inside and out. You got a good heart; that's a good thing. But don't let a good thing get you in a bad spot. Stay away from them bad boys. They're smoooooth talkers, probably tell you just what you wanna hear. But they're full of crap. How a boy treats you, that's what matters. Words are garbage; actions are gold. You're different. You're special. You hold out for a boy who sees it and treats you that way."

With tear-filled eyes, I pulled Clyde's covers back so I could straighten them for the night. There he was, naked from the waist down, his poop-covered brief wadded up next to him, slightly shredded, his poop-covered hand right in the middle of it.

"I think the dog crapped on the bed," he mused as he reached up and scratched his ear with his poopy hand.

"What on earth makes you think it was a dog, Clyde?" I laughed.

"Well, surely a person didn't take a dump on my bed!" he said as if I was as dumb as a rock, overlooking the purely obvious.

Gradually, it became harder to get Clyde to eat at dinnertime, and he became less zealous about his bedtime snacks, though he always managed to eat at least some of the sweet stuff. Nobody can say Clyde didn't maintain his priorities.

One evening, though, I was going through all the motions, rambling about anything and everything I thought might catch his interest. Clyde was intermittently opening his mouth and accepting spoonsful of food, grimacing each time he realized he had food in his mouth. Finally, he took a bite, froze briefly, grimaced, and swallowed. Then, still grimacing, he almost yelled, "*Please* don't make me do this. I don't *want* to. I *know* you mean well, but I don't *need it* anymore."

I listened. With all the love and respect in the world, I pushed that divided plate away, pulled Clyde's chair back from the table, took him to his room, cleaned him up, and listened to his familiar squeal as the aid helped me transfer him from his wheelchair back into bed.

Clyde grinned big and immediately tugged his freshly tidied blankets back into a wad, looking for that "hammer" he'd "just had". I switched on his television. Clyde laughed and said I "done that real good" as he continued his search, though he no longer recalled exactly what it was he was searching for. "It don't matter none," he said. "I'll know it when I find it." I left him contentedly searching.

Clyde left us that night. I hope heaven has candy bars.

Milly, his daughter, gave me the little, yellow, metal school bus that Clyde had kept on his shelf. I remember Clyde saying, "The doors open and close just like they did on *my* bus." Milly told me Clyde once took a butt-whipping for a kid. He had retained a bully on his bus until he'd dropped off every other child. Then he took the bully home and walked him to the front door. Clyde had kept his hand on the kid's shoulder, knocked on the door, and asked the kid's sister if he could speak to their father. Clyde calmly told the kid's father about the kid bullying other children, that he didn't tolerate such on his bus. The kid's dad reached out and pulled the kid inside the house by the hair of his head.

Clyde said, "Well, I'm guessin' that explains it. The boy thinks that's how a man is sposed to treat another. Ain't his fault, sir; it's yours. I done him wrong bringing him to you."

The kid's dad punched Clyde in his face. Milly said Clyde punched two holes in the wall when he got home. He'd told his wife, "I wanted to beat the crap out of that ignorant S.O.B.! But somebody's gotta show the boy right from wrong!"

Milly said Clyde had stood on that small porch and used the back of his hand to wipe the blood from his mouth and nose, wiping his hand on his jeans. He'd stood firm, looked at the kid, still standing behind his dad, and said, "Son, it takes a real man to turn and walk away from a fight that stems from stupidity and don't accomplish nothin'. Man only fights when he has to, not just cuz he might want to." Then Clyde had turned and walked away.

I wasn't at all surprised, and I was so proud of him.

Milly also told me Clyde hadn't recognized her for a very long time. We talked a bit about how painful that can be, for your loved one to no longer know who you are. Then Milly smiled and said she had visited one morning and found a Three Musketeer wrapper wadded up in Clyde's bed. She'd wiped a chocolate smear from his chin and sat with him awhile, though, as usual, he'd never acknowledged her. She then said that, on her next visit, she had brought him a Three Musketeer bar. Tears rolled down Milly's cheeks, pooling at the corners of her enormous smile, as she finished, saying, "I held that candy bar out, and Daddy looked me in the eye for the first time in years! He saw me! He smiled and said, 'My little Silly Milly.' Then, of all things, he grinned and shouted, 'Candy for Clyde!' I didn't have him back long, but that goofy candy bar gave me my daddy just for a minute, one last time!"

I hugged Milly and told her how much I adored her daddy, how delightful he had been. I told her how much genuine joy that man had added to my world and what a valuable role he'd played in my life. I'd learned a lot from Clyde. I filed away his advice, like he told me to. I'm still holding out for that "boy" who will appreciate me and treat me special. I think Clyde might get a big kick out of how *long* I've been waiting, but I know he'd be pleased that I valued his input, his love. He'd be proud of me, too. And *that* means the world to me. Clyde was a good man.

I sincerely thanked Milly for the bus, which now sets on a shelf in my home. Every time it catches my eye, I grin and think, *candy for Clyde!*

I imagine that when I get to heaven, I'll hear a familiar voice say, "Hey, where you been? I been lookin' fer you."

Truth Hurts

My sincere apologies in advance. I truly have no desire to offend anyone. Unfortunately, sometimes the truth does hurt, and it often hurts in a variety of ways.

Hallie:

Hallie was a big girl. She was tall with big bones and broad shoulders. But her voice was a complete contradiction to her presence. It was as soft and sweet as a lullaby, as tiny as a newborn babe. Hallie said I reminded her of a doll she'd had as a child, but she was pretty sure the doll was a little bigger. She'd apparently "never seen a nurse so itty-bitty". As I said, Hallie was big boned, but she had a heart bigger than all her bones put together. Her face was as pretty and sweet as an angel's, with smooth skin, huge Hershey brown eyes and eyelashes that made you think you needed to duck every time she blinked.

Hallie had been a truck driver and loved every second of it, until the cancer metastasized to her brain. One minute, Hallie was fully present, as mentally functional as you and I are now. The next minute she was lost, confused, even combative. Sometimes she recalled fragments of her behavior after an episode of confusion, and she'd apologize profusely. I think I hurt more for Hallie in those moments than at any other time. She was mortified. Consolation wasn't even possible. I think it's undoubtedly harder to be cognitively in and out than to just be out.

Hallie was loved. In fact, when she told me that she had been a truck driver, I immediately expressed concern for her safety, out there all alone on the road in that enormous truck, often at night.

"Don't worry about me!" She laughed genuinely. "We take care of each other. And every trucker that knows me watches out for me. I'm safer than a secretary!"

I readily believed every word. Hallie was easy to love. And Hallie loved back intensely. She worried herself sick over her sons. I walked in to give her some pain medication one evening and found her in a panic.

"Give me a pen. Hurry! And some paper! Now! I'm going to forget this again! I have to tell my sons!"

I grabbed a pen and pad from my pocket, then slapped both on her overbed table. "Write!"

Hallie began a fast scribble, then stopped, wilted, and cried. "It's gone. I can't remember!"

"Leave it right there, Hallie. Pick it up when it comes back. It'll come. Calm down."

Cancer had first taken Hallie's cervix and uterus, then her bladder; thus, Hallie had nephrostomy tubes. Nephrostomy tubes are sutured into the kidneys, exiting one's body on each side of his or her back, to drain one's urine into drainage bags that serve as the bladder. Emptying the bags timely and maintaining infection control are critical.

Hallie was distraught, literally devastated, and scared because, no matter how hard she tried, she could not recall what she so desperately wanted, needed, to tell her sons. I leaned down over her, reassuring her and stroking her hair, and then I realized my knees, which were against the side of the mattress, were soaking wet. I kept quietly talking to Hallie as I felt around with my free hand. My heart literally ached as I realized Hallie was lying on a dry pad covering a soaking wet bed. Upon closer inspection, I saw that one of her nephrostomy bags was open, the other bulging full. I disinfected and closed the open one then emptied the other while Hallie fell asleep with a tear-stained face.

My anger peaking as I scrubbed my hands, I stomped back across the building to find the nurse aid. Unable to find her, I did finally manage to find her partner in another resident's room. Let's call the partner Chief, as I was most accustomed to seeing her sitting across from the nurses' station, looking much like an Indian chief, her face solemn and her arms crossed, propped atop her enormous belly. I quietly requested that Chief step out into the hallway for a moment. I explained that Hallie needed help and described what I'd seen. Chief rolled her eyes and told me the other aid had Hallie that night, and that aid had gone on break.

"We make rounds, you know," Chief then sneered. "She'll find it on her next round. We make one round at the beginning of our shift and another one at bedtime."

Before I could speak, Chief added dryly, with a sarcastic glare, "In fact, she already knows. She's like me. She ain't gonna argue with nobody.

Hallie refused to let her get her out of bed. So she slapped a dry pad underneath her and went on break. So, you see, she already knows. She'll take care of it. Maybe Hallie will be a little more cooperative next time."

Fire burned in my heart. "I'd say that I'm going to forget everything you just said, but that'd be an outright lie. I think your words will forever be seared into my brain. What I will say is this: You just told me that these folks are only getting incontinent care twice in your eight-hour shift."

Chief interrupted. "It's not like they drink enough water to pee more than that. Most of 'em stay dehydrated." She said this as if I were wholly stupid not to have realized that myself.

"Thank you. I'll add the fact that you aren't encouraging fluids to the list. Now then, if you would be so kind as to allow me to finish without interruption. You also told me the other aid left even though Hallie was lying in a pool of urine, even though one nephrostomy tube was exposed to any germ that wanted to crawl in and one drainage bag was so full that urine was backing up into her kidney. You then told me that you *also* knew this, and you also had every intention of leaving Hallie in that predicament even longer. You see? I'm a bit like you, too. I ain't gonna argue with nobody, neither. So I'm telling you that it would no doubt be in your best interest to help me with Hallie just as soon as you're finished with Ms. Liza. And I expect you to have a smile on your face while you're helping. I'll see you shortly in Hallie's room."

I wrote them both up for everything while both smirked and chortled with one another, saying, "Don't nobody care about no write-up. It's not as if anybody is going to fire us. There ain't nobody to take our places."

The next day I insisted Hallie be moved over closer to the nurses' station. However, I didn't have an empty room on my unit, so she was under the care of my co-worker. It wasn't my preference, but at least I could check on her more easily and frequently. I moved her pen and paper with her, placing it on the overbed table in her new room, but she never got to finish whatever it was she so desperately wanted to write down for her sons.

Hallie's cancer was aggressive. She was tumbling downhill at a gruesomely rapid pace. But Hallie fought hard, and she still had occasional lucid moments. While checking on her one day, I found the notepad I had given her lying next to her on her bed. She'd drawn a goofy picture of me, giving me an oversized smile and a lopsided heart, the words *my angel doll* written beneath it. I taped it on her wall, then drew a picture of her (if you can call it that), giving her long, sweeping eyelashes. I taped it on the wall next to angel doll.

"I look like a cheap hussy!" Hallie laughed when she later saw it.

"Well, if the shoe fits." I winked.

Hallie laughed.

Ultimately, Hallie's cancer took her from us altogether, cognitively speaking. It left her with nothing but pain. I found her moaning one day, literally writhing in bed to the extent that she was almost falling over the edge. We had to lower Hallie's bed to just above the floor so she wouldn't get hurt if she fell out or off. Then we placed cushioned mats beside the bed.

Nurses are very territorial, but I had to know. I politely asked my co-worker about Hallie's pain management: What did she have for pain? When was her last dose? My co-worker informed me that she had administered Hallie's hydrocodone but that she was not going to give her any morphine.

"I'm not going to be the one that gives her the medication that causes her to take her last breath. Oh no. Not me!" she announced, smacking her gum.

I took a deep breath. "The morphine is not going to take her life. The cancer is going to take her life. You feel better letting her moan and writhe in pain up until her last breath? Or would you feel better if she slept peacefully and *possibly* took that last breath a few minutes sooner than she would without the morphine?"

"Gum smacker" walked away. I called my supervisor at home and requested that Hallie be reassigned to my unit immediately, despite the location of her room. Of course, my supervisor wanted the rationale, so I told her. Hallie was reassigned and medicated immediately. I then monitored and addressed it as needed to ensure the nurses on other shifts were keeping Hallie comfortable.

A few days later, on an drizzly afternoon, Hallie passed peacefully, with her sons at her bedside. I will forever remember Dan's face and his words after his mama passed.

"Thank you. Thank you all for taking care of our mom. Living thousands of miles away, I just couldn't get here to see to her care." Tears welled in his eyes. "And Joe," he glanced at his brother, "is always on the road, all over the country. I – we - are so grateful that Mom wasn't in pain. That was our greatest fear. Before the cancer spread to her brain, that was *her* greatest fear. She feared pain more than death."

Tony:

Tony was an outgoing guy, energetic and outspoken. Most memorably, he was loaded with integrity, chock-full of life, and royally ticked off that his doctor had "forced" him to come into a nursing home.

"Rehab, my ass," he said emphatically the first time I met him. "Doc just thought I was abusing my pain medicine, so he figured he'd fix that. I mean, I never took more than I had, and it lasted as long as it was supposed to last. So, you tell me!" He shrugged.

"Oh, Tony, I don't know. I wasn't there, and I certainly can't speak for anyone else. I get into enough trouble when I speak for myself." I chuckled, trying to lighten the mood. Tony was hot. Unfortunately, his doctor had documented his suspicions about drug "misuse" in his progress notes, thus all who accessed Tony's records could read about it. Most unfortunately, many automatically judge, and convict as opposed to thinking for themselves, observing, and giving one the benefit of the doubt.

Tony continued venting. "That home health nurse came by one day when my buddies were there. She gave me a big, looong speech about drinking beer while I was taking the pain medicine. We tried to explain to her that it was a rare deal. My buddies had come to see me from all over the country. We were in the Marines together." His eyes sparkled as a grin spread from one ear to the other. "We were celebrating our reunion! We were supposed to meet in Kansas, but my leg went bad, so they regrouped and came here. Now *that's* loyalty!" Then, frowning, he continued. "She embarrassed all of us that day. I felt bad for my buddies. They started pouring their beers down the sink like a bunch of kids who'd been busted by somebody's mama. We'd only had one or two. We weren't hurting a thing. Next thing you know, she left, and my doctor's nurse called me, said I had to go to a nursing home, or Doc wasn't going to give me any more pain medicine. Shit! My leg is messed up again! I got to have the pain medicine! So here I am. Oh, I argued, but Doc said I needed therapy to strengthen my good leg. Bullshit, that's what that is."

I smiled. "Speaking of your leg, let me have a look."

Tony had lost his foot while in the service. Recently, the circulation had "fouled up," and he had undergone a subsequent surgery, losing more of his leg. At the point I met him, his stump ended just below the knee with a large, bruised, but clean incision covering the base of his stump.

Tony proved to be correct about not needing therapy. The man got around better on one leg than most people do on two. But being the *man* that he was, after his initial venting, Tony never mentioned it again. He just went along with the program, enjoyed his scores of visitors, laughed often and seldom complained.

His third day with us, I was getting report when Adrian, the nurse I was relieving, commented, "Tony always wants pain medicine, but I'm not going to help him misuse it. That man watches the clock to make sure he gets every dose he can have."

Having heard this kind of judgmental stupidity from many a nurse over the years, I had long before developed a fixed response. So, without any thought what-so-ever, I replied wearily, "Well, you aren't the pain pill police, so if he has a doctor's order for it, and you have no factual health-related rationale against it, give him his medicine and shut up about it."

Adrian's eyes grew wide, and she huffed dramatically! She did! She actually huffed!

"What?" I laughed when I saw her expression and heard her huff.

"I can't believe that's your attitude," she snipped before scooping up her belongings and huffing her way to the break room to clock out. I shrugged... chuckled. A couple of weeks later, when I returned to work after two days off, the PTA (physical therapy assistant) asked me to talk to Tony. "For some reason he's started refusing therapy. He won't tell me why. He won't even look at me. He just holds his stump up in the air and stares straight ahead. He trusts you. Maybe he'll talk to you."

I went in to see Tony and found the social butterfly/energizer bunny moaning in semidarkness as he cradled his stump midair. Tears began streaming down his face as soon as he saw mine. His shoulders shook, and my heart broke as he sobbed. I stood quietly, waiting. Finally, words poured out like a raging river as he wiped repeatedly at his eyes and his, then snotty nose. "Please help me! It's throbbing! They are making me wait for my pain medicine. I don't understand it. I don't. What have I done to them? They keep telling me they will go get it, but then it takes two or three hours for them to come back with it! Adrian even sighed and rolled her eyes at me! Then I tried to explain that I didn't mean to be a problem, but the pain is reeeal bad. She rolled her eyes again and said, 'Oh, I'm sure it is.' She did! Like I was lying to her! I don't lie! Not to nobody!" He slammed his fist down on the bed. "I know they're busy, but I just can't take the pain so long! I try. I do! But I can't! I don't mean to be a problem to nobody. Hell, I was taking care of myself just fine at home! I didn't want to come here! It's throbbing! I can't take it! Chop the damned thing off! I just-"

"Tony!" I yelled to get his attention. His eyes popped open wide, and his lips snapped shut. I almost felt guilty for having raised my voice. "It's going to be okay. Breathe deep. I'll be right back with a pain pill."

I hurried back out of his room and up the hallway. Upon looking, I found that Tony hadn't had a pain pill since seven that morning. It was then near three in the afternoon. His pain medication was ordered every four hours as needed. I took him a pain pill immediately.

An hour later Tony was feeling better but still hurting. I took him another pain pill four hours after the first dose, and was relieved to see that his pain was getting back under control a short while after the second timely dose. I then made time to look back in his records. Tony was right. He was ordered as many as six doses per day. During my two days off, he'd received four doses one day and three the next.

Over the next two days, I discovered we had several "pain pill police" on diligently active duty. Finding Tony in severe pain on my arrival at work two days in a row, I hurriedly administered his pain medication. The second day, I called his doctor; the doctor who had insisted on his coming to us for "rehab," and spoke with his nurse, Julie. I explained Tony's pain level, stressing that he had exhibited no signs of substance abuse tendencies, and requested that the doctor make his pain medication routine to ensure adequate pain management, as it was "currently indisputably inadequate". Ultimately, post Julie's exasperation with me, Doc called me back himself and I told him the same. Per his approval, I then discontinued the order for as needed pain medication and entered the order to make it routine. Later that evening I informed Tony of the new order, explaining this meant he would get the medication every four hours without having to ask for it.

Tony grabbed my hand. "Oh, dear God, thank you! You are my *hero*! I was dreading your next day off!"

Laughing, I cried, "I'm no hero! Good grief." I rolled my eyes dramatically. "I'm just doing my job, Tony. No big."

Tony laughed. "Well, you're no Marine, but you're still a hero." He winked. I laughed, turned, and walked back out the door. All was well for a quick minute.

One week later, again after a few days off, the treatment nurse, who had stepped into the position without any formal wound care training, asked me to look at Tony's leg. I hadn't seen it since that first day, as it was always dressed by the time I arrived at work. I readily agreed and went in with her to see Tony. Tony was moaning, again cradling his stump midair, his eyes closed.

I slapped my hand over my mouth to stifle a gasp, immediately grateful Tony's eyes were closed. Tony no longer had a slightly bruised stump with a nice clean incision; his stump was covered with hard, black tissue that extended a couple of inches above his knee. I glanced at the treatment nurse.

"What do you think?" she asked.

"He needs to be sent out immediately. No 'thinking' to it. And do not send him to a local hospital. He needs to go to the hospital where he had his surgery done. Go, make arrangements now, please." I hadn't had formal wound care training, either, but I've always held the firm opinion that common sense goes much further than all the books in the world. And common sense told me that Tony should have been sent out long before then.

"I'll be right back with some pain medication, my friend," I told Tony as I turned for the door.

"I already had it," he forced through gritted teeth.

"Let me worry about that."

I called his doctor, telling him that Tony's stump was necrotic; and that I was going to give him an extra one-time dose of his pain medication prior to sending him out on the bumpy ambulance to ride the eighty miles to see his surgeon. Maybe it was my tone, maybe it was guilt; regardless, Doc readily agreed.

I got the pill and hurried back to Tony's room. As I gently wrapped fresh gauze over and around his stump, Tony was mumbling, "I should have been looking. I should have been watching..."

"What do you mean Tony?"

"The pain was so bad when they wouldn't give me my medicine, that I started closing my eyes and holding my breath when the bandage lady did my leg. I should have been looking! I should have stayed on top of it! I should have been tougher!"

"Tony!" I cut him off again. "*This* is not your fault! Anybody else would have been *screaming* long ago. *This* didn't happen overnight. Now stop holding that pill in your hand and put it in your mouth. Your hand ain't hurtin'." My desperately clumsy attempt to make him smile.

Grinning, despite his pain, and still cradling his stump midair, Tony popped the pain pill into his mouth and swallowed. "And you say you aren't my hero. Darlin', I been begging all of 'em to call the doctor for three days. I don't know a lot of things, but I know the pain suddenly tripled, and now that I've seen it, I know this leg is gonna have to come off. I know that black stuff means it's rotten. I cried all night. I was angry, hurting, and scared. I don't think I've been scared since I was a little kid. But I was. I was scared shitless, until I saw your face. Yeah, you're my hero... and my friend. Thank you for everything, and I mean that."

"Oh, stop it. I'm just doing my job." Blinking back the tears threatening to flow any second, I turned to leave so I could check on the status of Tony being sent out.

"Hey," Tony called out. "Do I have the right to retract my previous statement?"

I turned back to face him. "Okay, okay." I sighed dramatically. "Right granted. Retract away."

Tony grinned. "See there? Tough as nails and bad to the bone, yet tender hearted and good as gold . You'd make a great Marine!"

"You couldn't leave without making me cry, too, could you?" I asked as tears filled my eyes, and I walked back to give Tony a hug. "I'm honored. Thank you. Now go get that leg taken care of!"

I never saw Tony again. I checked on him. He lost the remainder of his leg, but he was healing well. And Tony went home!

I did get a surprise visit from a local Marine recruiter laden with a huge bouquet of flowers and a thank you note. I wish I'd thought to take a picture of that big, tough dude blushing behind that bouquet of brightly colored flowers. He'd met his obligation to his fellow Marine, but he thrust those flowers at me as if they'd been burning his hands. Tony would have gotten a big kick out of that. He would have added that "a Marine handles what has to be handled, no matter how much it may hurt!" I would have readily agreed, having seen it with my own eyes.

Ole Joe:

Joe had been in the Navy and later the Coast Guard. I found this out one day while his son, Todd, was visiting him. Todd had brought with him some old pictures he'd found in his dad's things. Joe remained as soft-spoken as always, but his pale gray eyes lit up like stars as he recalled, precisely, the moments those pictures were taken, relaying even the smallest details.

"Tell her the story about the little blonde, Dad," Todd teased.

Turns out, ole Joe had met a little blonde girl while docked, and the old codger had switched ships so he could go where the little blonde was going. Joe shrugged and added, "I just told 'em I'd made a mistake and got on the wrong ship." He chuckled softly, his pale eyes dancing merrily.

I'd often seen and heard Joe requesting his "pain pill", but I'd never had any cause to think much about it until the afternoon Joe shuffled to my office door. "Will you take a look at my ears?" He blushed. "I can't hear too good all of a sudden," he added as he poked a finger into his right ear. "Sure, let me get my flashlight. But for starters, get your finger out of your ear. That might help." I laughed. Joe smiled, then looked at the floor. "Ear wax. Your left ear is full of it, but that right one is completely occluded." I turned my flashlight off and set it down. "I'll get you started on some wax removal tonight, but you tell me if your ears start itching or burning, okay?"

Joe blushed. "Okay. You're right. I can't hear a thing out of this right ear." Joe turned to shuffle away, then stopped and turned back around. "Uhh, ma'am?"

"Yeah, Joe?"

Joe smiled big and blushed as he shuffled the few steps back to my office door. In whispered conspiracy, he confided, "Them pain pills aren't workin' like they used to, and them nurses keep tellin' me that's all the doctor is going to give me. They're nice about it, but that's all they say." He shrugged. "But that one last night, I asked her for my pain pill, and she said I was grouchy. I guess I might be ma'am. Truth is, I'm feeling downright ornery. I hurt all the time. I don't know why them pills aren't workin' no more. I don't mean to be grouchy."

"Oh, Joe, constant pain will make anybody feel ornery." I smiled. "Some people are ornery just to be ornery! At least you have a reason for it." I laughed.

Joe chuckled softly, blushed, and shrugged.

"Let me look at your meds. I'll get back to you in a little while."

Joe bowed his head. "Thank you, ma'am. I appreciate it." He turned and shuffled away.

I finished my immediate responsibilities and opened Joe's chart. It was a simple fix. I called Joe's doctor and informed him of Joe's pain medication no longer being as effective as it had been. I also informed the doctor that Joe wasn't taking any kind of anti-inflammatory medication and that Joe had no known drug allergies. The doctor gave me an order to start a daily anti-inflammatory medication to facilitate the effectiveness of his pain medication.

As I was writing the new order on the nurses' twenty-four-hour report, the charge nurse was reading as I wrote. She commented, "Oh, Joe?" She rolled her eyes, raised her hands in the air, and laughed. "Good! Maybe he won't be so grouchy! He been driving me crazy asking for that pain pill! Joe don't hurt no more than I do, and I feel fine. At least this one is routine, so he won't be bugging me about this one, too. The medication aid gives the routine meds."

The next afternoon Joe hunted me down, grinning like a kid and blushing like a new bride. "Ma'am, I feel better than I have in a long time. Thank you for your trouble."

"Wasn't any trouble, Joe. Just doing my job." I smiled, genuinely pleased for Joe. "If you have a need you feel is being ignored by anyone, you head straight up that hallway to the front office. Tell them you can't get anyone to help you, ya hear?"

"Yes, ma'am." Joe chuckled. "I hear you with my left ear. Thank you for them drops, too, by the way. Didn't nobody want to do nothin' about that, neither."

"Front office, sir. Don't forget it." I looked Joe in the eye. "Stand up for yourself like you stood up for this country, my friend."

"Yes, ma'am." Joe blushed, bowed his head, gripped his walker, turned, and shuffled away.

I watched Joe shuffle off with mixed emotions, glad he felt better but knowing there were many Joe's out there being ignored, hurting for no reason, miserably at the mercy of the system and those who work within it. I also knew the front office wasn't going to make much difference, if any at all, but it was all I had to offer.

Hickley:

Hickley's right leg had been amputated just above the knee due to severe infection in the bone. Hickley was extremely disagreeable. He didn't like anything served at any meal, nor did he like any alternative. He didn't like anything anybody said to him. He didn't like the weather, rain or shine. He didn't like the color of the walls in his room.

"I don't know who picked that color, but I have to look at it, and it looks like somebody vomited on the wall. Then y'all just smeared it over all of 'em, called yourselves painters." He grunted disgustedly.

Hickley didn't like anything about anything.

"George Strait's song 'I Hate Everything' was written for me, and, by damn, I do!" he readily professed.

Thing is, Hickley was actually a good dude. He was just weary of pain. He would probably argue this, as he argued everything. But Hickley had been in such pain for so long that his whole personality had changed. He no longer realized he yelled out almost constantly. He'd moan loudly, then follow it with expletives. Then he'd quickly yell out an apology. Expletives, apology. Over and over, all day, every day. All night, every night. All of this happening as he writhed in pain.

Everybody knows that being cold can make one's bones hurt, but to get him closer to the nurses' station—so there would be quicker intervention related to falls and yelling out—Hickley was moved to the coldest room on the unit. I heard him moaning in his sleep one night. He was curled up in a ball, his blanket bunched and hanging over the side of the bed, his sheet bunched up next to him, goosebumps freckling his skin from his neck to his ankles. Tiptoeing around his bed, I gently spread his blanket back over him, at which point Hickley screamed out, his eyes popping open from a sound sleep when the weight of one blanket touched his stump.

"Oh, Hickley, I'm so sorry!" I cried. "You looked so cold! Please forgive me!"

Wiping tears from his sleepy eyes, Hickley mumbled, "It's okay. I'm freezing. Thank you for covering me up. It kind of helps just to know someone cares. Don't feel bad. I'm going to hurt no matter what. No point freezing, too, right?"

"Thanks, Hickley. I'm truly sorry. I'll make sure to leave your stump uncovered next time."

Hickley wiggled to a different position, his eyes closed. As I tiptoed toward the door, Hickley, having grown more alert in his shifting, grumbled, "I don't like these blankets y'all got, anyway. They itch."

The next day I brought Hickley a large, soft, super lightweight blanket. I'd looked at every color in an attempt to find one he might like, as if that were even possible. After clocking in, I went straight to Hickley's room. "Hey there." I smiled. "I got you a new blanket. It's warm but really lightweight," I chattered as I removed the heavier cotton blanket from his bed, spreading his new, lightweight, hunter green blanket over him. Finishing, I looked up and saw the cutest jack-o-lantern grin I'd ever seen.

Seeing me looking, Hickley quickly scowled. "I hate green."

"I figured you would."

I heard Hickley laugh for the first time. The sound didn't last long; he saw to that. The feeling, however, will last forever.

In the five weeks Hickley stayed with us, he fell out of bed twenty-three times. While writhing in pain, he'd inadvertently roll off the bed. I'm guessing that leg hitting a "fall mat" hurt almost as bad as it did when it hit the floor prior to the fall mats being placed at the bedside. But he didn't break anything when he fell. For whatever that is worth in his world of pain.

Me being me, I got it. I did. The doctor wasn't ordering anything stronger. So I called the surgeon who'd cut Hickley's leg off, and asked for more effective pain management. I described Hickley writhing in pain, yelling out, and falling out of bed onto the stump with the ongoing and severe bone infection, for which he was still receiving two IV antibiotics. The surgeon's nurse interrupted. "Ma'am, we don't order anything stronger than Tylenol four anymore, either. Just too much paperwork required to order anything stronger. I'm sorry," she said before hanging up without allowing me time to say another word.

"Too much paperwork." I sighed heavily. Lifting my face skyward, I asked God to help me stop wishing that the doctor and surgeon would develop severe bone infections that would require amputation. I'm ashamed to say how hard I had to pray to stop wishing that every time Hickley screamed out.

I wish I could write about a happy ending here, but the only thing I can say is that Hickley finally went home once his twenty-day Medicare stay was completed. His pertinent IV antibiotics were to be continued via home health. Hickley could not afford to pay even part of the costs to stay, having long since gone broke with medical expenses as the infection was no new thing. He had started, years before, with the loss of the foot. This was his third amputation on that same leg. And, though he had no one at home to help him - no pay, no stay.

Food for thought on a larger scale:

Hickley is writhing in pain, suffering beyond adequate description, and the drug addicts still have their drugs.

Result? The innocent suffer.

Similar to guns. I don't have a gun, but I have a load of common sense. Common sense tells me that if you take guns from citizens, that is all you accomplish. The criminals still have their guns.

Result? The innocent suffer.

Point? Taking something from all to control a few is ... a habitually humanistic knee-jerk reaction, completely void of not-so-common-at-all common sense.

I was speechless the first time I had an elderly man tell me that he had to see his doctor monthly to undergo a urine drug screen, solely to have his pain medication refilled.

Firstly, the man was literally twisted with rheumatoid arthritis, unable even to straighten his torso, unable to walk, unable to grasp a glass of water. That man had to have someone take him into his doctor's office monthly to urinate in a cup, that someone also having to hold the cup for him while he urinated into it because he couldn't do it himself.

Second of all, urine drug screens are completely unreliable; they are *not* one hundred percent. I know this to be fact. I pointed it out to authorities, and provided evidence, but I heard absolutely nothing in response. The *authorities* do not *want* to recognize, not to mention *admit* to, the fallibility of their overused, blatantly abused, handy dandy *tool*.

Amelia is proud, dignified, and determined. Her entire spine literally degenerated to such an extent that her neck is now backward, so she is in constant pain. To top it all off, she, too, has rheumatoid arthritis. And yet one would never know by watching her that she hurts relentlessly. She is too determined to fight, to live her life, to choose happiness. In addition to her pain medication, Amelia tries every natural remedy she can find. She exercises *through the pain* to strengthen her muscles, thus taking the work-load off her bones and joints.

Amelia was angry, to the point of tears, when she visited her father on a Wednesday afternoon. When we were talking, she informed me how "dirty" the pharmacy staff makes her feel when she gets her pain medication refilled. Amelia looks healthy, she doesn't appear to be hurting, things for which she should be admired, if anything at all. However, these are not things that should cause her to be deemed pain-free, silently labeled, judged, and blatantly treated as a drug abuser.

These are words I have heard from many, not all, but way too many nurses, way too many times:

"He/she watches the clock to make sure he/she doesn't miss a dose."

"He/she doesn't look like he/she is in pain."

"I don't see any signs of pain. He/she ain't hurting."

"He/she doesn't even have a diagnosis for pain medication."

"Oh yeah, he/she is hurting so bad (eyes rolling), but he/she can still go play bingo and go out on pass."

"I'll get 'em the pill when I get 'em the pill. They don't need it, anyway."

I could go on forever. Sadly, I truly could.

Pain that gets out of control is much harder to get back under control. We "teach" that to our patients. Well, we are supposed to. We used to. Lack of pain management *used* to be something the state took seriously.

Everybody handles pain differently. Everybody handles every-thing differently.

You want a diagnosis for the pain pill? Pain! There, now take that poor soul his or her pain relief.

This is the red flag of truth waving in the wind: *You don't know the accurate diagnosis for ninety percent of your patients' medications, and you aren't concerned about those.*

It is only the individual and the individual's doctor who should decide if an individual is in pain or if an individual requires pain medication. *That* is not the business of the government, insurance companies, pharmacists, or, when it comes right down to it, nurses. In reference to an inpatient setting, that decision should include the input, as applicable, of the patient; the family, if any; the nurses that provide care; maybe even the aids that provide care, and the therapists that provide care. But that decision should ultimately be made by the doctor and that patient *only*. *Period.*

Fully cognizant of the widespread drug related crime issues in the world today. I humbly suggest we leave the doctoring to the doctors and leave the crime solving to law enforcement.

It is wholly wrong to make innocent people suffer when relief is available.

Gina:

Gina was seventy-four years old and a mother of seven children, all of whom she'd already seen "lowered into the ground", in addition to her beloved husband of fifty-six years. Gina was bitter, irritable, and hard to like. Oh, but she was easy to love. Gina was one of those rare genuine souls who tells it like it is, and I respect that. I find it refreshing.

I did not find it refreshing when I discovered Gina was hoarding her medications. I happened to walk in as she was adding her morning meds to the cup she kept in the drawer on her bedside table, caught her stuffing a wadded napkin on top of her collection, "just in case one of them with dementia happens to get into my drawer". Gina explained. "Some of'em ain't with it enough to know that swallowing all them pills might kill'em. Lord knows I couldn't live with that."

One of the many reasons nurses and med aids should stop handing people meds and walking away. "Talk to me Gina." I sat on the edge of her bed, waited.

"Hell, I don't want to keep living in pain, and nobody is going to do a damned thing about it." She shrugged. "So I'm going to. I'm gonna take all them pills just as soon as I'm sure I have enough to do the job. This pain isn't *life*; it's a never-ending nightmare. I'm going to end the nightmare," she said emphatically, and void of expression.

I called her doctor and requested a pain management evaluation, explained Gina's related desperation. Huge mistake. Unfortunately, there are requirements for such things, and this particular Doc merely focused on the legalities, asking only if I thought she was serious. I knew very well that if Gina said it, Gina meant it.

Live and learn, stupid, I thought to myself while making arrangements to send Gina to an inpatient geriatric psyche facility for "suicidal ideations." As opposed to doc simply managing Gina's pain, I had to send her to the care of Frito Dude! My heart was broken. I was ashamed, *guilt-ridden*, for not thinking that one through more thoroughly before calling the doctor. In retrospect, I should have told Gina to say the same words *to* the doctor. I'm just short of one hundred percent confident the outcome would have been much different had the doctor stood in the "hearing" shoes, looked into the "speaking" eyes.

So Gina went. She could have refused; she had the right. Sadly, Gina "hurt too bad to put up a fight about it." Just as sadly, she'd have eventually gone anyway most likely; unless she lied and said she hadn't meant it. Gina wasn't the lying kind.

So Gina went. Gina returned, still in pain. However, she had gained three things: an antidepressant, an anti-anxiety medication (also potentially addictive, I might add), and the confidence that she could trust no one. The latter being my fault. Knowing such, I was more determined than ever. Contacting her doctor at least daily, I cringed my way through multiple butt-chewings before finally persuading him to refer Gina to a pain management specialist. The specialist ultimately did the required paperwork, and she got Gina's pain under control. Of course, Gina then had to go pee in a cup monthly.

A ludicrous waste of time, energy and money, but it's better than Gina living a life of pain.

Gina was a new person! I wiped tears from my eyes when I saw the relief on Gina's face after her first dose of effective pain medication. Gina will always be one to shoot straight, but her arrows are less like daggers and a bit more like Cupid's. She wouldn't allow me to keep apologizing, and I love her even more for it.

"Let it go, little one," she barked. "It was just as stupid of me to say them things to you as it was for you to repeat them, though that *was* stupid!" Gina chortled. "You really had no choice, and in the end, you fought like a champ for me. I have no regrets and no hard feelings, only gratitude. You got me relief."

"Well, thank you for forgiving me," I said as I turned to walk out.

"Hold up, shorty. I have something for you." Gina leaned over and opened her bedside drawer, then took out a cup with a napkin stuffed into it and handed it to me.

Baffled, my mind racing, I pulled the wadded napkin from the cup and stood gazing upon a collection of Gina's new psyche meds, both the antidepressant and the anti-anxiety. I looked questioningly at Gina, who grinned like a Cheshire cat.

"You can tell Doc to shove them pills where the sun don't shine! I took'em the first time they brung'em. She brung'em so early in the morning, I was too sleepy to think to dig'em out. They taste like that crap we had for lunch." Gina hung her tongue out dramatically. "After that, I remembered to dig'em out. You can tell that smarty-pants doctor I never took them pills at that damned hospital, and I ain't gonna take 'em here. Thanks to the pesky little nurse being a thorn in his side"—she cackled— "my body ain't throbbing like an abscessed tooth no more. I can think about something besides pain for a change, and I got things ta do!" She winked in dismissal.

Gina's cackle followed me down the hallway as I headed for the phone. I couldn't resist grinning as I informed the doctor that the psyche meds were never taken and were now discontinued per resident request. I miss Gina something fierce, but I'm told she is calling bingo, has independently formed a resident "fix the food" committee, and is president of resident council. Better look out! Gina don't play!

What about all the other Gina's out there? Who is fighting for them? Is anybody noticing? Does anybody care? Will they literally throb in pain until the day they die? Will that day be sooner rather than later?

Consider all the tax dollars wasted on the additional doctors and the additional doctor's additional lab work, scans, x-rays… the additional appointments requiring additional time and transportation. Why can't the doctor simply treat his patient effectively and be done with it? Why all the extra hoop jumping? Why all the extra doctors, expense, effort, time, and money?

Yet another mess on which to waste tax dollars. Meanwhile, the druggies are off getting high somewhere while the innocent suffer significant pain, sometimes indescribable agony. Knee-jerk reactions are not the answer. It is past time to stop and think. The effects of chronic pain trickle down and cost the individual and the taxpayer in an endless variety of ways.

Unrelieved pain leads to suffering, depression, and decreased appetite, which leads to decreased intake, which leads to a vast variety of health problems resulting from nutritional deficit.

Unrelieved pain leads to decreased movement and activity, weakness, impaired balance, decreased joint mobility, falls, and need for a higher level of assistance. In fact, increased pain exacerbates all the secondary issues. And the cycle continues, grows, all because the doctor isn't allowed to simply treat his patient effectively.

Pain is a slow, relentless killer.

Daniel:

New to the facility, my neck was bent, and my head was spinning as I tried to acclimate myself. Finally, after a couple of weeks, I was beginning to learn the facility and those within.

Pushing a medication cart is much like trying to shove a rickety old school bus with square wheels and no steering wheel up a steep hill... through the mud...with no brakes...in the dark. As a shorty, I didn't have the world's greatest view over the top of those things. Thus, I had to observe my path in advance. That's how I first glimpsed him, from a distance. He was slowly propelling his wheelchair into the dining room as I manhandled and corralled the cart in that direction. At a glance, all I saw was a lean, long-legged elderly man with thinning white hair and a, somewhat large, white bandage on the side of his face. Nothing unusual in the world of long term care.

He must be on Elsie's unit, I thought to myself briefly. *I've not seen him before.*

Banging the cart through the doorway, I quickly braced every muscle in my body, gripped the sides of the cart, and jerked back on it with every ounce of strength I could muster, attempting to slow the cart's momentum and keep it from slamming into the wall as I parked it. Panting, puffing the stray hairs from my face, and feeling much like Sylvester Stallone in '*Rocky*' as the cart nestled gently against the wall, I turned victoriously, ready to prepare for the dinner hour.

Pale blue eyes snagged my gaze as I turned. Translucent like glass, set over an aristocratic nose and a large white bandage, the pale blue eyes had been quietly observing my struggle from the back side of the large dining room. Smiling, I dipped my chin to say hello. The eyes widened almost imperceptibly.

Surprise? I wondered as the eyes briefly crinkled, sparkling deeply, like the sea rippling in the light of a full moon. A heartwarming smile spread like soft butter, half concealed by the white bandage, as the observer dipped his chin ever more slightly in return, then turned shyly away.

"Excuse me." Patsy jutted her indignant chin into the air once the hustle and bustle of serving was done. "I didn't get my apple juice."

"Let me get that for you." I forced a smile, clearly recalling that Patsy had declared a pure hatred for apple juice just the day before, insisting she be served milk instead.

Hurrying back with the juice, my gaze was drawn to a table in the back. After setting Patsy's juice next to her milk, I straightened, stood, unconsciously observed as a large bony hand tediously scooped a bit of pureed food from a plate. Tremulously, the hand then slowly raised the spoon, clumsily maneuvering it even as the spoon tilted, threatening to drop its meager contents. Finally, the pale hand slowly passed the spoon between lips half covered by a large white bandage.

So…determined…so alone…my blue-eyed observer.

The spoon then hovering midair, he gripped the table with his free hand, bracing himself for the obviously strenuous task before him. Practiced, he bowed his head slightly, his shoulders hunching as he stared into his plate. Seemingly oblivious to all around him, he focused on his efforts to move the food to the back of his mouth. Ultimately, his chin dipping a small parenthesis, he swallowed.

Exhaling, I realized that I had been holding my breath and swallowing with him. Blinking the tears from my eyes, I watched him slowly raise his face, take a long, deep, purposed breath before lowering the spoon to his plate and beginning the process once more, for another small bite.

Suddenly weary beyond words, I sighed heavily.

"Well, if it's too much trouble, never mind," Patsy snapped. "Don't heavy sigh me! I'll just choke on my food so you can stand there in a daze."

"I'm sorry, Patsy. I didn't realize I had sighed. I was thinking." I resisted rolling my eyes. "What did you need?"

"Milk. I need milk. Milk, milk, MILK," Patsy sassed. "I've only said it a hundred times while you stood there ignoring me."

Glancing at the full glass of apple juice, I headed over to get Patsy some milk, milk, MILK.

That Saturday I covered a shift on the opposite unit. Kelsey, who was covering as treatment nurse, asked me to assist her with Daniel's wound care. "I'm not sure I can do it," Kelsey exclaimed, her face twisted with horror. "It makes me shudder just thinking about it."

Having no clue who Daniel was, I laughed at Kelsey's dramatics as I followed her into the room. Standing beside the bed, a smile grew all the way from my toes and exploded across my face as my copper-brown eyes met pale, translucent blue.

"Daniel." I grinned. "It is indeed a pleasure to officially meet you."

Again, his eyes widened almost imperceptibly. *Why the surprise?* Again, the half-smile spread like soft butter toward one ear. This time he didn't look away. His pale blue eyes locked on mine, speaking things I could feel, but couldn't yet hear. Daniel shifted his gaze to observe Kelsey's expression, the half-smile vanishing in a blink.

Kelsey removed the dressing, revealing a cavernous wound on Daniel's cheek and mouth. More precisely, half of Daniel's lower face was gone, a gaping hole in its place. Kelsey hesitated and glanced at me, dangling the old dressing midair with her thumb and forefinger; almost as if she were afraid the wound might be contagious.

"You a football fan?" I smiled brightly at Daniel, whose brow creased with confusion as he nodded his head slightly. Rolling my eyes dramatically, I continued, "Oh Lawd! Not you, too. Well then, let's get this finished before the game starts."

A smile winked across half his face as Daniel closed his pale blue eyes.

Nodding at Kelsey, I scooted into her position as she backed out of it, taking my place so I could perform Daniel's wound care.

A couple of weeks later, I met Daniel as he was leaving the dining room after dinner.

"Hey, Daniel." I smiled.

His pale blue eyes widened, again almost imperceptibly, then locked on mine with a palpable intensity. I listened. I know. But it's true. I listened. Even more amazingly, I *understood*. "Of course, I see *you*, Daniel. You aren't your wound. You are Daniel, who happens to have a wound." I shrugged. Daniel's eyes grew as big as quarters. "And I appreciate that you, too, see *me*," I continued. "You are the first person in yeeears of nursing to notice how near impossible it is for one my size to maneuver those bulky, clumsy carts." I chuckled, and Daniel smiled, both of us recalling my scene. "You see me, you speak to me, and you acknowledge my existence as a person, not just as a nurse. When I look at you, Daniel, I see *you*, another soul who, like me, is trying to get through this earthly trial. I see you, not your bandage. I see it now." I shrugged again, chuckled. "Cuz it has food on it. Let's go change it."

Daniel's eyes crinkled, sparkled, and spoke. "I know, right?" I said, laughing out loud. "We now know we are gifted. You can speak clearly with your eyes, and strangely, I can hear you. I'm not sure what that says about us, but hey, it works!"

Daniel chuckled, grimacing as his bandage tugged with the movement of his remaining cheek muscle.

"Oh crap! Don't laugh!"

Daniel laughed, then grimaced. I grabbed the handles on his wheel-chair, mentally zipped my lips, and headed down the hall to his room. Removing his dressing, I willed myself to keep chattering, maintaining my casual expression as I cleaned the large, gaping hole, which had then progressed to the side of his nose, exposing his nostril completely. The wound was slowly progressing upwards, threatening to consume his eye.

Silently I prayed, *Dear Father in heaven, please don't let this eat away Daniel's eyes. Please, Lord, spare his eyes. In Jesus' name!*

Daniel had developed a basal cell carcinoma on his upper lip years before, as he had worked outside, farming his entire life. Unfortunately, he'd ignored it, thinking it to be nothing significant, just a mole. Ultimately malignant, it was consuming Daniel's face, literally eating it away, leaving a massive hole in its wake.

"So, I met your wife the other day." I continued my chatter as I cleaned Daniel's dinner from the many pits and crevices of his wound, contemplating the related risk of infection. "How'd you land a looker like that?" I laughed.

Daniel grinned, revealing food deeper in the wound. Looking Daniel in the eye, I explained the risks of his continuing to eat by mouth. Daniel agreed, communicated that it was becoming too painful to do so, anyway. Daniel got a g-tube/stomach tube for nutrition and hydration, so he no longer ate by mouth. But the cancer relentlessly ate away at his face.

Just a couple of weeks later, I went over to check on him, having noticed the treatment cart outside his door. "Hey, Daniel." I smiled. "Haven't seen you in a while."

Daniel immediately locked his eyes on mine. Again, that palpable, track-stopping intensity. Paula, the treatment nurse, looked back and forth between Daniel and me, then proceeded with his wound care. She looked up, puzzled, when I spoke.

"Okay, my friend." I smiled. "Paula, Daniel needs better pain management. It's not holding anymore. Will you see to that as soon as you're done, please?"

Daniel watched Paula's face closely.

"Umm, okay," Paula stuttered at me, then looked at Daniel. "Is that right, Daniel? You told her that?"

Daniel remained expressionless, nodded his head slightly, then closed his eyes.

God, please don't let it take his eyes, I prayed silently.

A week later, on Wednesday, I asked Paula about Daniel's pain management. I found out Daniel had been admitted to hospice. It wasn't the fact that Daniel had been admitted to hospice that bothered me; it was *why* it had happened. Hospice hadn't come up until Daniel requested stronger pain medication. Daniel's more than justified request brought two things to light.

One: Daniel had been suffering severely, as he was given one hydrocodone twice a day while cancer literally ate away at his face. While they put a nebulizer mask on that half-eaten face, the mask smashed against the wound, the elastic stretched over more of the wound. Even once doc increased it to one tablet every four hours, and even when he received it every four hours (which was only the days on which I worked that unit), his pain was relentless.

Two: Daniel had to sign on with hospice to get appropriate, effective pain management. He could not get it otherwise.

I stopped everything and went to see Daniel, who was in bed in a dark room, his blinds having never been opened that morning.

"Hey, Daniel," I said, opening the blinds. "How's your pain medicine working?"

Spinning back around, I hurried to Daniel's bedside. Daniel locked his eyes on mine, but with less intensity. The bandage was now just beneath his right eye, covering the lower lid.

Dear Lord, please don't let it take his eyes! I cried silently, then struggled to maintain focus, to hear Daniel.

The sparkle was gone; the intensity was weak. But the insistence remained. Before I left the room, though it took more attempts than in the past, I understood clearly that Daniel wanted pain management only. No more nebulizer treatments. No more life sustaining medications. Daniel was ready to just be as comfortable as possible.

The next day I arrived to find Daniel's wife, Carolyn, sitting with him. Carolyn disagreed with Daniel's wishes, so everything was continued, as Carolyn was Daniel's POA and had coerced Daniel into going against his own wishes. Daniel was angry, but he loved his wife. He had a horrible cough due to secretions pouring down his throat, as, with little remaining facial structure, they had no other place to go. His wife insisted on the nebulizer treatments despite the mask and elastic pressing against Daniel's wound. I stood and held Daniel's gaze while his nurse put the mask on him, my heart breaking. But I knew he needed me to stay.

I checked a few minutes later, and Daniel had not yet received a single dose of morphine, which was his strongest pain medication and the very reason he had signed with hospice. When I asked his nurse, I was told, "I'm not gone give it. I'm not gone be the one that helps him take his last breath." Furious at the ignorance, I explained to Daniel that he had stronger medication available if he wanted it. I explained the related effect of depressing respirations. Thus, if respirations were weak enough, there was potential for taking the last breath as a result. Tears formed in his eyes, his only facial feature still whole, and he nodded his head vigorously, causing pain so intense that tears poured from his eyes, soaking into his dressing.

Carolyn started to speak, and maybe she was going to say that it was a beautiful day. Who knows? I interrupted and said, "Carolyn, I'm so sorry. It will have to wait a minute. Daniel needs his medicine now." I hurried out.

His nurse thrust his morphine in my face. "You give it, then. I'm not."

Carolyn could not recall what she'd been about to say.

I spent the next two weeks watching the tissue beneath and to the side of Daniel's eye disappear, praying, monitoring his pain medication administration, and advocating for him with the nurses who essentially refused to give him his morphine. I never put that nebulizer mask on his poor little face again. Instead I simply held it near his face. For once I found myself grateful that nebulizer treatments are most often documented but not actually done; thus, it was likely no one was smashing the mask against Daniel's wound, which by then consumed almost the entire half of his face as far back as his ear. After reviewing Daniel's pain medication administration, finding he was still not being given his morphine, I spoke with hospice and requested that Daniel's anti-anxiety medication and morphine be made routine. I did this after he asked me to do so—asked with eyes at imminent risk of being eaten away.

Dear God in heaven, please don't let it take Daniel's eyes. Please bring him home to you with his eyes intact! I prayed silently one afternoon as I watched Daniel fidget painfully in his sleep.

Looking much like a stick figure with a mummied head, Daniel opened his pale blue eyes and stared into mine with his old intensity. The only visible corner of his mouth slid like melted butter toward his ear as his eyes crinkled, sparkled, said, "I'm going to be okay," and then closed again. I couldn't help noticing the cancer wasn't spreading to the eye as it had the mouth and nose, just bulldozing straight through, taking everything in its path. Instead it was working itself steadily around the eye. The hole had begun consuming his brow, but his eyes were still intact.

"I know," I whispered with a teary smile. "You're in His hands, my friend."

Later that evening an aid rushed into the dining room at dinnertime. "His nurse ain't here. She went to lunch. Daniel needs you! We think he's done died!"

I hurried to Daniel's room and grabbed his hand. Daniel opened his eyes just long enough to crinkle the corners and say, "Thank you for being my friend." Closing his eyes again, Daniel took a deep breath and sighed as if settling in for a nap long overdue. Within fifteen minutes he took his last breath. I held mine, waiting, and squeezed his hand as I felt it go limp. The aids thought I was completely bonkers when I checked Daniel's pulse, found none, grinned, and whispered, "Thank you, Jesus!"

Daniel left for heaven with his eyes intact. I felt sure he was talking some heads off, talking about all the things he'd been thinking all that time.

Daniel's story was worth telling simply because Daniel is worthy. But the point here is that even with the man's face being slowly and painfully eaten away, effective pain management was overlooked! Then, once pointed out, it was difficult to obtain. Then, once obtained, it was difficult to get the nurses to administer it.

Personally speaking, I don't understand. I'd feel much better about myself if the individual in my care was comfortable. What is quantity without quality? I wouldn't want "another day" if that day was spent in excruciating, thought-consuming pain.

What matters here, though, is Daniel's perspective. Daniel was no longer able to speak for himself. I believe that is why I picked up on Daniel so quickly and easily. The man was about to burst. He needed to tell somebody he was hurting. He "felt" that I "saw" him, and this surprised him. But once he had confirmed it and accepted the possibility of being *heard*, he used his eyes to scream for help.

Macy:

This happened just yesterday.

Macy, not quite sixty years old yet, is a precious soul who has suffered from two bone diseases since birth, in addition to painful, twisting rheumatoid arthritis and painful, mystifying fibromyalgia. Due to her disease processes, Macy has two artificial hips and knees, along with multiple joint deformities elsewhere.

Most outstanding about Macy is her purely adorable spirit and her light-the-room-up smile, which was glaringly designed by God's own hand. That lady could melt the heart of Hitler with one smile. Unfortunately, thanks to…well…us, Macy's been smiling a lot less these days, because Macy's been sleeping a lot more.

When I say sleeping a lot, I mean nearly twenty-four-seven, sometimes falling asleep while lifting the spoon to her mouth at mealtime. That is *if* Macy stays awake long enough to pick her spoon up in the first place.

That's how I first met Macy. I walked by her open doorway and noticed her fast asleep, her dinner tray sitting untouched on a table beside her. After that day, I checked on Macy at dinner from time to time, always finding the same thing, except for the day I found her holding her jello in one hand, her eyes closed, chin resting on her chest, drool pooled at the corners of her mouth. Macy had obviously been about to remove the plastic covering from her jello and had fallen asleep again in the process.

Everybody—the nurses, aids, therapists, and administrative staff—was concerned about Macy's newly developed and ongoing lethargy. I don't see the same people twice very often, so the first time I met Macy, I had no clue she was any different from her norm. I did know that she scared the poop out of me, as I thought she was dead. I did. For a few interminable seconds, I thought I was about to call a code. After checking, however, I realized Macy had a pulse, and though shallow, she was breathing. Ultimately, I awakened her with firm physical stimuli, at which point she smiled at me so angelically that I almost thought she'd died and taken me with her to heaven. She got an enormous kick out of having scared me. Again, I had no clue that was not her norm. As I said, I just happened by and saw her sleeping instead of eating, then went into her room to wake her.

I became actively involved in the situation several weeks later, when the charge nurse asked me to see Macy and try to "figure out" what had caused the drastic change. "She was alert and active when she first got here," the nurse explained. "She was going to the dining room for meals, doing therapy, and getting out of bed with assistance to use the toilet, but now she is completely incontinent and seldom gets out of bed at all."

After assessing Macy and reviewing her records and medical history, which were provided by her previous and longtime doctor, this is what I found: Macy had been taking an antidepressant, and we didn't have her on it. Macy had been taking a sleep aid as needed (meaning she took it only if she found she couldn't sleep), which we had her taking every night, routinely. Yes, we were concerned about severe lethargy and sleeping incessantly, yet we had her popping a nightly sleeping pill that was supposed to be as needed.

Macy had been taking her pain medication every twelve hours; we had gotten it increased to every six hours. Macy's previous doctor had specified every twelve hours in order to prevent over sedation in light of the potential sedating effects of Macy's strong antipsychotic medication. But then, one would only know this if one had reviewed Macy's records. (If a prudent and thorough admission process had been in place)

And I discovered Macy's blood pressure was persistently low, which can also contribute to or cause lethargy.

All the things I'd discovered could be contributed to and/or cause lethargy.

I also discovered that, like the charge nurse had informed me, on her admission to our facility, Macy had been alert, chirpy, and active, like a friendly, bright-eyed butterball turkey with a halo. However, a few days later Macy had complained that her pain was not fully controlled. So, the nurse had called Macy's *new* doctor and asked if we could increase the frequency of her pain medication from twice daily every twelve hours to four times daily every six hours. So, it was done. A quick, easy fix. No research or further consideration necessary.

In light of what I'd found while reviewing the records, what I'd learned after speaking with Macy, and what I'd noted while assessing Macy, I prepared a communication to the doctor requesting that Macy's medications be changed back to what was previously ordered, which would include resumption of the pain medication at every twelve hours, plus the addition of Tylenol every six hours, as needed, for breakthrough pain. After all, Macy had several significant pain-inducing disease processes, and yet over sedation was a big consideration in light of her other necessary medication. We had checked basic bloodwork, and Macy's results were better than mine, possibly yours. All I needed was to check Macy's heart rhythm and sounds, and I was ready to communicate with her doctor. So, I trekked down the hall and did just that, at which time Macy asked softly in her child-like voice, "Would you please get me something better than Tylenol for pain?"

I almost said, "You don't take Tylenol; you take a pain pill." But my gut said, *Hush. Wait. Go talk to the nurse on duty. She doesn't even have an order for Tylenol. Why would she mention it specifically and request something better when she isn't even taking it to begin with? She doesn't even have a doctor's order for Tylenol yet.*

After I hurried back to the nurses' station, the charge nurse, Willy, informed me that (a) they'd held the pain pill for twenty-four hours and given Tylenol instead, resulting in Macy being more alert; and that (b) Willy had already contacted the doctor to see if we could discontinue the pain pill altogether due to lethargy, and just use Tylenol. Willy further informed me that Nilly, the assistant director of nursing, had then contacted the doctor with the same request because the doctor hadn't responded to Willy.

Nilly came out of her office after overhearing this conversation. She stood across from me, just a tad annoyed. I readily rattled off all that I'd found during review of Macy's records, including the persistent low blood pressure, as well as the *as needed* sleeping pill that someone had changed to every night. I watched Nilly roll her eyes and sneer.

"I changed Macy's sleep aid to every night because it is classified as an anti-depressant, and the state says psyche meds can't be as needed," Nilly said; that meaning the state required psyche medications to be routine. I couldn't help but wonder about all the as needed, non-routine anti-anxiety medications in the long-term care world. (However, on that note, the state's lack of individualism only allows as needed anti-anxiety medications for fourteen days. After that, one's recurrent anxiety is supposed to be resolved in the state's across-the-board, authoritative opinion.) Nilly stood, arms crossed, head cocked to the side, waiting for my reply.

"So you're giving a nightly sleep aid to a woman you are concerned is oversleeping," I quipped. Nilly sneered, rolling her eyes. I continued, "And back when Macy was perky and active, simply needed a bit more pain management, why did some ninny get her pain pill doubled instead of simply adding Tylenol for breakthrough pain?"

Willy stared at me, her arms crossed like Nilly's. Nilly crossed her ankles, sneered again, and sighed heavily.

"So, since you two have already muddied the water with a request that will inevitably leave the sweet lady in pain, while you're getting your order for Tylenol only, talk to the doctor about her low blood pressure, which none of her nurses have ever noticed." I rolled my eyes and shook my head.

"No!" Nilly nearly yelled, her arms uncrossed and flailing. "I was just trying to do something about the lethargy! You can handle it if you've already found all *that!*" She stormed back to her office.

Biting my tongue, I returned to my office and contacted the doctor. Three minutes later the doctor returned my call. I received an order to discontinue the pain pill and start Tylenol instead. I suggested reconsideration based on Macy's inevitable pain exacerbation, at which time I was cut short.

"That's what they asked for," the doctor barked.

"Yes, sir, I'm aware of what they asked for. Did you want to do anything about the blood pressure?"

"Oh, yeah," the doctor replied, then gave me an order to decrease the dosage of one of Macy's blood pressure pills, the only thing with which I agreed.

Genuinely concerned about Macy's pain and lack of effective pain management, the knee-jerk reactions vs prudent, assessment and review of her records, I went to speak with the director of nursing. The director replied, "Well, all we can do now is give it a try, see how the Tylenol works for her."

Bless Macy's heart. She is going to be awake alright. Awake and in pain, I thought to myself as I headed back to my office. *Sadly, after getting a sleeping pill nightly, considering her other medication, pain may be the only thing keeping Macy awake, but, by dang, she'll be woke!*

Two weeks later Macy rolled up to my office door after she'd come from therapy. Half smiling up at me, she squeaked, "Could you help me get something besides Tylenol for my pain, please?" Her eyes flooded with tears, and the half-smile vanished. "My shoulder hurts so bad, and I wake up every morning in pain all over. I hurt all day, every day."

Nilly heard every word from her office just across the hallway. "Hey, what about an anti-inflammatory?" she called out to me.

I held my finger up, indicating to Macy to give me just a minute, then stepped over into Nilly's office. "Pardon?"

"What about an anti-inflammatory?"

"Has anyone ever gotten her pain medication reordered at every twelve hours?" I asked nicely.

Nilly rolled her eyes at me. "No, that's why she's not zonked out."

"So she's still getting nothing but Tylenol?" Biting my tongue, I stepped back over to Macy.

"I have rheumatoid arthritis," Macy whispered, peering up at me with big blue eyes that flashed once toward Nilly's office door.

"I know, darlin', and that hurts. I get it. Trust me. Yours is advanced, too, so I can only imagine how badly you hurt. I am so sorry. I'll call your doctor and let you know what he says. I will not forget about you, okay?"

Macy smiled, her pudgy cheeks plumping up like pillows. "Okay," she said as she rolled away toward her room, fully confident that I'd do just that.

But I didn't. Completely against my grain, but near desperate to avoid stepping on toes, I held off that day, hoping Nilly would step up and take care of it. Knowing I would get grief if I did what I knew needed to be done, I gave Nilly the opportunity to right their wrong.

The next day was Friday. That evening I suddenly remembered I hadn't checked on Macy's pain medication, and on doing so, I found that nothing had been done. I checked on Macy, and the first thing she did was ask me if I'd gotten anything to "help the hurt." I was not going to leave Macy in pain, so I called her doctor. Ultimately, Macy's original pain medication order was resumed—same medication, same strength, given at the same frequency of every twelve hours. The only difference was that I asked the doctor to keep Tylenol as needed for breakthrough pain. I went home knowing Nilly was going to be pissed off but also knowing Macy would no longer be suffering.

The charge nurse sent me a text in the wee hours, telling me she'd called Nilly to get her to phone the order for Macy's pain medication to the pharmacy. She told me Nilly had said, "I don't agree with it, but I'll call it in."

Oh, how I dreaded Monday morning. But Monday came at the end of that Sunday night like indigestion after Thanksgiving dinner. Sudden, miserable, onset, with no relief in sight. Solely in attempt to keep peace, I stopped in Nilly's office after arriving at work. I told her the doctor and I could think of nothing else for pain management, as something stronger would for sure zonk Macy out, but we could not leave her in pain. I added, "If you have any suggestions, please share."

Nilly popped off, "No, I don't have any suggestions. *I'm* not the doctor."

Easily catching her drift, I thought, *Well, you readily had a suggestion when you doubled the pain medication. You had a suggestion when you changed the as needed sleeping pill to every night, routinely. You had a suggestion when you got the pain medication discontinued altogether. You weren't "the doctor" then either.* But I said nothing. And I didn't add, though I wanted to, that Nilly had had every opportunity to take care of the problem herself the day before… but didn't.

Nilly sneered at me, said, "I haven't been down there today to see if she's knocked out."

Again, I caught her drift. Again, I said nothing, walked out, and went to my office.

Two days ago, I was asked to see Macy's roommate. Macy smiled radiantly at me as I sailed into the room. After assessing her roommate, I stopped to say hello to Macy on my way back out. Before I could say a word, Macy grinned and said, "Thank you for helping me. I knew you would." Her eyes grew wide with wonder. "I know I don't know you, but I can tell you care. You listen. I see you listening, and you hear what we say. And you fussed at me for scaring you that day when I was sleeping so hard you couldn't wake me up." She giggled.

"I sure did, and don't you do that to me ever again." I laughed, recalling the horrifying moment as if had been yesterday. "You feel better since we got your pain medicine back?"

"Oh yes! Sometimes I take Tylenol in-between, but sometimes I don't even need it. And I'm not sleeping all the time. I eat my food when they bring it instead of after it gets cold, and I'm doing my therapy, too!"

"Wonderful! I'm so glad it's all better now."

"Me too! What a relief! And now I won't be scaring you anymore." She grinned.

"That *is* a relief!" We both laughed as I hurried out.

Down the Tube

Grayson:

Grayson was just plain ornery. Six feet, three inches of authority, with a shiny bald head and piercingly unwavering gray eyes. Highly educated, Grayson was intelligent, interesting, and inquisitive, but Grayson was equally ornery, demanding, and stubborn. He had a head like a rock. I'm guessing it was a combination of these things that led to his getting a highly respected physician to place a g-tube in the first place.

A g-tube is a tube inserted externally into the stomach through a small incision in the abdomen. Its purpose is to provide a means of nutrition, fluids, and medication for those who are no longer able to swallow normally, or safely. The mind boggler here is that Grayson was perfectly capable of swallowing; he simply didn't like the taste of his potassium. The tablets were too big and chalky, and the liquid form "tasted like shit." So, somehow, some way, Grayson convinced his doctor to place a g-tube solely for the administration of his potassium. Now, potassium is crucial for the functioning of the heart. One's potassium level must be within therapeutic range; it can't be too high or too low, or the heart will not function properly, if at all.

That said, without a doubt, it was pertinent that Grayson take his potassium. However, Grayson should have been told, "Buck up, buttercup, and take your potassium like a big boy, or find yourself a new doctor." Unfortunately, Grayson wasn't told that; Grayson got a g-tube instead.

Over time Grayson started receiving a nutritional shake (similar to Ensure or Boost) to supplement his intake. His taste buds were so finicky that he didn't eat enough to provide adequate nutrition. And of course, Grayson didn't like the taste of the nutrition shake, either, so down the tube it went, as opposed to down the hatch, which is where it should have gone. What it boils down to is this: The g-tube was surgically placed because Grayson was stubborn.

His wife, Rose, was as sweet and gentle as a lamb. She used to come up and spend the night with Grayson; bring her things and sleep on the second bed in his room. I was administering his medication one evening, just after nine p.m., when Grayson called Rose and told her he wanted her to come up and spend the night.

"Grayson!" I fussed. "It's raining and cold outside. You should have called her before it got dark!"

"I didn't think about it before it got dark," he replied without looking my way.

"You can't ask her to come out on this cold, rainy night."

Grayson turned his head and stared me in the eye as he spoke with Rose, and up she came, within the hour, smiling at me as she dripped by. Rose acknowledged her husband was a stubborn man, but she adored him, anyway. Rose said, "Grayson has a way of sneaking into your heart when you least expect it. And in Grayson's case, nobody ever expects it!" She laughed.

In retrospect, I have to agree with that. The ornery coot snuck right into mine, and I sure as heck never expected it!

Amazingly, Grayson liked me. "You, I like. You tell me what's best for me, whether I like it or not. And I usually don't. You care about what you're doing, and you do it right. I trust you. The rest of 'em? They don't care, and they're dumb as rocks."

"Well, thank you, Grayson. I think."

Grayson had been a professor at a large university. He would often share his thoughts and opinions on various subjects and/or television programs while I provided his care. He liked that I was outspoken and had "intelligent input" vs. the "stupid crap most of the others would say." Ornery. He was just plain ornery. And as particular as an OCD poster child!

Every single time I walked into the man's room with cups, water, a nutritional shake, and medications, it was the same thing.

"Sit that right there." Pointing.

I sat everything where I always did.

"Now, wait a minute."

I stood, unmoving, and waited like I always did while Grayson picked up the towel he kept at his side and spread it out over his abdomen, all but ironing the thing.

"Okay, now you gotta put a little bit of that shake in first so my stomach isn't empty when you put the medicine in."

I stared him briefly in the eye, then proceeded with the task at hand, just like I always did.

"You got my sleeping pill in there? I don't want my sleeping pill yet. I want my sleeping pill at nine o'clock. Not before. Not after. Nine o'clock."

"Yes, Grayson. I know. Nine o'clock. Just like always."

"You have gloves?"

"Yes, Grayson. You watched me put them on. Just like always," I replied, holding my gloved hands in the air, wiggling my fingers.

"Yeah, well, some of the nurses don't wear gloves."

"Okay, ornery." I chuckled. "But you watched me put them on, just like always."

Grayson shrugged and began telling me about the CSI episode he was watching, and then he moved on to the latest news on the upcoming election. But the constant questioning and instructing resumed when I began to clean and dress the tube insertion site.

One evening, after I returned from a glorious seven days off, Grayson and I were starting our usual routine. But as he was placing his towel on his belly, I noticed the skin around his g-tube was a deep, intense red.

"What's up with this redness, my friend? It didn't look like this when I left. Does it itch?"

"No, it kind of burns sometimes, and nobody is putting anything on it. I've been asking the idiots. That one nurse…Vivian. I like her, too. She put some cream on it one time. She said she'd called the doctor, and he ordered the cream, but nobody has put a damn thing on it since then, not even Vivian!"

"I'll check it out when I'm finished here, and we'll get it taken care of."

I proceeded with Grayson's care, and Grayson proceeded with Grayson's instructions. It started out normally, until I poured his bright orange potassium into the syringe. As it flowed in via gravity, I literally watched it seep back out around the base of the tube at the same rate it flowed in. It wasn't the same bright orange once mixed with gastric contents, but it was undeniably potassium.

"Grayson, how long has this been happening?"

"Several days now. I need that cream."

"You need to see the doctor. I'm going to call him now. I'll be right back."

Grayson's doctor informed me, a bit irritably, that a little seepage is normal. I stressed the fact that it wasn't a little seepage, then described the contents coming back out at the same rate I put them in. I added that the seepage was breaking his skin down. The doctor insisted it was fine and ordered an ointment for his skin. I, in turn, informed the doctor we wouldn't use the g-tube again until he'd seen Grayson, and we'd be scheduling an appointment the next morning. Then I went back to inform the king of Stubbornville.

"Grayson, if you want this medicine, you're going to have to swallow it. I'm not putting anything else in that tube until the doctor has seen it himself. And we're going to schedule you an appointment with him in the morning."

Grayson argued and demanded, but eventually he swallowed select pills, refusing everything else, including his potassium.

I cleaned his abdomen, put extra gauze around the base of his tube, and applied some ointment.

The next day I arrived to find out they'd used the g-tube for both medication passes and shakes, and no appointment had been scheduled. I was told transportation would schedule it as soon as possible.

I notified the doctor about the medications Grayson wouldn't swallow, then told him that the other nurses were continuing to use the tube but that I adamantly refused. The doctor chewed me out and said to administer the medications via tube. "With all due respect, sir, I am utilizing good nursing judgement, and I will not use that tube until you have seen it for yourself. And, sir, I stand firm on my decision." I then made a grand, but predictably futile attempt, to persuade Grayson to go to ER.

With diligent and meticulous wound care, and large amounts of gauze around the base of Grayson's tube, I managed to narrow the skin breakdown to just the area beneath the gauze. There was simply no way to keep that area dry.

Grayson eventually took his medications for me via mouth. I pleaded with him to refuse use of the g-tube, for any reason, until he could see the doctor. Apparently, the doctor had thought about it more after our conversation, and he referred Grayson back to the surgeon who had actually placed the tube. Unfortunately, it takes time to see a specialist. Grayson wasn't going to be able to see the surgeon for nine weeks.

"That's unacceptable!" I cried to the director of nursing.

"That's the best they can do. We can't make them see him sooner."

"Did you call the office? Did anyone tell them how bad it's leaking? Have you told the other nurses to stop using the damned tube?" I cried in desperation.

Of course, she had not. I called the surgeon's office and begged for an appointment immediately, telling them how severely the tube was leaking. Grayson was referred to the emergency room. Grayson refused to go, again. I called the surgeon's office back and told them Grayson refused ER, as he wanted to be seen by the surgeon. Grayson was scheduled for the following week.

Returning to work after my three days off, I found that Grayson's stoma, the hole through which the g-tube was inserted, was twice the size it had been. The nurses were then wrapping a towel around the base of the tube in attempt to soak up the seepage. Yet they still used the tube. Grayson's entire upper abdomen was tomato red, and the skin right around the tube was sloughing, the top layers of skin peeling away, much like a burn. The stoma had developed an odor, and there was purulent drainage indicative of infection.

"Grayson! Please! That potassium just is not that bad, my friend! Stop using your tube! Please! I've told you the risks. You're an intelligent man. Don't let a little thing like a bad taste cost you your life."

"I'm going to the surgeon in four days, and it's not costing my life. It's costing my abdomen."

Shaking my head, I sighed heavily. "As I have explained, my stubborn friend, the abdomen is the only damage you can see. You are risking your life. Think on that again please. I'll be back. I'm going to call your doctor. It looks and smells like your stoma is infected now."

After hurrying back to Grayson's room with the antibiotic the doctor had ordered, I found that stubbornness can indeed get worse.

"Swallow it."

Grayson stared at me for a moment, baffled. "You really care! I don't mean to upset you. The other nurses are telling me it's fine to use the tube, that the doctor said so," he explained in genuine consolation.

"Yes, Grayson, I do. I really care. And the doctor hasn't seen it. I have. You see it. It's really not rocket science. This is serious, Grayson. Like you said yourself, I know what I'm doing. If I'm wrong, I'll apologize for you having to suffer through a little bad taste. But, my precious, stubborn friend, I'm not wrong on this." As an afterthought, I added, "And I truly hate to encourage your grumpiness, but you do realize that you are going by the word of the ones you yourself call idiots. Think on that."

Grayson looked as if I'd slapped him, then stared at his abdomen. It was the very first time I had ever seen him silent. Frustrated, I directed my focus on trying to heal Grayson's abdomen.

Five days later I arrived to work. The first thing I asked was what the doctor had said about Grayson's tube. I was told his appointment had been rescheduled due to a "scheduling conflict". I went to the director of nursing again, who was fully aware the appointment had been rescheduled and told me to calm down. I pointed out the related risks for Grayson. She pointed out that he refused ER. I pointed out that refusal or not, the nurses were still using that tube. She pointed out that the primary doctor had said it was okay. I pointed out that we, as nurses, were supposed to use our good judgement and that it wasn't okay, as the doctor hadn't seen it. She again told me to calm down, saying that Grayson had an appointment in two weeks. She dismissed me, literally saying, "You're dismissed. This conversation is over."

Three days later, on a Friday evening, I was doing wound care on Grayson's abdomen when I saw it was distended and firm.

"Grayson, dude, please, you gotta go to the emergency room. You cannot wait any longer. I'm calling an ambulance."

Grayson grabbed my hand. "It's my right to refuse to go."

"Yep. It is, my friend. But I happen to care about you despite your being the most ornery, stubborn man I've ever met, and I have a right to call. You can tell them you're not going."

Grayson was wheeled out on a stretcher within twenty minutes, grumbling the entire way. He winked at me on his way past, still grumbling at the EMTs. "Think you can make this ride a little rougher if you try, young man?"

"I'm proud of you, el presidente' of Stubborn-ville!" I laughed, then noticed that Grayson was looking feverish.

"Stop," he ordered the EMTs. "There is a human being on top of this cot on wheels!" Grayson turned to look at me. "Don't go anywhere while

I'm gone. I need you when I get back. I believe I'm going to listen to you from now on." He grinned.

"That would be really nice, my friend. But I'll have to see it to believe it."

Grayson chuckled, then addressed the poor EMTs once more. "Hurry up! We're going to the hospital, not church."

Seventeen hours later Grayson was gone. He never came back to listen to me nor anybody else. The peritonitis had become so severe that it caused massive edema, sepsis, and organ failure. Grayson had gone into shock in the emergency room, and he never came out. Grayson was dead.

Suddenly everybody wanted to talk about how stubborn Grayson was, which was an undeniable fact. But no one stood accountable for continuing to use that tube, for rescheduling his appointments and delaying treatment, or for dismissing my every voiced concern, my every plea. No one. Grayson's third day gone from this world forever, just after Rose left with his belongings, the director mandated that we never discuss "the unfortunate incident" again. Grayson was tucked way back in the closet to await the settling dust.

Elisa, aka Leese:

At only thirty-two years of age, Leese's life was forever changed. She had an accident while riding her beloved motorcycle. Exactly what happened is forever locked away in the mind of one who is no longer capable of sharing. Leese was the only person known to have been present when the accident occurred. All anyone else knows is that, for some reason, Leese and her bike went down. Her bike was fine, just a few minor scrapes, but Leese suffered a fractured skull. Her helmet, having somehow come off, was found lying beside her on the pavement. After being in a coma for months following her accident, Leese had come out of it without any use of her legs, very little use of anything else, and mentally disabled. Leese's vocabulary was severely limited. Seldom speaking at all, when she did speak, it was simply "yeeeah", "noooo", or the F bomb. Most often, if Leese spoke at all, it was the F bomb, though completely without malice, or even expression.

By the time I met Leese, she was fifty-four years old.

An easy roommate, Leese was shifted around like an old couch, at management's convenience. The latest move had put her in my care.

While getting her settled in, I noticed her g-tube feeding was ordered at 75ml an hour for eighteen hours per day, off for six hours per day. No times for starting or stopping were specified on the administration record, so I went to seek clarification from Suzanne, her previous nurse.

"You don't stop it." Her brow crinkled with confusion. "You just hang a new bottle when it runs out." She shrugged, turned back to her task.

"But... the order states 'for eighteen hours per day, off for six hours per day'. So it has to be stopped at some point. Is it on the night shift, maybe?" I was baffled.

"It don't say that."

"Yes. It does."

"Let me see." Suzanne followed me to my medication cart to look at the administration record herself.

I stood by, watching her face as her eyes grew wide. "Shit! We been running it round the clock!" Suzanne cried. "I've been working here for over a year and ain't nobody ever said it was sposed to be stopped! Girl, I don't know what to tell you." She waddled away, waving her arms in the air to indicate she was washing her hands of the whole thing. Leese wasn't her concern anymore.

Later that evening, I dug through the Dietician's progress notes and confirmed the order for Leese's feeding was indeed 75ml per hour for eighteen hours a day, off for six. Leese, who wasn't able to burn any calories outside of basic metabolism, was receiving 675 extra calories per day, and had been for a long time. And Leese was so big that she required a special bariatric bed.

It was then that I recalled overhearing the words of Leese's mother, Cheryl, as she had spoken with Suzanne one day: "Elisa would have a fit if she could see herself today. She was meticulous about keeping herself up, keeping her figure. Elisa always said, 'If you want to keep your man, keep being his girl.' She'd be mad as a hornet if she had any comprehension of how big she is now!"

My mind then flashed back to my second day on the job, "Here, we go to Meesha, the assistant director of nursing. Never go to Sheila Faye, the director. Meesha handles everything." The nurse had informed me.

Meesha's words then reverberated in my brain, as she'd later told me herself, "If you find a problem or have one, bring it directly to me and I'll fix it. We not gonna have no problems get past me. And, sugar, I can fix anything."

Thinking I wanted this corrected, not just "fixed," I called the registered dietician for advice. The problem was corrected with a new physician's order, identical to the original order. I then clarified the order on the administration record, specifying that the feeding was to be stopped each day at eleven a.m., and resumed each day at five p.m. The dietician then spoke with Meesha, but nothing was ever said about the longtime, ongoing error. Another thing stashed in the closet.

Grabbing the phone, I called Cheryl, Leese's mom, and informed her of the 'new order', and further explained that the 'new order' should result in gradual weight loss which would hopefully get Leese back within a healthy weight range.

"Oh, that would be wonderful!" Cheryl cried. "I know she's busy, but I've discussed Elisa's weight gain with Meesha many times. She has always assured me that you all were working on it!"

Well, we weren't. But we are now, I thought to myself as I hung up the phone.

Five weeks later, to make "an appropriate spot" for a pending new resident, Leese was moved again. That move landed her in the hottest room in the building. Even with a fan blowing directly on her from two feet away, Leese was sweating like a farmer in July. So I had dipped a small towel into ice water to cool her down. As I laid the cold towel on her forehead, Leese blurted, "Ah LUUUUV yew!"; with emphasis on the love, and her twang so thick that she sounded much like one from deep in the Carolina mountains.

"Ah luv yew too." I grinned.

A short while later I headed back out of her room and heard myself say, "I love you" as I always had. It struck me then that Leese may well have learned that phrase from our routine interaction. My heart ached as the next thought slammed into my head: *So... who the heck did she pick up the F bomb from, and how? Why?* Returning to Leese's room a short while later, I wiped her face down once more, then put the towel away before hurrying to the dining room.

They put an enormously obese lady, who is completely dependent for every-thing, into the stuffiest room in the building, I thought, once again irritated with the system.

Not at all surprising at that point, within the week, a roommate crisis on the other end of the hall resulted in Leese being moved again. Two warring roommates had demanded to be separated, so Leese was rolled to her newest domain. Again, I wholly disagreed with the reasoning, but I was relieved to find that Leese had been moved to the coolest room in the building. The move, however, having taken Leese out of my care and placed her back in the care of Suzanne, meant I that had to make a point to go check on Leese from time to time. I was always pleased to find she wasn't sweating. But I wasn't pleased the afternoon I walked in and found the lights out, drapes pulled, and Leese slumped down in the bed, her entire body and head pressed against the wall.

"Girl! What are you doing all crumpled up against the wall like that?" I laughed as I stopped her feeding tube, grabbed the pad beneath her, and tugged with every ounce of muscle I had in attempt to get Leese back toward the center of the bed.

"I don't... knooow." Leese smiled up at me, her blue eyes blinking innocently.

Panting, still grasping the pad beneath Leese's hips, I stood gaping at Leese, speechless.

She just understood my question and responded appropriately!

"And I didn't budge you even a centimeter." I laughed, once I'd wrapped my head around Leese's newly discovered cognition.

"But, listen at you! Leese! You understood my question! You answered my question!" Grabbing Leese's hand, I bumped her fist before walking out to get help pulling her back over and up in bed.

Three weeks later the "old couch" was shoved again. Leese was coming back to my unit and Suzanne was coming with her. Suzanne would then be working the day shift on my unit. This move returned Leese to my care, and she still wasn't at the stuffy, afternoon-sun-drenched end of the hall. So, once again, though I did not at all agree with the motivation for the move, I was pleased with the outcome. Hanging Leese a new bottle of formula, I wrote the date, time, and my initials on the bottle, as is required, while Leese busily fiddled with the tubing. Her hands certainly burned a calorie or two each day. If Leese was awake, Leese was fiddling! So Leese was in her new room, fiddling contentedly. She was starting out with a new bottle of formula, fresh sheets, and a fresh gown. Having noticed her lips were dry and cracked, and a thick white coating on her teeth and tongue that would have gagged a maggot, I performed oral care that won me another "I luuuuuuv yew," her blue eyes blinking as she smacked her lips.

The next afternoon I went to administer Leese's five o'clock medications.

Reaching up to press the stop button on her feeding pump, it struck me. The feeding is supposed to be turned back on at five, I thought to myself. It's supposed to be turned off at eleven a.m. The schedule was specifically set up so that from eleven in the morning until five in the evening, Leese could be gotten up into her special chair, therefore allowing her to sit out in the lobby and be exposed to life, as opposed to lying in bed, isolated from the world twenty-four hours a day. Dammit, Suzanne!

The following day, at shift change, I discussed this with Suzanne who said she was overwhelmed with learning the new unit and would do better.

Suzanne's "better" proved to be worse than bad. Now, I give her credit for one thing: After several 'discussions' Suzanne started turning that pump off at some point during her shift. No doubt about that. I never found it running again.

However, it wasn't long before I noticed that I was having to hang a new bottle of formula every single day, to replace the bottle I, myself, had hung the day before. Now, stay with me here. Each bottle of formula holds a thousand milliliters. Leese was to receive seventy-five ml an hour for eighteen hours per day. This amounts to one thousand three hundred and fifty ml each day. Therefore, one bottle cannot possibly last an entire day. And yet there I was hanging a new bottle to replace the bottle I had hung the day before, which was not even empty! I was having to replace it simply because our policy dictated a bottle and tubing change every twenty-four hours. In other words, a bottle I hung at five in the evening should have run empty at around six the next morning. Then a new bottle should've been hung to continue running until eleven a.m. The pump should've been stopped at eleven, and then I should've been able to resume that partial bottle at five p.m. That is how it should have gone.

Leese, who was supposed to receive 1350ml each day, was not even receiving a 1000ml.

My educated guess is that I was taking down and replacing my own bottles because Suzanne came in at six a.m. and stopped the feeding pump for the day to ensure she didn't forget to stop it later. Thus, Suzanne likely blew off Leese's two o'clock seizure medication altogether. After all, who would know? I started taking pictures of the bottles with the date, time hung, my initials, and the amount of remaining formula. I started monitoring Leese's weight. Leese had lost thirteen pounds in three weeks. That is a lot for somebody whose only activity is fiddling. That was far from the gradual weight loss we had intended. That was completely unacceptable. Bypassing Meesha, 'the fixer', I went straight to Sheila Faye, who instructed me to write Suzanne up. It was not something I saw as my responsibility as a charge nurse, to write up another charge nurse, but I did. Honestly though, coming from a co-worker, who really cares? But to be fair, Sheila Faye really didn't have time to do it herself. She was never in the building. Well, I say never. She was in the building for a few minutes each weekday morning, looked over the report sheet before zipping off to her real career and leaving the facility to Meesha. Corporate was fully aware that our Director of Nursing was only in the building for a total of approximately three to six hours a week. The regional director of operations was buddies with Sheila Faye, and he had hired her with an 'understanding'. So… there you have it.

The important thing is this: Leese is a joy. She is a human being who has absolutely no control over any aspect of anything. Leese is far from the only one wearing those shoes; others may wear a different style, but the shoes tread the same vulnerable path.

Sadly, Leese had come to that facility from a large city. She had been raped twice while in a facility there, and her family thought she would be safer in a smaller town. She was safer, in that aspect. Our only crime was making her morbidly obese and then starving her.

Note:

1. Nobody but me seemed to find this atrocious. I kid you not. Nobody was astounded, nobody got "all worked up".

2. I worked a lot of overtime, and much of it was on the other unit. One weekend, just after the Leese incident, I came in on a Saturday morning.

I found Ms. Laverne's bottle of formula empty, pump off. Okay, the bottles do run out. I took it down to replace it, but as I was about to throw it away, the date and time caught my eye. The bottle had been hung on Thursday at 5:20 a.m. Ms. Laverne's order was for fifty ml an hour, continuously. That is a total of twelve hundred ml a day. A bottle would last twenty hours. This meant Ms. Laverne would have run out of food at approximately 1:20 a.m. on Friday morning. I was taking it down on Saturday at 7:10 a.m. Ms. Laverne went twenty-eight hours with no nutritional intake.

3. Again, I could go on and on, but I'll leave this here. I once went in to work overtime on a Sunday night, and I found every g-tube fed resident in the facility with an empty bottle, all of which had been hung at some time on Friday. They had all gone much, or even most, of the weekend with no food, maybe without water. Were the meds given? If so, why wouldn't you also hang a bottle of formula and start the pump, you know, while you're standing there with their g-tube in your hands?

Granny G and Sandra:

"Just call me Granny G," she said the first time I met her. Her actual name being a horrific challenge to pronounce, Granny G was fine with me!

Granny G was a feisty, energetic little woman with a quick mind and a quicker tongue. Skinny as a toothpick with a tight gray ponytail topping her knotty little head and size twelve feet tipping her knobby little legs, Granny G looked much like an aged Olive Oyl. Regardless of her big feet, the biggest things about Granny G were her heart and her mouth. Both were as big as Texas. She was into everything and stopped at nothing.

Granny G was fired up, "hot as a wood stove," when I walked into her room one afternoon. Apparently, Granny G had overheard a conversation between the day shift nurses, which resulted in Granny G marching herself into another resident's room to see things for herself. Not good, but it was too late.

"What the hell does that daughter of Sandra's think she's doing?" Granny G fired at me. "Selfish! Selfish is what she is! She ain't thinkin' of her mama; she's thinkin' of herself!"

And on she raved while I cleaned and dressed her wound.

"Are you finished yet, Granny G?"

"I'll let you know when I'm finished, missy!" I waited briefly. "Okay, I'm finished. I'm sorry. But what matters here is what you're going to do about it." She crossed her bony arms.

"I can't discuss another resident, or their business, with you, Granny G. Just the same as I can't discuss you or yours with anyone else. You can understand that."

"Yes, ma'am, I can. I'm not an idiot. So, don't discuss it with me." She shrugged. "Fix it!" Granny G stared me down for a full minute before she cracked and reached out to give me a hug. "I love you, ladybug. I'll hush. I know you care as much as I do. And if anybody can fix it, it's you. That's what you do best, so get to it. I'll just go back to having fun and stirring trouble, which is what I do best." She winked and cackled.

A grin escaping, I hugged Granny G, then headed for the door.

"But I'm watching now," Granny G added, far from surprisingly, as I turned to head down the hallway.

Granny G was right. I knew this. I had already gently encouraged Sandra's daughter to consider hospice. I had gotten nowhere, but the seed was planted at least. In a way, I understood both sides all too clearly. It was indeed a pickle. A pickle I had no desire to bite. My hands were tied. The decision was Tammy's, Sandra's eldest daughter.

Tammy's love for and devotion to her mother was undeniably clear, but Tammy was also a bit in denial, at least in my humble opinion. Tammy kept a wave machine at Sandra's bedside, which she wanted turned on at bedtime, and she wanted Sandra's television on, playing gospel music, during all waking hours. Tammy came to see Sandra daily, at all different hours. It depended on her work schedule, but she never missed a day. She bathed and moisturized her mama every day, then did her mama's laundry so it would smell like home. Tammy swore Sandra responded to her, though no one else ever saw any sign of awareness from Sandra whatsoever. Maybe Sandra did respond. I've seen many miracles. But that almost makes it even more sad. What would Sandra say if she could speak for herself?

One couldn't help but feel Tammy's pain. However, one couldn't help but agree—silently, of course—with Granny G.

A pickle. A big, fat, drippy sour pickle.

Sandra was an obese African American lady with a beautiful face and eyes that rarely opened. She had already lost one hand, three fingers from the other hand, and half of one leg to diabetes. Her remaining hand and foot were in the slow, painful process of rotting off, as well. The change in vital signs and reflexive muscle spasms during wound care clearly indicated that Sandra experienced significant pain. She was not a candidate for more surgery, as she wouldn't survive it. With advanced end-stage renal disease, Sandra had to be hauled from her bed onto a stretcher, then hauled to dialysis three times a week. Even the EMTs expressed that they felt guilty for putting her through it. We had to medicate Sandra with a mild sedative before dialysis, as all the move-ment caused significant agitation, which resulted in her blood pressure shooting sky high. We couldn't medicate for high blood pressure just prior to dialysis, as that would place her at very high risk of her blood pressure bottoming out during or after dialysis. Sandra didn't require the sedative at any other time, only before dialysis. She, of course, had a g-tube for nutritional intake, medications, and hydration, having long before lost her ability to swallow effectively. And of course, she was no longer alert enough to take a bite or a drink if she could. In short, Sandra was a hot mess, a lovely hot mess that stole every heart that came anywhere near her.

A pickle.

Later that afternoon, while administering Sandra's medications, I got just plain ticked. On top of everything else against her, they still hadn't arranged for her g-tube to be replaced. The tube was already so old that it was mushy soft, had black gunk covering its entire inner surface, and was constantly clogging no matter how diligently one flushed it. Gummy was the word I'd used when I'd last pointed it out to my supervisor. Her tube was literally gummy. One could squeeze the tube, and the sides would stick together, then slowly pull apart. I couldn't replace it myself because it wasn't the balloon type tube. Never mind the technical details. The point is, Sandra needed to go out to the doctor to have it replaced, and I had addressed this repeatedly for several months.

"I'm so sorry, Sandra. I'll go talk to them about your tube again. I promise I won't stop until it's changed," I said quietly while gazing at San-dra's innocent face with eyes closed.

"Well, get after it, then! That thing is dirtier than my old garden hose!" Granny G suddenly exploded into my right ear.

"Granny G, you aren't supposed to just bust up into other folks' rooms." I laughed, placing my hand over my racing heart. "You scared me to death! I had no idea you were standing behind me, gawking over my shoulder!"

"I didn't mean to scare you, ladybug. But I did tell you I'd be watching." She grinned mischievously. "And I didn't bust up in anywhere; I snuck." She grinned. "You need to work your magic for this sweet lady! She's got enough rottin' off! She don't need her stomach rottin' out, too! Now then, I'm goin' to win me some bingo while you fix this," Granny G said as she scurried back out the door, her scraggly ponytail swinging.

I stood and stared after her, then sighed heavily and headed for the administrator's office, having decided to give up on the director of nursing doing anything about it.

Getting nowhere quick, I returned to my unit, called Sandra's daughter, and sent Sandra to the emergency room. I called the ER and informed the nurse that Sandra needed her g-tube replaced, simple as that. Sandra was still out at the emergency room when I finally punched out late that night.

On Monday afternoon Granny G met me in the parking lot. Yes, in the parking lot. I swung my truck door open before turning the engine off, as Granny G had literally raised her knobby knee into the air as if she were planning to step her size twelve up onto the running board to open the door for me.

"That's it! I ain't a'lettin' this thing go no longer. I've been to talk to them idiots in them offices up there." She rolled her sassy eyes skyward. "Lord help! That's like trying to reason with the ass end of a donkey!"

"Calm down. And stay down, on the ground!" I laughed as Granny G again raised her foot.

"I can smell it now!" Granny G shouted as her tattered boot hit the pavement again and her hands swung to her bony hips.

"Smell what?"

"Her stomach a'rottin' out! That's what! I thought if I went and talked to them idiots, too, they might do something. All they done was tell me to talk to you!"

Granny G yapped at my heels the entire walk across the parking lot, through the building to the time clock, then to my unit, and then down the hallway to Sandra's room. She'd apparently gone to someone in every office in the building, then verbally assaulted the receptionist up front for "not calling the po-leese."

The odor was so strong, it was like walking into an invisible wall as you entered the room.

"She was supposed to get it replaced Friday," I said as I approached Sandra, noting, even from a few steps away, that what I could see of her tube was still black, so soft it folded over flat against her belly.

Granny G was busy opening the window. "That bubblehead y'all call a weekend nurse poured cokee-cola in Sandra's tube on Saturday when she got back from dialysis, 'cause it was plugged up," Granny G said as she reattached herself to my side. "She told me she did."

"I know you mean well, and I know you love Sandra, but you've got to go. I need to assess Ms. Sandra, please."

"Okay, I'm out." Granny G raised her hands in the air. "You do your thing, ladybug. I see it in your eyes."

The odor was definitely emanating from Sandra's tube, which didn't just collapse; it wrinkled up when I attempted to pull back on the syringe.

So we know that nobody is assessing gastric content before giving meds, I thought, but I wanted to scream it out loud. The base of the tube, where it entered the abdomen, wasn't just gummy anymore; it was wet at the insertion site. It was sticky, as if the tube was literally breaking down or, as Granny G said, rotting.

It turned out that Sandra's blood pressure had been up when she'd arrived in the emergency room Friday evening. They'd treated it, not stopping to realize it was likely because she'd been loaded onto a stretcher and hauled across town in an ambulance. The doctor told me when I called him that the nurse I called had never mentioned the g-tube replacement. I couldn't help myself entirely. I did resist asking if he was blind, but I proved unable to resist asking if he'd noticed the black crap coating the entire inner length of the tube. He, of course, hadn't even seen the tube.

I sighed, rolled my eyes, bit my tongue, and informed the doctor he was about to have another opportunity to do just that. I also informed him that we would not be accepting Sandra back without a new tube, and I requested a full GI assessment while they had her there.

Sandra was admitted to ICU with a systemic fungal infection, a systemic bacterial infection, and sepsis. She very nearly died, and she had to be intubated. But once the g-tube was replaced, her status began gradually improving.

The hospitalist caring for Sandra called the facility to chew me out over the fact that he "had to intubate someone in Sandra's condition". I tried to remind him that the decision is not mine, but he was too angry to think clearly. In a way, I understood completely, so I just set the phone down, walked away and let him chew.

Meanwhile, Granny G made me the most beautiful ugly sweater I've seen to this day! I'm certain it would win any ugly Christmas sweater contest. It was a green sweatshirt with a big, gold, satin heart on front. There was a big, felt ladybug in the middle of the heart, with the word HERO written just above it in silver glitter. To top it all off, she had added lopsided angel wings on the back, which were silver but had been outlined with gold glitter. I wore it once for Granny G. She laughed heartily as she grabbed me in a bear hug, sending silver and gold glitter twirling to the floor.

"Yep. Only a true hero would wear that gawdy thing just to make an old lady smile."

Sandra returned from the hospital a month later. She, too, suffered the love of Granny G in the form of an atrocious lap blanket, minus glitter, thank goodness. As Granny G spread it over the foot of Sandra's bed, I found myself grateful, for Sandra's sake, that she no longer opened her eyes.

"Well, ladybug? Ya done good. And now it's bingo time!" Granny G winked at me as she scurried toward the door. I was anything but surprised when she stopped and turned around. "Now get on that hospice thing. That lady deserves to get to rest in peace. Stop putting her through all this dialysis shit. Cuz that's what it is. SHIT! It ain't gone open her eyes or grow back her arms and legs!" She wiped her eyes fast, and I kept quiet. "Okay, now stop deterring me from whipping the old folks' butts in bingo! I got a reputation to uphold!" I heard her cackle down the hallway.

The nurse's words reverberated through my head. The nurse who'd called from the hospital to report about Sandra had said, "Y'all need to put her on hospice."

I shook my head, then looked at Sandra's beautiful face. "It is a pickle. I'm so sorry, love. You have dialysis in the morning. Get some rest."

Note: Facilities will keep g-tubes in place until they literally rot and disintegrate. The day they simply cannot administer anything more through that tube—when they simply cannot, no matter what—is the day the individual will get a replacement; or the day they pull it out themselves. Seldom one day sooner. G-tubes are absolutely, undeniably never changed on a routine, maintenance-type basis; g-tubes are frequently used long past the point of safety or wisdom; and g-tubes are sometimes used past the point of no return.

Side note: I'd like to take this opportunity to encourage all to consider quality of life priority over quantity. A little fantastic is better than a lot of nothing.

There are many people like Sandra.

Mobile Medicine

Mobile medicine is long-term care's answer to laboratory and radiology needs, both of which are frequent, though laboratory needs are nearly daily. However, Oaklyn just popped into my head. Puffing the stray hairs out of her pretty face, tucking the longer strands behind her ears, she wearily asks, "Okay, anybody else I need to see while I'm here?" in a desperate attempt to avoid getting fifty miles north, south, east, or west before receiving word that she's needed back here again. Oaklyn is one of our two x-ray techs. In fact, I've seen Oaklyn at a few of the facilities at which I've been employed, as the mobile x-ray company, for whom she is employed, serves a large area. Oaklyn would readily profess that our x-ray needs are fairly constant, as well.

Realistically, one simply cannot haul five to forty individuals over to the lab each day. Some are completely bed bound. Many are wheelchair-bound. Some are confused to the extent that they exhibit bizarre, disturbing, or unsafe behaviors. Some are in severe pain. Some are highly contagious. Some are all the above and then some. So a solution is no doubt necessary. I'm simply far from convinced that they've come up with the right one. I think what concerns me the most is the undeniable fact that they are fully, undeniably aware that there are significant problems with the services, yet they carry on as if the problems don't exist and everything is working out just fine. They, being the administrative personnel, the upper management, and the owners and members of the boards of long-term care facilities and corporations. Sadly, other than the "few," and the nurses who've heard me rant about it, nurses are clueless as to the discrepancies, quite frankly because they aren't really even looking at the lab results or comparing their clinical assessments with the x-ray results. Okay, if they performed a thorough clinical assessment at all. But hold up, they at least noticed something, or they wouldn't have ordered the x-ray. So... there is that.

If I've said it once (oh, and I have!), I've said it a million times. "Critical thinking. That is why nurses can never be replaced by computers. A monkey can be trained to perform a skill. A nurse is supposed to think! Critical thinking is the nurse's duty. It's what makes one a nurse!"

Saying such has not made me a candidate for winning a popularity contest with my co-workers, but it doesn't change the truth in what I said.

Nila, Jamie, and Heebie Jeebie (I shrug, chuckle, and roll my eyes.):

Nila had gone to the ER and returned with a diagnosis of Flu A. She'd taken Tamiflu and completed it. But her nurse asked me to see her because she just wasn't really getting any better. She still had a bad cough, and the nurse didn't know "what was the matter with her".

I'd never met Nila before. But I could easily see that she'd been through the ringer with that flu. Still on contact isolation due to having had the flu, Nila was in a room alone, coughing so hard that drawing her blood proved to be a challenge, as her arm was jerking with every cough. Lung sounds were horrendous, and Nila had developed a low-grade fever. There was no doubt in my mind that Nila was still sick … with something.

I ordered a mobile chest x-ray, though by then I'd lost all confidence in them. However, I had to get one done to show we took the appropriate steps. And goodness knows I couldn't continue to verbalize my complete lack of confidence in mobile x-rays, as the director of nursing was somewhat exasperated with my repeatedly voiced opinions. This seemed to be a pattern throughout my long-term care career.

Just a few hours later, having run Nila's blood to the hospital lab, I had Nila's lab results in hand. The results indicated a mild infection. Her white blood cell count was slightly elevated. I could have predicted Nila's chest x-ray results in my sleep. It was the same results, verbatim, that we received on many patients with acute and obvious respiratory, or lung illnesses. "No acute cardiopulmonary disease." This meaning there ain't a thing about that individual's heart or lungs outside their norm at that moment. Once again, I begged to differ.

Confident that the chest x-ray results were incorrect, I called the doctor. Informing Doc of all the results, I stressed to him that Nila's clinical picture, lung sounds, temperature, and labs did not correlate with the x-ray.

"Doc," I pleaded, "I don't care what the x-ray says. Nila has a respiratory infection, and she's going to get sicker without treatment."

Doctor Sikes said, "Thanks."

Nothing. I got nothing. No new orders were received.

Frustrated, I waded through the knee-deep remarks from my co-workers. "Someone who's had the flu is going to cough awhile," they said. "What do you expect? She just got over the flu!" They exclaimed, shaking their heads as I hurried by, taking Nila a specimen cup. In full agreement with the comments yet fully believing something else was in the mix, I gave no reply. I could have been wrong. I knew that, but my gut told me to keep digging.

"When you cough up some sputum, love, spit it into this cup and put the lid back on it. I'll be checking the cup from time to time, so no need to call anyone when you've spit into it." I smiled as I set the cup on her overbed table, then placed a cool damp cloth on Nila's forehead. "I'm sorry you feel so bad. We'll get to the bottom of this. Just hang in there and stick with me."

I asked the aid to ensure Nila had plenty of fluids to drink, including juice, at all times. A short while later I had the sputum specimen, which was so thick that it never budged from the spot on which it had landed at the top, inside of the cup.

I wrote sputum specimen to hospital on the nurses' twenty-four-hour report so that the nurses could be looking for the results. However, I knew full well that the nurses would not be looking for the results. But again, the motions… I wrote it on my calendar so that I would remember to look for the results. Just as predictably as the sun rises, the nurses did not look for the results.

Seven days later (it takes five to seven days to grow a culture) I called the hospital lab to obtain the sputum culture results.

MRSA, or methicillin resistant staphylococcus aureus, or multidrug resistant staph aureus. Essentially, it is a big, bad, highly contagious, hard-to-treat bacteria. I went first to inform Nila of her results, but Nila was no longer where I had left her. Nila had been moved out of isolation and back into her room with her roommate. I found her raised up on one arm to support herself during a coughing attack. I waited until she was breathing easy again, then glanced at her roommate to see if she was showing any sign of infection yet, as she was breathing the germs Nila so frequently and forcefully coughed out.

"Well, sister, I didn't know they'd moved you back into your room. I'm sorry. Your sputum culture grew MRSA. That means you still need to be in isolation."

Nila's double chin dropped, and her marble blue eyes popped open wide. "Back across the hall?"

"I don't know, love. I'll go find out."

Heading straight to the director of nursing's office, I filled her in. She said Nila was going to need to go into the room with Heebie Jeebie. Apparently, Heebie Jeebie had MRSA in her sputum as well. Same hall. Hmm...

"Oh no, you better get the social worker to tell Nila she has to room with Heebie Jeebie. I'm not telling her!" I laughed. "Not just no, but heck no! I like Nila!"

Heebie Jeebie was my term of endearment, which I used to prevent the use of her real name and, of course, to prevent myself from calling her what I really want to call her. She had gone straight through every single roommate she had ever had! In fact, there was one sweet little lady, who was mildly mentally challenged. She had sudden episodes of paranoia; it was just part of her disease process. And every time she became paranoid, she was convinced that 'they' were going to make her move into the room with Heebie Jeebie, her greatest fear! She literally sobbed, snot pouring from her nose, tears streaming from her eyes, her shoulders shaking. She was so incredibly fearful that she might have to share a room with Heebie Jeebie, that we had to jump through hoops to calm her. Having realized over time that I shoot straight, every time, she started seeking me out when afraid.

"They ain't gone put you in with Heebie Jeebie while I'm here. I'll move Heebie Jeebie up in they office! That'll fix that!"

Ultimately, she grinned and chuckled. "And you would do it, wouldn't you?"

"Abso-frickin-lutely, my friend. I would indeed. So rest easy and enjoy your evening." I'd smile facetiously and wrap her in a big bear hug.

Anyway, Nila flat-out refused to room with Heebie Jeebie. I laughed. I laughed hard. It turned out that Nila had once been roommates with Heebie Jeebie, and Nila was not going to relive that "nightmare".

I understood completely! I happened to be present the last time they'd stuck some poor, innocent soul in the room with Heebie Jeebie.

Jamie, the poor woman, had just arrived from the hospital at just before nine p.m. Jamie had burn wounds covering her legs from her toes nearly up to her "tutu," as she so eloquently termed it. She'd smoked a cigarette at home with her oxygen on, and the tubing draped over her legs had caught fire. Fortunately, she had jerked the tubing from the oxygen source in her wild attempt to put herself out. So, she was lucky. Her legs were no doubt fried, but it could have been much worse.

So, Jamie was discharged from the hospital, to us, for healing and rehab. On admission, the nurse is required to measure and describe any, and all, wounds. Jamie's wounds being so extensive, there were three of us in the room. Two of us were helping the admission nurse remove the old dressings, measure, clean, and redress the wounds. We had the curtain pulled for Jamie's privacy, of course; and Heebie Jeebie was on the other side of the curtain, lying in her bed, chattering like a crazed squirrel the entire time we were doing wound care.

To make things just a bit worse, Heebie Jeebie also kept her room like the Snow Miser's. We were diligently working, holding the dead weight of Jamie's painfully torched, obese legs in the air while the nurse dressed the weeping wounds, hands coordinating the wrap. In any other patient's room, we'd have been sweating. But, in Heebie Jeebie's winter not-so-wonderland, we were freezing. Thus, we all remarked occasionally about how cold it was.

All of a sudden Heebie Jeebie swooped the curtain back with her cane and thrust out her arm, in which she held a bulky blue sateen comforter.

As words of appreciation but clear declination poured forth from our lips, Heebie Jeebie proceeded to shove past us and spread that danged gawdy comforter over Jamie and her half-dressed wounds. I stopped her, which I feel certain only added to her hatred for me. I asked her nicely to retreat to her side of the curtain and not come back. She complied with her retreat, but she continued with her berating chatter from the other side as we started over, cleaning Jamie's wounds of the potential germs from the dreaded comforter.

Finally, I reached my max. I could take no more.

"No, ma'am, she doesn't want a sweater. Thank you, though. And she doesn't care what's on TV, nor does she want to know what your daughter said yesterday about the president. Ms. Harris is getting her wound care done, and it's very painful. Could you please just watch TV and let her get through this with as little stress as possible?" I kept my voice even, pleasant. "I'm certain she appreciates your welcoming her so abundantly, but she could not possibly feel up to chitchat right now. I know you understand. Thank you."

Like talking to a brick wall.

"Well, I understand. I just—" Blah, blah, blah. Heebie Jeebie rambled on.

A few seconds later, the curtain ruffled wildly as Heebie Jeebie headed to the bathroom, her chatter ever louder as she passed. Then her voice became muffled after she closed the bathroom door, and it grew loud again once she finished her business and ruffled her way back to bed.

Finally, we completed Jamie's wound care, through which she had been a real trooper. But just as soon as the other two nurses walked out and I pulled her blankets up beneath her chin, Jamie's face wadded up like a child who had just been told to go get a switch.

"Are you finished?" A voice suddenly climbed up my spine.

Turning, I saw Heebie Jeebie in her long, cream-colored sweater, cane in hand, nose in Jamie's business, standing just inside the still-pulled curtain.

"No, ma'am. That's why the curtain is still pulled for privacy." I struggled to maintain composure. "Please do not disturb Ms. Harris again tonight. She is exhausted."

"Oh, I understand. I won't bother her a bit. I mind my own business and don't bother anybody." Blah, blah, blah. She continued as she disappeared once again to the other side of the curtain.

Tears welling up in her eyes, Jamie whispered, "Could you please move me to another room?" She pleaded, "I can't take it in here with her. I know I can't. Not for one minute. I'm sure she means well, but I can't do it. Please!" She grasped my wrist in desperation.

I leaned close to her ear. "Give me five minutes to get some help, and we'll rescue you." I chuckled.

Jamie clung tighter.

"I promise."

She reluctantly released my wrist as tears ballooned from her eyes, rolling down her cheeks and sopping her pillowcase.

I could not walk out. Even knowing that I'd return, I could not do it. After all, Jamie didn't know me yet. Jamie had no way of being certain I'd return. I released the lock on the foot of the bed, and like Superwoman in scrubs, I began inching that bed around in that tiny space, ultimately rolling Jamie out into the hallway as she wiped the tears from her eyes and grinned with relief. I think she would have readily remained in the middle of the hallway as opposed to remaining in the room with Heebie Jeebie for another second.

Yes, I digressed severely. But since I'm there, anyway, let me tell you what I found out the next day as I continued to vent my astonishment at Heebie Jeebie's lack of consideration.

Katy, the medication aid, whom I adore for her purely amazing heart, was neighbors with Heebie Jeebie prior to Heebie Jeebie moving into the facility. Katy's kids had given her some pretty plants for Mother's Day, and Katy had lovingly placed them on the back patio of her apartment that evening. The next morning Katy went out to water her beloved plants, but they were nowhere to be seen. Baffled, Katy stood, hands on hips, repeatedly scanning the small patio within the black, wrought-iron fence.

Later, after picking her grandson up from school, Katy pulled into the parking lot of her apartment complex and spied all of her pretty plants displayed beautifully on Heebie Jeebie's front doorstep! Katy was shocked! She said she just stopped mid-drive and stared until her small grandson said, "Meemaw?" Then she snapped out of her shock. Ultimately, Katy parked her car, took her grandson's hand, walked over, and knocked on Heebie Jeebie's door.

"I'm so sorry to bother you." Katy smiled radiantly. "But someone has taken my plants and put them here at your front door! I'm just going to take them back home now. I wanted to let you know what I'm doing outside your door."

Heebie Jeebie ducked her chin in disbelief. "Oh no you're not! You're not taking my plants anywhere!" she huffed. "You've lost your mind! Get on out of here right now, or I'm calling the police!" she shrieked before slamming her door in Katy's face.

Katy, her grandson in tow, walked straight to the manager's office. The manager returned with her to Heebie Jeebie's front door, where the manager proceeded to explain that Katy was going to retrieve her plants.

Gasping in genuine offense, Heebie Jeebie proceeded to blurt obscenities, during which she proclaimed, "That lady is crazy! These are all my plants, and she's not going to touch them!"

The manager bent down, plucked a card from one of the plants, and read it aloud. "Happy Mother's Day! I love you to the moon! Renea." He raised fuzzy brows at Heebie Jeebie. "Do you know a Renea?"

"I do not! She put that card in my plant!" She flailed her free arm. "I told you she's crazy!"

The manager bent over, plucked a card from another plant, and opened his mouth to read it, but Heebie Jeebie had reached her limit.

"ENOUGH!" she yelled. "If you don't leave right now, I'm calling the police on both of you!"

The manager glanced at Katy, then smiled down at Katy's wide-eyed grandson. "Yes, ma'am," he said quietly. "You do that while we get Ms. Katy's plants back home where they belong. Oh, and I don't expect them to be moved again once we get them there. Would you mind informing the police about the plant bandit?" He chuckled as he grabbed a plant with each hand.

Katy released her grandson's hand to grab a plant, and her grandson double fisted the last one.

Heebie Jeebie looked wildly at the child. "You're as crazy as your grandmother!" She slammed her door once more, the large front window rattling with the jolt.

Katy's plants flourished under her lovingly watchful eye, and one glorious day, after being off work for a couple of days, Katy realized she hadn't seen Heebie Jeebie at all during the entire two days. Katy grinned when the manager confirmed Heebie Jeebie had moved out. There was not a mean bone in her body; Katy was simply relieved that there would be no more issues now that Heebie Jeebie had moved away.

The next day Katy returned to work. Early-morning, while passing out medications, she looked up and saw Heebie Jeebie walking toward her, waving like a long lost friend, an enormous smile plastered across her face.

Katy told me she shook her head and rubbed her eyes. Then, with her heart thumping wildly, she held her breath and looked again. She was just sure it was a horrible hallucination, her mind playing a nasty trick on her.

I laughed at Katy's unabashed sincerity in describing her horror.

"But then the hallucination hollered my name!" she continued. "Girl, I gasped! I waved back, hid my face, and ran to find the nurse!"

"Yeah, that's our new resident," the clueless nurse had explained to Katy. "She came yesterday. You're going to like her. She's really sweet."

"Oh boy. You're in for an ugly surprise!" Katy had laughed sarcastically as she hurried, disheartened, back to her cart.

Heebie Jeebie is the only resident in the building to whom the nurses are required to administer routine oral medications. Why? You may wonder. I did. I wondered. Because the medication aids, all of them, ultimately refused to administer Heebie Jeebie's medications. According to them, they'd rather be unemployed and starve to death.

I've been a nurse for twenty-eight years. I've successfully managed to find a way to be lovingly effective with thousands of people who have thousands of varied personalities and thousands of assorted preferences and habits. But I have successfully managed without fail ... until this moment. Having been given no heads up, I was to IV push a medication on Heebie Jeebie. She was my seventh IV push that day, and all others took about five minutes start to finish. Heebie Jeebie's took forty minutes, and ultimately, she did not get the medication at all. She refused to allow me to perform venous access. She wanted to direct me on the who, how, when and where of both the previous injection three months prior and the injection she was about-to-but-never-did-receive. For the first and last time in my professional life, I gave up. I threw my hands up. I quit. I refused to ever, even, consider sticking that lady again, for any reason. Period. I further refused to ever attempt medical intervention on her again aside from sheer emergency need. And I felt no shame, remorse, or humiliation. I, too, would rather be unemployed and starve to death!

Side note: I was the one recently sitting at Heebie Jeebie's bedside, wiping her down with a cool cloth, giving her sips of ice water to help reduce her fever after suspecting a bad case of pneumonia and having the charge nurse call an ambulance. Goes to show that God will teach you to love. Might as well do it from the start, regardless of their… personalities.

Back to mobile medicine:

So, Nila's chest x-ray was dangerously inaccurate, which is something that continues to happen often. What if I hadn't thought to obtain a sputum specimen? What if she, like many others, hadn't had the lung power to cough any sputum up? We rely on the x-ray to tell us what we need to do. Just as importantly, it's our tax dollars paying for these useless x-rays. In fact, our tax dollars pay for many useless and unnecessary things and services. Someday, I shall tell you about the annual garage sale you fund. For now, lab and x-ray.

Robearto:

Sick, pale, weak, debilitated - grumpy, spoiled rotten, demanding, and adorable. All this rolled into a taller than average, soft spoken gentleman with stark white hair and teal blue eyes.

Mobile lab drew a complete blood count (CBC) on February 3, and Robearto's white blood cells (WBCs) were high at 11.2. Because I noticed a sudden unexplained shift in multiple lab values, I redrew the same day, then took my specimen to the hospital lab. WBCs were 13.57. That's almost a three-point difference.

Mobile lab drew a CBC on March 16. WBCs were high at 14.0. I redrew, and WBCs were high at 15.53. Hemoglobin (oxygen level in the blood) according to the mobile lab was 8.5. My draw was 7.7. (Seven or below indicates immediate need for a blood transfusion. It matters.)

Eight months and three days after rolling through the front door for the first time; after the facility finally determined to draw and locally process all of Robearto's labs and x-rays, Robearto got better went home!

In fact, since I had started working there—I was just under a year of employment—eight different individuals had been transported from the facility to the hospital for blood transfusions, only to arrive there, have blood drawn, and be sent back due to their hemoglobin levels being significantly higher than the mobile lab results had indicated. Thus, no transfusion was needed. Three individuals had been transported and had received transfusions. Those three individuals' blood had been drawn and processed at the hospital lab.

I discussed the mobile lab discrepancies with the director of nursing. I began providing her copies of the mobile lab's results and copies of mine from the hospital lab. This was for comparison purposes, so she could address the problem with the lab and avoid paying the mobile lab for the pointless lab draws with the inaccurate results. After I brought her approximately the twentieth set of results, the director sighed heavily when she looked up from her desk and saw it was me, papers in hand. Eventually, she began telling me to set the copies on a stack on her desk. I happened to go in one afternoon as she was "cleaning up her office." I watched as the "stack" went into the shredder pile. I stopped providing the copies, hoping she would then at least ask me if the issue was resolved. I had previously, and bluntly, recommended that all hemoglobin levels be re-checked via an in-house draw prior to contacting the doctor, and certainly prior to sending the poor people out for a blood transfusion. Not only were some of these people confused, scared, and in pain, but they were also being exposed to germs. It made us look just plain stupid, and again, our tax dollars paid for every related expense, including the unnecessary ambulance ride to and from. Have you priced that lately? I've still not heard a word from the director, and I won't. Lab results are still frequently inaccurate, yet treatment is based on them, and we are still sending people out for blood transfusions only to have them sent right back due to not needing one, after all. That's at least better than the guy who went for one and was admitted to ICU because the 7.3 the mobile lab reported was actually a 5.9 on the hospital lab draw. What if the doctor had decided to recheck in a day or two instead of sending the guy out for a transfusion at 7.3?

Side note: Our tax dollars also pay for all these inaccurate blood tests, and for the redraws. Unless the patient is skilled, which only lasts a short time, the facility only pays the lab to come perform the draw. We taxpayers pay for the processing and, of course, any related treatment. If they are accurate and necessary, no problem! But when they are not, there is a problem. There are a lot of problems.

Minerva:

Minerva was a quiet lady, but she loved her some dominos. I had to interrupt her game to draw her blood. Sailing around the corner into the dining room, I laughed heartily as the four ladies chimed, "Uh oh!" in unison when they saw me coming.

Joeann, the leader of the pack, spoke for all, asking, "Which one of us is going under the knife?" Giggles bubbled around that table like champagne.

Seeing my eyes dart reflexively to Minerva, Sally squealed with delight, clapping her hands as if she had won a prize. "Oh good! It's not me this time!" She pointed her purple, glitter-tipped finger at Minerva. "It's you!" Sally rocked gleefully back and forth in her seat.

Without word or expression, Minerva began shifting and bumping around in an attempt to scoot her chair back. I helped her get up, then walked with her back to her room after asking the other ladies to hold the game for about ten minutes.

Minerva needed to go on dialysis. In fact, as I was drawing her blood, she said softly, "I was supposed to start dialysis, but I still haven't. I don't know what happened to that." She frowned, shrugged, then gazed innocently about the room.

I knew, but it wasn't my place to tell Minerva that her family had opted to decline dialysis. I didn't have the details, the whys, or the wherefores, but I felt strongly that Minerva had a right to know. I asked the social worker to address Minerva's concerns. Minerva still, to this day, has no clue. If Minerva had no recall of the fact that she needed dialysis, no problem. But Minerva did have recall. It troubled her, so in my humble opinion, there was a problem.

Lolly, Minerva's nurse, had brought Minerva's lab results to me just a short while before, questioning their accuracy. Minerva was to receive an injection each week if her hemoglobin was below a certain level, and the Nephrologist (kidney specialist) also had a chemistry profile done weekly to monitor kidney function and potassium level. Lolly had noticed that Minerva's White Blood Cell count was unusually high at 16.9, yet Minerva wasn't having any symptoms of any type of infection. Minerva's WBCs were usually within therapeutic range, she didn't run high. And she wasn't taking a steroid for anything, so that couldn't explain the increase. Scanning the lab results, I pointed out to Lolly, "Well, look at her creatinine. The three previous weeks were 2.8, 3.2, and 2.9. Then this week, out of the blue, it's perfectly normal at 0.8! It would take God Himself reaching down and touching Minerva to heal her kidneys like that, and if He did, I don't think He'd jack up her WBCs while He was at it!" Patting Lolly on the back, I praised her, saying, "You go, girl! That is what I'm always preaching about! That is thinking. That's real nursing! I'm so proud of you!"

Ultimately, I got the results of my blood draw and took them to Lolly. Minerva's results:

	Mobile lab	vs.	My draw (hospital lab)
Sodium	127		142
Chloride	89		113
Creatinine	0.8		2.9
BUN	14		49
WBC	16.9		6.87

The differences were astounding. Most, if not all, of the other nurses would simply have faxed the mobile lab results to the doctor and based the decision to give or not give the injection on those results. I see it all the time, in every facility.

Occasionally, I run across a nurse who really wants to *be* a nurse, like Lolly. I'm on it like white on rice! I love to teach those nurses!

So, that was a couple of months ago. Time flies. Earlier this week, therapy reported that Minerva was a bit confused and that her balance was off. She was normally able to walk with the therapist just behind her, but on that day, she had nearly fallen twice, and had run into a wall.

I started to draw some labs but remembered Minerva had basics drawn every Friday. So I got a urine specimen and reviewed her labs from the previous Friday, April 24. It appeared God had once again reached down and healed Minerva's kidneys. However, nobody bothered to even get the results until April 27, when Daffy, the fearless leader on that unit, noted the labs (meaning she initialed and dated, then stamped "MD Notified" at the bottom) and faxed them to the doctor. Obviously, she then tossed them into the to-be-scanned stack. Surely, had she been a *nurse* and actually reviewed the labs, she'd have noticed the miraculous shift in the kidney function as well as the ongoing, dangerously high potassium level. Surely.

To muddy Minerva's water further, her lab draw had been missed altogether on April 10, and it wasn't until April 13 that somebody noticed and actually obtained a lab draw. Of course, there was no nurse note to facilitate one following the nasty trail, which would have explained what was or wasn't done in order to help one get the 'big picture'. The nurse working on April 13 simply blew off Minerva's Procrit injection, which boosts her hemoglobin level, likely because she had no lab results to go by, yet she did nothing to see to it that the error was corrected. The nurse working on April 13 simply noted the lab results and faxed them to some doctor. It didn't specify which doctor, so it was most likely the primary care physician, who never looks at faxes anyway, and the nephrologist was the ordering physician. On April 17, the weekly labs were drawn timely. That nurse initialed, dated, and faxed the results to the nephrologist. She got the doc right, but either didn't look or didn't care, as she never obtained orders for the elevated potassium level of 5.8, nor did she pay any attention to the fact that Minerva's hemoglobin had quite naturally dropped even more after the skipped injection on April 10.

In a proverbial nutshell, Minerva was… let's say… screwed.

4/10: Weekly lab draw was missed. Hemoglobin-boosting injection was subsequently missed or skipped.

4/13: Labs drawn in place of the missed draw on April 10. Potassium dangerously high at 5.3. Nothing done.

4/17: Lab results reflect Minerva's potassium level at 5.8, meaning it had jumped five points in just four days, but still nothing was done. Additionally, Minerva's hemoglobin level had dropped lower after the April 10 injection was skipped. This nurse faxed the lab results to Minerva's nephrologist. Nothing was done.

4/24: Lab results were obviously jacked up and inaccurate. Kidneys appear to be miraculously healed, but thank goodness the fearless leader was the one to process those results. Being an RN and the unit supervisor, she could be expected to be prudently on top of things. Nope. Not. The unit manager, Daffy, failed to notice the impossibly improved levels. Probably not having looked at them at all. Daffy simply noted and faxed Minerva's lab results to her primary care physician.

5/1: Prudence, the night nurse, looks at lab results. She readily noticed the potassium level that had elevated to a heart-stopping 6.2. She asked me to draw blood on Minerva, then told me she'd given her kayexalate to bring her potassium level down. The doctor wanted a repeat level four hours after the dose was given to ensure it was effective in bringing her potassium level down. It had brought it down to a high but at least less dangerous 5.4, so Prudence was giving a second dose of kayexalate as I left for home.

We can all rest easy now, however. Prudence got Minerva's potassium level back within the safe range, and of course, Minerva didn't have a heart attack during the two weeks her level was so high. Oh, and Daffy *suddenly recalled* that she herself—the one who refused to learn how to do any nursing *skills*, proclaiming it had "been yeeears" since she'd done any "patient care"—had given the injection on the tenth. She made a late entry and signed that it was given, so all is well *now*.

A nurse reviews lab results, thinks, and obtains related orders immediately. A nurse does not robotically receive and fax lab results, then toss them into the 'to-be-scanned' stack. I've seen many individuals wearing the clothing of a nurse do the receive, fax, toss thing. Even worse, I've seen many of them totally disregard and never even pick up lab results. I did not say they did not *see* the lab results; I said they *disregarded* the lab results. I've seen many nurses never attempt to obtain results not received. And I have seen many more not even aware that they should be expecting to receive any lab results. To top it *all* off, one never knows if the mobile lab results are even going to be accurate … or not.

Freddie:

Glucose (blood sugar) at 4:53 a.m. according to mobile lab: 59

Glucose at 5:06 a.m. according to glucometer: 223

59! And thirteen minutes later his BS was 223 without any food or drink intake. Not possible! It would not be possible *with* intake. It's certainly not possible without.

Same lab draw according to mobile lab:

Hemoglobin dropped from his usual 14s to 9.1.

Serum albumin dropped, protein dropped, sodium dropped, GFR dropped, potassium shot up, and alkaline phosphatase shot up.

That same day, on January 20, *every single individual* who had labs drawn by the mobile lab required a redraw *due to sudden significant drops or elevations in critical levels. Every single re-draw prevented ineffective and/or unnecessary treatment based on inaccurate lab results, and/or ensured needed treatment, which would not have been received had we not redrawn.*

Topper? Yeah, believe it or not, there is a topper. Because the nurses paid so little attention, I spent the next three days intervening as to prevent orders from being carried out that were based on the inaccurate lab results that the nurse(s) robotically faxed over on the 20th, *despite* the fact that I'd informed them all that I was having to re-draw everybody due to significant discrepancies. It would have helped if the lab would just send one copy. For a service so lacking in adequacy, they sure go overboard with the faxing. However, in the end … had the nurses been being nurses…

I called the lab myself and spoke with Ivory. I informed her I was having to redraw every individual and told her why. Ivory replied, "I don't understand that. I used to be the lab tech for your facility, and we never had problems like this."

Or did no one notice? I thought to myself.

"I'll talk to my supervisor about it, and we'll get the problem resolved. I assure you," Ivory promised.

I called her back on two additional occasions. I spoke with my supervisor on all three occasions. Nothing has changed. I fail to see what more I can possibly do. So I'm telling you.

Flennin:

"Ma'am, I sure don't feel good." He said it as if he felt guilty having to admit such things. "I'm sorry, but I don't feel good at all."

Flennin, who normally used his walker and took himself to the bathroom, was so weak that I had to get the aid to help him. I simply wasn't big enough to do it myself. The man was that weak.

I listened to his near constant, forceful, wet-sounding cough as the aid assisted him to the toilet.

After Flennin returned to his bed, I assessed him and found his lung sounds diminished in both lower lobes. There were just faint, scattered crackles, and in the remainder of his lung field, it sounded like someone scrubbing a washboard with a brick as he breathed in and out.

Chest x-ray results? "No acute cardiopulmonary disease." His white blood cell count, though, was through the roof at 18.3.

I contacted the doctor, stressing the fact that Flennin's lung sounds did *not* correlate with the x-ray results. Thank goodness Flennin's doctor was one of those who paid attention, and trusted my assessment. He listened and started IV antibiotics.

Flennin was sent to the ER later that evening due to shortness of breath and low oxygen levels. He was admitted to the hospital with double pneumonia.

I'm going to say this: Flennin didn't get that weak, that sick, overnight. It should have been caught by both the aid and the nurse. But, by dang, the chest x-ray was absolutely, undeniably, and uselessly inaccurate.

October: I had five individuals whose chest x-ray results said, "No acute cardiopulmonary disease," and all five proved to have pneumonia, infiltrates, or effusions once admitted to the hospital. Five in one month. All five x-rays useless. Strangely, sometimes the x-rays were accurate and correlated with the clinical assessment. But one never knew which one he or she was going to get, accurate or inaccurate. Yet onward we march with the mobile x-rays, and as sure as I sit and write this, nobody seems the least bit concerned, except me and two doctors: one from this current facility, "Doctor C," and one from a past facility, "Doctor K." I tell you this, as both will come up again. In fact, Dr. K will always and forever be in my heart. He is not only an excellent doctor, but he also is a good man.

I should add here that it has always been my practice to write vital signs and details of my assessment on the x-ray or lab results. I did this to summarize the issue at hand, simplify the doctor's job, ensure that the doctor was thoroughly informed, thus facilitating and expediting effective treatment. I would then call the doctor and discuss the information I had faxed over. If x-ray and lab results were involved, I also wrote any related, significant lab results on the x-ray result. On the five x-ray results referred to above, I also wrote *Lung sounds/clinical assessment do not correlate with x-ray results.* Not only was I instructed not to write that on the results, but I also found, upon looking, that the results - the ones on which I had written - had disappeared. A new copy of the same results had been obtained or printed, and *that* copy was scanned into the resident's records. *MD notified*, was at the bottom, along with the initials of someone who had not, in fact, received the results, *nor* notified MD. This was in place of my original copy which had notation by me, one who *had* received the results and notified MD.

Me being me, I wanted to know *why*, "why were my lab/test results being pulled and replaced?", so I asked. The director of nursing responded, "Well, it has just always been our practice here to scan in clean, noted results; you know, with nothing written on them. I don't know *why* really. It's just how we do it." She chuckled innocently.

It's just my opinion—please allow me to stress that—but this is the way I see it after much consideration:

My practice of writing the assessment on the results provides thorough information to the doctor. All efforts are made to ensure prudent and effective care. Having been a director of nursing myself, I would have appreciated the documentation aspect of it, as well as the prudency. I'd have used it as an example to my other nurses. But...

I was told, "You can put all that in your nurse note."

"Yes, but Doc doesn't see my nurse note. My nurse note doesn't ensure Doc is fully informed of patient status, needs and allergies. Furthermore, I can put anything I choose to in my nurse note. Any nurse can do the same. But that faxed, detailed information backs up my nurse note. In essence, it's undeniable proof that Doc was notified and fully informed of all pertinent data. As such, I cannot fathom why you would prefer it not be scanned into the records." I shrugged, smiled. "But okie dokie. Won't do it again. I'll make a copy of the results and write on the copy."

"Good idea!" She exclaimed, smiling grandly, as now everybody could be happy.

The only rationale my little brain can come up with is this: My writing "clinical assessment/lung sounds do not correlate with x-ray results" clearly indicates a problem with the x-rays. Thus, it clearly indicates a need for the problem to be resolved ASAP.

Clearly, no one desires to resolve the problem.

I'm open to any rationales anyone may have that may differ from my own.

Dardorff:

Samson was a short man with a voluminous voice. A loner, he spent much of his time in his room and paid little attention to his roommate. A dignified fellow, he was always polite, his manners impeccable.

The nursing world being short staffed is simply a common thread running throughout the fabric of the entire profession. That being what it is, a PRN nurse (meaning works as needed) worked my two days off, as the position opposite my rotation was vacant yet again. When I returned to work on Wednesday, March 17, I got nothing in report about Samson.

On Saturday, March 20, I heard a rowdy commotion from down the hall. I readily recognized Samson's voice, and there was a higher, squeakier female voice begging, "Please! Let us help you! We're trying to help you. I promise!"

"No, no, no," Samson irritably demanded. "Now, go on away from here, please, and let me get down there and fix that thing!"

I rounded the corner of the hallway and saw Samson, who was as naked as a newborn, an aid on each arm struggling to assist him back into his room, obviously so he could put some clothes on. Samson was trying desperately to jiggle the aids from his arms, every bit of his old jingle just a-jangling with every jiggle.

Suddenly, jerking both arms free, Samson took a step forward. Both aids reached out to catch him, as he immediately began a fast, downward descent.

I ran the last few feet and thrust my body in front of his. With timely teamwork, we managed to keep Samson from hitting the floor face first, but I must admit that I wasn't too crazy about having a naked old gentleman lying on top of me. My first thought was, *Oh Lord, please don't let him pee on me!*

The aids quickly assisted Samson to a standing position, and I popped up like a pop tart, checking my clothing for moisture. Samson resumed his struggle to free himself from the "nuisances" so that he could "go get some damned groceries." I'm guessing that whatever had needed fixing just moments before no longer needed fixing.

"You bought groceries yesterday, Mr. Dardorff," I blurted. "Remember? You bought me some of those cheese crackers you like so much. I sure did appreciate it, too. They were delicious! You still have some of those? I didn't get to eat dinner."

"I sure do, little lady. You can't go hungry. Come on in here and get you some." He turned and walked bowlegged to his snack shelf, the aids beside him. They dressed him while I opened some crackers (His son kept him supplied with cheese crackers), and he and I had a picnic. (Lord, I hate cheese crackers!) I babbled on about the pure deliciousness until Samson was fully clothed. Noticing the color and odor of his urine in a urinal sitting on top of his overbed table (on which he eats), I told him I needed a urine specimen, thinking a urinary tract infection just might be the cause of his sudden bizarre behavior. I asked the aid to move the urinal and disinfect his table while I went to grab a specimen cup.

Rora, the night nurse, arrived just as I was about to grab a cup. She asked for whom I needed the cup, and I told her I needed one for Mr. Dardorff. Rora casually informed me that Gabby, the PRN nurse who had worked while I was off, had gotten an order on March 15 for a UA (urinalysis) on Samson.

"We sent the specimen to the lab, but she always dreams up problems when she works. She documented that he was exhibiting strange behavior." Rora rolled her big brown eyes. "I haven't noticed any behavior."

"Maybe because you work at night, when he's asleep," I snapped. *Is that why it was dropped off report? Because the night nurses haven't noticed anything, so they felt it was insignificant?* I wondered to myself as she spoke. *Things are notoriously dropped off report, lost in the shuffle.* I shook my head.

"Why are you shaking your head?"

"I was just thinking."

"Yeah, but what? What were you thinking?"

"Well, if you're going to push it, I was thinking that I'm sure Gabby put the UA on report, and that nurses should stop dropping things off report simply because they are either lazy or don't find whatever it is relevant."

"Oh, okay." She laughed.

I snatched up the phone and called the lab. It turned out that the lab had lost the urine specimen. The guy told me we needed to collect another specimen.

"Oh, okay then." I was maxed! "So the UA was ordered, and the specimen was collected and sent to you on March fifteenth. It's now March twentieth at ten-fourteen p.m. So, when, exactly, were you planning to let us know you had lost the specimen and needed another one collected? Not to mention the fact that I still wouldn't know if I hadn't called *you*!"

I slammed the phone down and glanced up at Rora, who turned and hurried away. A few minutes later she stuck a cup of urine under my nose. "I got the specimen."

"Good. Thank you. Send it out tonight, please."

On March 24, we finally had Samson's urine culture results—not the final, but the preliminary—and they were sufficient enough for us to treat effectively. (strangely, the mobile lab is capable of processing urine correctly) So, *nine days* after a problem was determined and a cause suspected, laboratory confirmation was finally received. So Samson was placed on contact isolation to protect others and was finally started on antibiotics to protect him.

Of course, his roommate ended up with the same bug in his urine. As did Margo, the lady in in the room next door. The aids told me after Margo was diagnosed that Samson had gotten confused on several occasions. He had come out of his room and gone to Margo's room to use the toilet.

It was like beating my head against a wall as I attempted to educate on proactive care. "So, anytime you see something such as that, make the effort to prevent cross contamination and go disinfect the bathroom. Please and thank you."

Danella, aka Ella:

"Who's that in the window?" Ella strained to see better. "Good Lord, he's ugly!" She cackled most uncharacteristically.

"Oh, that's just my reflection." I laughed, wondering, *What the heck is she seeing?* My mind flashed back to the little lady who kept seeing people outside her window just before they'd pass away. The mind is a mystery.

"Well, your reflection looks like an ugly old man!" Ella roared.

"Chill!" I could not help laughing. "You're going to roll right off that bed, Ella! How about we get you up so you can sit in your wheelchair awhile?"

"How about we don't and just say we did?" Ella snickered like a naughty child.

"Just try to be still for a minute, please. I'll be right back. No wiggling!" I laughed.

Closing the blinds, I turned and hurried to the linen closet, grabbed blankets, and stuffed them between Ella and the tiny side rail the state allows us to utilize in long-term care. Then I stuffed rolled blankets at the edge of the bed beneath the fitted sheet, hoping that would keep Ella from rolling out as she continued restlessly straining to see the window. (I knew full well that the great state would probably consider this a restraint, but then, the great state wasn't there to keep Ella safe, were they?)

After my assessment, during which Ella suddenly thought I was "Gaynelle," and suggested we skip school Friday to meet Jason and Bill at the park." I called the doctor.

"So, we now know a bit of Danella's history." I laughed with Doctor K. "I simply cannot find any overt symptoms. She's really pale. Her respirations are a tad more rapid at twenty-two, but then she's talking and giggling incessantly, which also prevents thorough lung sound assessment. All I can tell you for sure is that they aren't breezy."

The doctor wanted STAT labs, and I requested an order for a STAT chest x-ray. I got them ordered at 2:20 p.m. STAT means right now, more or less, and the mobile services have four hours in which to complete STATs.

At 2:50 a.m., I had the chest x-ray, which indicated no problems, but I still didn't have lab results. I'd called the lab multiple times and been promised results "any minute" each time. So I blew a fuse.

"Okay, it's been over twelve hours. I get off work at ten, but I'm not leaving until I have those results! I don't care what you have to do, or stop doing, in order to process Danella's blood, but get it done. Let me find out she has some critical level that you've taken over twelve hours to process, and I promise you I'll shut you down!" I slammed the receiver down.

The night staff sniggered from their seats behind me, some from beneath their blankets.

Five minutes later a pudgy little dude banged his way through the front door, slapped a strange-looking machine on the counter in front of me, and thrust the cord in my face.

"Would you mind plugging this in so I can spin some blood down?" he panted.

"Huh?" I grinned. "You want to spin somebody else's blood down here? In our facility? Is that not crossing the lines of infection control?" I couldn't help laughing, though it wasn't at all funny.

Rora stood quietly next to me. I could feel her waiting for my response.

"I need to spin it down within a certain time frame." He stood holding the cord, his face a splotchy red picture of desperation.

Shaking my head, I grabbed the cord and plugged it in. "Well, I have to say, *this* is a first." I chuckled. "But I can't let some other poor soul go without their lab results."

While the blood was "spinning," I asked, "So, is this…uhh…is this, like, routine for you guys? I mean, do you carry your little spinner there into other facilities? Do you stop at gas stations? I'm sorry." I laughed. "I'm truly curious!"

Kevin, the little dude, proceeded to explain that he was not even a lab tech. He worked in the office but had been called to pick up and transport some specimens. It turned out that Kevin had been given a few minutes of "training" over the phone, and then he was sent to the lab to pick up the spinner, and he'd hit the road running.

I gave Kevin a cup of hot coffee and called the EMTs to come pick Ella up and take her to ER. I then called ER and told Tracy, the nurse, that I was sending Danella over to be checked out due to bizarre behavior with no other overt symptoms, but largely due to an unreliable mobile lab service.

Ultimately, Ella had three critical lab values: hemoglobin, ammonia, and carbon dioxide. She was placed on a ventilator for two days. She received a blood transfusion and she was treated to lower the ammonia level. It turned out that her CPAP hadn't been put on the entire week I was off, and she'd received no nebulizer treatments. Rora told me about the former, saying, "Well, the two o'clock to ten o'clock nurses didn't put her CPAP on her all week long." *I'm guessing the ten o'clock to six o'clock shift nurses couldn't put a CPAP on a patient*, I thought to myself. And I had already discovered the latter earlier in the evening, when I had grabbed a dose of the nebulizer treatment medication from the fridge and noticed my initials and date still on the packet in use. No doses were missing, except the one I'd taken out of the same packet a week before. Unfortunately, it also turned out that Ella had a new diagnosis of liver failure to add to her list of complications. We finally received Ella's lab results from the mobile lab some time the next morning. I'm not certain of the time, as I wasn't there. However, I did ask about them upon my arrival that afternoon. Looking them over, I was naturally quite relieved to see that all was well. According to those results, the lady on the ventilator, right that minute, was as fine as sweet red wine, not a problem in the world.

I was reprimanded for chewing the lab guy out on the phone. I apologized. It was unprofessional, I readily admit. No excuses.

But I still politely suggested we obtain alternate lab services.

We didn't.

I could go on forever on this. It is a major thorn in my side that pokes me frequently. I see this in every facility. I address this in every facility. Nobody seems to want to fix the problem. Heck, nobody seems to want to admit that there *is* a problem. I sit here now, baffled. What do they tell themselves that allows them to find peace while doing nothing?

Please understand me: This is widespread, ongoing, unaddressed, and in the records. One must first want to see. One must first open one's eyes, and one must look.

In the Beginning

I'm no contractor, but I would think that when building, one would first want to ensure a solid foundation. What good are solid walls if the foundation crumbles? Right?

As a nurse, I do know that when devising a plan of care, one must first know the patient's status and needs. Therefore, it is pertinent that the admission assessments, orders, and documentation be thorough, accurate, and timely. That is the foundation on which you build your plan of care, with the intention of ensuring a positive outcome for your patient.

And yet admissions are literally slammed. Every admission, every facility. I kid you not. In fact, a basic admission entails the completion of twelve to fifteen varied assessments (each assessment ranging in length from one to ten pages), reviewing and entering all the orders (a patient with zero medications, which has happened only once in my twenty-eight years, will still have roughly thirty orders), and three to six consent forms that must be reviewed with the patient and family and then signed. This is in addition to settling the patient into his or her room, answering the patient's and his or her family's questions, and familiarizing the patient with the room, call light, and facility. The nurse must ensure all basic need items are provided. God help us if there are multiple or complicated wounds, as all must be uncovered, measured, described, and redressed. A lab requisition must be completed for admission labs. An initial care plan must be completed. And so on and so forth.

A comprehensive, legitimate admission, which ensures a solid foundation, takes about four hours of hard, fast, and focused work. _Zero_ extra time is allotted for admissions. In fact, in many facilities, multiple admissions are completed simultaneously by the same nurse. An admission adds so much work and stress that in all facilities across the board, it is an ongoing issue, and those multiple and varied assessments are about as useless as a tick. They are _busy work_ for the overworked with maybe a whopping two percent of them actually being 'done' as opposed to merely being 'filled out, signed and dated'.

I was just recently asked to see a gentleman due to his consistent complaints of knee pain. It turned out that he had fallen at home. The knee, wrist, and ankle were x-rayed in the hospital due to complaints of pain. The ankle was documented as swollen and warm. The wrist was swollen and tender. All three had limited range of motion. All this per the hospital records at the time of his discharge from the hospital to us. However, our admission 'Joint Mobility' assessment? The admitting nurse documented all joints "within normal limits", thus functioning normally. Hmm, this man's joints completely healed during the ten minute ride from the hospital to us.

Useless. Useless, time-consuming crap. If you don't need it, chuck it. If you need it, do it right.

At the first LTC facility for whom I was employed, I worked the skilled hall, and the admission system was as clear as mud. It was *verbally* divided up between the first three eight hour shifts starting with the patients arrival shift ; there was *nothing* in writing. Dividing the workload between the first three shifts was intended to prevent, thus avoid paying, overtime while still ensuring the admission was completed within the required twenty-four hour time frame. Yet the next two shifts, of course, did nothing, so ultimately, it was that poor sap who was on duty the moment the patient arrived who was hunted down and questioned about why the admission wasn't complete. Therefore, this person was also the one instructed to complete whatever hadn't been done. It only took one time for me to learn that the next two shifts wouldn't do any of it. Thereafter, I completed the entire admission(s) before going home. I was there until the wee hours, but it was finished and done with, and I would challenge anyone to find an error, omission, or oversight. I combed through the records; put everything in the report that one needed to know in order to provide prudent, effective care for that *individual*; and I actually conducted the assessments as opposed to simply filling them out. But it took the full four hours or more to do it, and I worked hard and fast.

The point is, the nurse struggles to complete this admission while performing his or her usual duties, and in many facilities he or she is managing multiple admissions at the same time. The admission process is slammed. The admission process is sloppy. The admission process is dangerously ineffective.

At one particular facility—a big, beautiful place—one of the office nurses was responsible for entering all the orders on admissions. The concept was good, as it split the load, but the outcome was horrific. If I've said it once, I've said it a million times: "You have to get this right. It matters."

I reviewed the orders once they were entered. One hundred percent of the admissions on my unit had errors. I'm fairly certain this was the case for the entire building, but I can only say for a fact that it was the case on one hundred percent of those admitted to my unit. Sadly, I can also say, as a matter of fact, that I am the only nurse who reviewed the orders. Every other nurse simply assumed they had been entered correctly, counted themselves lucky to have help with at least that much, and clicked on as if all was right with the world. I get it. Desperation. But still, no excuse. Fix the system. Don't let the overload affect the people. It's not their fault.

Lana:

Lana arrived on a Wednesday evening. I, however, did not meet her until the following Monday, which was my first day back after my biweekly five days off.

Lana was just forty-one years old. She'd slipped in some water at home while reaching to pass a tool to her husband, who was working on a plumbing problem beneath the kitchen sink. She broke her leg in three different places and had already been through two surgeries and a lengthy hospital stay. Finally, she had made it to us for rehab.

I walked into Lana's room—the last room on the right—just before seven a.m. to check her blood sugar. After introducing myself, I set my things down on some wax paper and then told her what I was about to do.

Lana swiped loose strands of blond hair from her pleasantly plump face. "Well, I can tell you now that it's going to be high." She stuck a finger out for the test.

"You right about that. Five hundred and sixteen." I glanced at Lana, then held the glucometer so that she could see the reading.

"It's been like that. They won't give me my Lantus," she yelled, suddenly (and understandably) irritable. "They are doing the Humalog with the sliding scale, but no matter how many nurses I tell, no matter how many times I tell them, and no matter how much I beg, they will not give me my Lantus!" She raised both palms into the air, exasperated.

"What did they say when you told them?" I was already as frustrated as she was, as I could easily imagine the nurses' responses. This was far from my first rodeo.

Rolling her eyes dramatically, Lana replied, "We don't have an order for Lantus. I keep hearing that same thing over and over. I told them to call my doctor! I have to have it! But I'm still not getting it."

"Well, let me take care of that right now."

"*Finally*, somebody listens!" She threw her head back. "Hallelujah!"

True to her word, Lana was supposed to be receiving fifty units of Lantus every morning and thirty-five units in the evening. I knew this by reviewing her admission paperwork from the hospital. So, grabbing some Lantus from stock, I took Lana her injection. Then I reviewed her records, during which I found that Lana's blood sugar had gotten as high as five hundred and seventy-two. The records indicated that her doctor had been notified, as ordered with all blood sugar checks with results over five hundred.

Yet no one bothered to ask her doctor about the Lantus while they were notifying him about the blood sugar level? I wondered.

As I lived in the real world, I was all but sure the doctor had never been notified. The records showed that Lana had been receiving the maximum dose of her Humalog every single blood sugar check, still staying around five hundred every single check.

"Three hundred and two." I smiled at Lana just before lunch. "It's coming down, my lady! But I still get to give you another shot, which, as you can probably tell, is my favorite part of the job." I winked.

Lana's pink-tinged cheeks plumped like tiny pillows when she smiled. "I was really worried about how my leg was going to heal with my blood sugar staying so high. I've been begging for a shot for four days! Poke me all you want!"

Late that afternoon Lana's doctor stopped in to see her. Looming over my head at six feet, seven inches, he asked for a copy of Lana's admission lab results. While they printed, he locked his sage green eyes on mine.

"You're the nurse who called me this morning. I recognize the voice, though I expected you to be bigger." He chuckled. "I thought about things after we hung up. So, for clarification purposes, you indicated that Lana had not received her Lantus since last Thursday. Is that correct?"

"Yes, sir, it appears to be correct… last Wednesday was the last dose of Lantus Lana had received, prior to this morning." I glanced at the floor.

"Please print me a log of her blood sugar readings." He forced a smile.

Handing him the copies, I simply could not bring myself to look him in the eye.

"So, why did you wait until today to call me?" he asked quietly, scanning the log and shaking his head.

"I'm sorry, sir. I have been off. Today is my first day back, and I called you just as soon as I checked Lana's blood sugar."

He looked up, a scowl consuming his otherwise handsome face. "I need blank orders, please. Lana's room number?"

"Three-twelve." I handed him a blank doctor's order form.

He took the form, stretched out his other hand, grasped mine, and shook it. "Thank you." His eyes sparkling as he spun around, he began making long, fast strides to the last room on the right. Less than ten minutes later, he loomed over my head once again.

"Excuse me," he said quietly. "Thank you again. Lana said you are terrific. I tend to agree." He grinned as he handed me his written orders for Lana.

I picked up the orders as he strode toward the door, read what he'd written.

"Discharge to alternate rehab facility of choice - effective immediately."

Lucas:

Quiet, soft-spoken, easy-going, and as compliant as a nurse could ever hope a patient could be. The man was truly as easy as Sunday morning.

Post open-heart surgery, Lucas had an incision running down the middle of his chest, along with three tiny incision sites on his right upper abdomen. The mid-chest incision looked perfect, but the three tiny incision sites, which were more like puncture sites, were gunky and red-rimmed. He had doctor's orders for the application of Bactroban and a dressing change twice daily. Lucas also had a venous graft site on his left lower leg, which needed to be kept clean but left open to air.

The way I saw it, once daily was better than none, so I didn't make a fuss about Homer, the day nurse, not doing the wound care on the mornings he worked. Instead I made a point to do it early in my shift so I could check the dressing again later and see if it needed to be changed a second time before I left. It was working. The sites were looking much better. But then Lucas was re-admitted to the hospital with chest pain.

Homer admitted Lucas upon his return to our facility from the hospital, but Homer completely overlooked the wound care to the right upper abdomen incision sites, and he failed to reference the venous graft site to the lower right leg. The incision mid-chest was healed, the staples having been removed while Lucas was back in the hospital. I had been off a few days, so I hadn't seen Lucas in almost a week.

"Hey, congratulations!" I told him when I assessed his heart sounds and saw his chest. "You graduated! Staple free now!"

Lucas grinned shyly.

However, I noticed that the dressing on the upper abdomen was the same dressing I'd last put on before Lucas went back to the hospital five days prior. He'd been back with us for two and a half days. *That explains the odor*, I thought to myself.

The hospital had fallen short, as well, as they hadn't changed the dressing, either, so I called the house supervisor and simply pointed out that, with a diagnosis of chest pain, somebody had surely placed EKG leads on the man's chest, somebody had surely assessed the man's heart sounds, and somebody had surely seen the dressing at some point while doing those things.

His surgical sites were bigger and more infected than they had been when he had arrived the first time. He now had tenderness that he hadn't had before. I performed his wound care, put a clean dressing over the wounds, wrote wound care orders to ensure it was done from that moment forward, added it to report, and then called the assistant director of nursing. After informing her that Homer had completely omitted wound care orders for Lucas's surgical sites, and that the sites were now larger and more infected than they had been to begin with, she asked, "What surgical sites does he have?"

She did not know. She was the one designated to review all admissions. I'm going to leave that right there.

I will add that Lucas healed up and went home, and Homer still works there. Homer saunters around and slips into certain rooms to talk sports. He's easygoing and well liked, probably a pretty good kid. He once said about me, "No need to get all worked up." I get it. I do. I get frustrated quite often over the lackadaisical crap I see every day, everywhere, by most everybody. And I tend to shoot pretty straight. I admit I have a low tolerance for lack of give-a-shit. I need to work on that. But frankly, I'd like to see Homer get "all worked up" once in a while.

Willow:

Willow was a bit strange. She had thin, scraggly hair that hung almost to her knees; and dyed it coal-black, though, naturally speaking, it was so mousy gray that the resulting color more closely resembled old cast-iron than coal. Truth is, Willow looked much like a manic version of Casper the friendly ghost. Tiny as a Smurf and pale as a sheet, Willow wore almost perfect circles of neon pink blush on her cheeks, and she put as much deep red lipstick on her lips as possible with as much around her lips as on them. She meticulously applied long false eyelashes each morning, which she topped abundantly with black eyeshadow. This, though, helped hide the lopsided aspect of her sweeping lashes. Willow smiled from the time she woke each morning to the time she fell asleep at night. The only time I ever saw her frown was the one time an aid was foolish enough to suggest Willow wear her hair up for a change. Flabbergasted, Willow readily insisted that all ten of her hairs were to "hang free like my spirit".

All that said, though Willow somewhat startled people upon first meeting—she even scared a few with advanced dementia—Willow was special. It was ultimately those with dementia who loved Willow the most, though everyone eventually loved her. Willow had a way of genuinely finding delight in everyone. She just didn't seem to notice people's not-so-good stuff. I had the pleasure of being present the day the facility grouch barked at Willow for being in his way of the coffee pot. I watched in amazement as Willow spun around, green eyes sparkling beneath the black eyeshadow, looked up at Grouchy, and said, "Oh my goodness, your voice is so resonant. I bet you sing!" She smiled, then flittered out of his way, going over to say hello to little

Alice. I almost grabbed the counter to hold on, expecting the earth to shake any second as I watched the corners of Grouchy's mouth twitch as he resisted a smile.

Grouchy almost smiled! I thought, glancing about to see if there were any other witnesses. *Nobody is gonna believe* this. *That woman has been here just a little over a week, and she's already touched more hearts than all of us put together.* I smiled to myself. *We should all be so strange*, I thought, glancing toward Willow once more before I hurried down the hallway.

Later that night, while covering a ten to six shift to help out, I was looking through Willow's records to find the appropriate diagnosis for her *antibiotic*. "Infection" simply didn't give me enough to go on regarding assessment of symptoms and documentation. I needed just a bit more specific information. She'd already completed the antibiotic, but we were to be doing the follow-up documentation. I had no clue if the medication had been effective or if the infection was resolved, as I had no clue what kind of infection she'd had. Of course, glancing through the other nurses' notes only told me there was "no adverse reaction" to the antibiotic.

Ultimately, I found in the hospital records that Willow had been prescribed the antibiotic for a urinary tract infection, which was discovered while she was in the hospital with an acute exacerbation of congestive heart failure. So, I added "for UTI" on the report. Upon further review, I found that Willow had steroidal eye drops ordered indefinitely. The diagnosis/indication for the drops was "lubrication." That being so ludicrous, I simply *had* to look to see who the admitting nurse had been.

"Homer." I rolled my eyes. *I should have known.* "You need to call the doctor today, Nara," I explained to the day nurse during report at shift change. "We have to have an accurate diagnosis for Willow's eye drops. A steroid is not a "lubricant." Nara laughed. I continued, saying, "We also need a stop date. Steroidal eye drops cannot be used indefinitely. It would damage the eyes. Heck, an ophthalmologist would tell you not to use allergy drops indefinitely. But a steroid? Come on! Common sense."

"Well, I'm glad you said something. I didn't know that, either," Nara said.

"I get it. I didn't know it myself until I got my first order for steroid eye drops and *looked them up*, so that I'd know about the drug I was administering, I hinted. But, I mean, they're a steroid. We all know steroids are hardcore."

"Yeah, yeah, I'll call the doctor for sure," Nara said, eyes wide.

Frustrated, I added, "The Amiodarone? That's for atrial fibrillation, not hypertension. The Levaquin was for a UTI, though I suppose nobody other than myself wondered what it was for. And the Lactulose is to rid her body of excess ammonia, not for constipation. Would you please make sure the day shift medication aid is aware of that so that she will stop holding it because Willow has diarrhea? The diarrhea is an inconvenient but desired effect. The diarrhea is the only way to rid the body of excess ammonia, so if the med aid stops the diarrhea, well, I'm sure you know this. And, by the way, ask the doctor if we can do a monthly ammonia level, please."

Nara stood gaping.

"Thanks, Nara. Sorry to throw so much at you so early in your morning." I smiled. "I don't mean to sound ugly. It's not intended that way, but to be safe, you guys best be checking behind Homer on his admissions. In fact, I personally check all admissions and prefer for someone to check behind me. That's actually how it is supposed to be done. That's the only way to be safe."

"Uh, yeah, I guess so."

I figured I'd said enough, so I didn't mention the fact that Willow was an APS referral for long-term admission after her skilled days ran out. Willow had been noncompliant with her Lactulose at home, resulting in an elevated ammonia level, causing her to exhibit bizarrely unsafe behavior as a result of the inevitable altered mental status. So APS mandated she be admitted to a safe environment in which she would remain in compliance with her medications. We blew that right quick and in a hurry.

Topper:

Just three days ago, on Friday night, I was entering some new orders, during which I reviewed the resident's medication list to ensure I wasn't duplicating anything. That was when I noticed the man had glaucoma and was seeing a specialist in a large city. Apparently, back on March twelfth, the specialist had ordered Prednisolone drops twice daily for inflammation. The nurse had failed to obtain a stop date.

Then, in April, the resident saw that same doctor again, at which time a different, less potent anti-inflammatory drop was ordered, also at twice daily. The nurse failed to obtain a stop date; and failed to get the first drop discontinued.

In a nutshell, both drops were still being administered two months later. Due to the late hour, I had to call the primary care doctor, who discontinued both drops, effective immediately, as "neither should be used longer than two weeks".

Having heard back from the doctor on my cellphone, after leaving the facility, I had to call the charge nurse to inform her of the new orders, then request that she add the orders to report so that the other nurses would know the drops had been discontinued.

Frustrated and angry about the risk of damage to the man's already-at-risk eyesight, I commented to the charge nurse, "Those robotic, non-thinking nurses are going to kill somebody someday." The charge nurse, who is a dynamite nurse with a good, caring heart and a conscientious manner, said, "I didn't know, either. I learned something today."

I could feel her smile, and I almost commented but found myself speechless.

I just drove home, wondering, *What made me immediately ask "how long?" the first time I had a patient for whom steroid drops were ordered? Why do other nurses not immediately wonder the same thing? If they saw their eye doctor and were started on drops for inflammation, I feel certain they would wonder, and ask, how long they needed to use the drops. So, considering the nurses are there to ensure prudent medical care for their patients, why do they not wonder and ask the same thing on their patients' behalf?*

I recalled my daughter, who has allergies. At one point, her allergies resulted in inflammation of her eyes which caused the inner lids to literally peel. Her eye doctor ordered steroid drops. My daughter is not a nurse, yet I clearly recall her saying, "*I asked him how long* I'd have to use the drops. He said until they stop peeling, but no more than two weeks. I have to go back to see him if they aren't better by then. But they already itch less."

Point is, my daughter knew to ask, and she's not a nurse. It's common sense. It's paying attention to what you're doing. It's thinking. It's *give-a-shit*.

As for nurses, it is being a nurse instead of simply going through the motions to get a check. It is doing your job despite the overload. Nurses, it is your obligation. The man's vision is already at risk, and you increased the risk.

The man's *wellbeing* is in your hands. His vision *matters*.

Hank:

Seventy-one years old. Hair still black as night. Eyebrows and beard as fuzzy white as the cotton balls on a child's construction paper Santa Claus. For that matter, Hank was every bit as merry as Santa, and Hank's wife, Verna, would have made a great Mrs. Claus. She stopped in frequently, bringing a smile to every patient's face in every room she passed as she waddled down the hall to her beloved "Hanki." And she brought home-made cookies to the nurses every Monday.

Hank was with us for rehab. He'd been admitted to the hospital for three days due to hypotension, which was caused by dehydration. Verna fussed, saying, "It's because he's too stubborn to realize he's got too old to spend these hot days on that danged tractor!" She then bent down and pressed her chubby little cheek against Hank's, and Hank rolled his merry eyes. "I keep telling him to drink more water when he's out in that hot sun."

A therapist had asked me to see Hank because his blood pressure was "always high" when they checked it prior to doing his therapy. Obvious to me, the first thing to do was look at his blood pressure record. So, doing just that, I was shocked (though I shouldn't be by now) to find that the therapist was not only right, but Hank's blood pressure was actually at stroke level ninety-five percent of the time. Hank had been with us for seventeen days. His blood pressure was checked, according to the records, once daily by the medication aid prior to administering his medications.

First: This popped into my relentless brain: *So, are the nurses simply using the medication aid's blood pressure reading? Are they not assessing themselves?*

Second: Did no one realize that a man with hypotension caused by dehydration wouldn't likely be hypotensive anymore once hydrated?

Again, obvious to me, I next looked over Hank's medications and made some notes. After reviewing the hospital records, I saw that Hank's blood pressure was back to normal and was inching toward high the day he was discharged from there to us. In fact, the hospitalist had written the following in his progress note: *Dehydration resolved. Secondary hypotension resolved, as well, with blood pressure at 154/87. Okay to discharge today to rehab facility.*

However, the hospitalist had not considered the fact that it would likely be a good idea to resume Hank's blood pressure medication. Maybe he thought the 'nursing facility' to which he'd discharged would be on top of that.

Hank, having learned his lesson, was doing just what Verna said and drinking plenty of water. He said, "She was right. I don't drink enough water, even when I'm not out in the hot sun." Raising his cotton ball brows, he grinned, "I hate the hospital, and I love my tractor! So I plan to be a good boy from now on." He winked at Verna.

It was an easy fix, and yet in seventeen days and thirty-four nursing shifts, no one had noticed this dude's blood pressure was at stroke level? Even though his admission diagnoses were blood pressure related? I mean, the diagnosis itself pointed out the need to be looking at his blood pressure. Forget the fact that vital signs are a basic part of assessment.

Had Hank's admission been prudent, thorough, thus effective, Hank would not have spent seventeen days at risk of a stroke. Dehydration would not have been the sole focus. But all is well, and we can rest easy. Hank did not have a stroke!

But what about the next Hank? There will no doubt be a next Hank. Will he be okay? Has the next Hank already had a stroke somewhere else?

This is only one example out of a million. Admissions matter. The foundation matters. In fact, someone with the access needs to conduct a study on rehospitalizations from nursing facilities. That someone needs to determine how many of those rehospitalizations would likely have been prevented if a prudent, comprehensive, and effective admission had been completed in the first place.

I stand behind all nurses everywhere on this issue, though in most cases it is simply consideration of themselves that inspires their speaking out about the admission process, or severe lack thereof. However, many are just as concerned about the negative effect on the patients as I am. Regardless of the specific concerns of the nurses, the admission process must be taken more seriously. Time must be allotted to complete them effectively, and staff must be provided to do so. Admissions is simply not a task that can be prudently added to a nurse's usual load.

Further, the report the admission nurse passes to the other nurses involved in the patient's care must me thorough. At most facilities they give the patient's name, room number, admission diagnosis, and anything good or bad they may have noticed about the individual, which is usually a report regarding whether the patient is predicted to be pleasant or a pain in the neck.

The reporting process is every bit as lacking as the admission process, but then, in all fairness, if one must slam the admission, all one has is a slammed report. One doesn't really know much to pass on.

Another angle on admissions: When one is admitted to the hospital, one is acutely ill or injured in some way. Thus, temporary changes are often made in one's home medication regimen due to the acute issue. Said changes needing to be reviewed and often revised once the acute issue is resolved. Additionally, hospital nurses are slamming their admissions, as well. Thus, errors occur. Unless one reviews the records, one will not be aware of the changes made or the errors that occurred. Thus, one cannot ensure the safety of one's patient. If one reviews, one knows many things one will not otherwise know. One knows things to watch for.

You would be amazed at just how little those caring for you truly know about you or your needs. In some cases, you would be devastated.

Medication:
Medley of Miracles & Madness

Medication administration in long-term care is much like a five-star magic show, never ceasing to amaze me!

In some facilities, nurses administer the medications in addition to their other tasks. In other facilities, medication aids administer the medications as their only task. In still other facilities, the task of medication administration is swapped back and forth as staff is cut, reinforced, and cut again. This keeps the corporate bottom line where corporate desires it to be.

Regardless of who is administering the medications, the show still goes on, and the show is amazing!

Elisa, aka Leese:

Remember Leese, my little friend who wasn't so little due to the nurses running her eighteen-hour feeding for twenty-four hours a day, causing her to be severely obese? Leese, my friend who had the motorcycle accident? The one known to spout a certain obscenity, but who learned to spout, "I luuuv yeeew," when she felt love received from you?

Well, while Leese had been making her latest move to her new room back on my unit, my co-worker Suzanne simultaneously moved to the day shift, which landed *her* on my unit, as well. Thus, Suzanne would be the nurse I relieved each day instead of the nurse I worked with each evening. Suzanne had been working there for several years and was considered one of their best nurses. An older African American woman who was still pretty, she was openly determined—hell-bent, in fact—on finding herself another husband.

"I even tole my son to find me a man," Suzanne said emphatically, further explaining that she felt she'd been shafted in her divorce and wanted a man to take care of her for a change.

I respected Suzanne. She hustled, appeared to be on top of things, always got her documentation done, and always got out on time! I, on the other hand, was no doubt on top of things. In fact, I am known for and have been awarded for excellence in clinical practice and documentation. I was even commended by the state for my documentation. However, I was nearly always late getting out. Naturally, Suzanne amazed me!

But then, it didn't take long at all for me to find out I had been wrong about everything except the fact that Suzanne got out on time. The first day I relieved Suzanne, I started having to pull medications from the backup supply. I didn't think anything about it initially; I just figured Suzanne gave the last pill, tablet or capsule from the blister pack and didn't restock the medication as we're supposed to because she was new to the shift, still learning the unit and running behind.

However, it continued. And it didn't take long for that to get old. I found myself having to stop repeatedly, lock my cart, and run down the hall to the medication room to get medications that weren't available on the cart. Patience was not at all a virtue. I readily admit and stand accountable for the fact that I grew extremely frustrated, and it was because I lack patience that I noticed the pattern pretty quickly.

I wasn't looking to find an issue. I didn't have the time or the desire to do so. Suzanne herself waved a big red flag in my face, bringing the issue to light through her own laziness.

Thing is, one remembers. It's instinctive. When one deals with the same group of individuals day after day, giving the same medications to those same individuals day after day, one's brain simply files the information innately. One memorizes the individuals' medications without trying. One not only innately remembers the medications, but one also recalls how many are remaining when one gets down to the last few.

As I said, I stand fully accountable for my frustration and related actions. I stopped restocking, too. I thought, *Okay, Suzanne, you don't want to restock when you give the last dose? Fine. I won't, either. You can run up and down this hall just as many times as you make me run it.*

(I know it's childish. I told you I'm just me. I'm no saint!)

Ultimately, I found that Suzanne didn't run back and forth at all. Suzanne simply gave medications that weren't on the cart to give.

Yes, I know you're wondering how that is possible.

I wondered myself. I pondered the matter extensively. After all, Suzanne had signed that the medications were administered, and yet they were not available on the cart to be administered. Upon glancing, I noticed that some of the medications taken only in the morning were also signed as given. However, not only were those medications not on the cart, but they weren't even in the building. It was a mystery.

Knowing the pharmacy was only going to send a month's supply—no more, no less—and that the nurse must request the refill or nothing is received, it was easy to solve the mystery. It took a bit of physical effort, but no mental effort was required at all.

When I gave a twice-a-day medication and trashed the empty pack, I didn't restock, meaning Suzanne would have to grab the new month supply in order to be able to administer the morning dose.

She didn't.

I would have to grab the new month supply to give the next evening dose. Finding the medication not on the cart, I trekked to the medication room, purposely popped the dose I needed from the blister pack, left the blister pack in the medication room, and administered the dose.

Suzanne carried right on, signing that she'd given or administered the medications while those blister packs sat in the medication room with the same amount of pills/capsules I'd left them with, always having the same amount when I came back to them to give the next day's evening dose.

Like 'Doublemint', 'two mints in one', I solved two mysteries at once. Suzanne wasn't giving the medications that weren't on the cart. And Suzanne always got out on time because she was just skimming the surface, drawing a check, and doing the things she knew could be pegged, like signing for the medications. Suzanne knew that management sometimes checked for missed initials, looked to make sure there was a nurse note for each shift, but they never actually counted the medications or randomly checked feeding pumps/bottles, nor did they ever check much of anything, with the exception of documentation. By dang, if the state might check it during survey, they would check it from time to time. Otherwise, they didn't give it a thought. Suzanne operated on this knowledge.

I let Suzanne know that I'd be counting the medications from that day forward. I smiled, adding, "Give my people their medications,

Suzanne. I don't want to cause you any grief, but for their sakes, I'm watching." I felt I had been fair, as I'd given her a heads up.

She got better about seeing to it that there was nothing I could catch her in. But, try as I might to prevent it, Suzanne's sloppy ethics ultimately had a grave effect, as I'd feared from the moment I discovered Suzanne was cold and conniving enough to skip medications so she could get off on time.

As a result of Leese's accident and related head injury, Leese had a seizure disorder. Seizure activity has repeatedly proven to be a red flag regarding missed or skipped medications. And liquids are more difficult to monitor than tablets.

One evening the aid ran up to me and said, "Something is wrong with Elisa!" As her nurse, I hurried in and readily identified that Leese was having a seizure. Her body was stiff, her extremities were spasming in tiny jerking motions, and her eyes were darting rhythmically from side to side, seeing nothing. Placing pillows at Leese's sides, I glanced at my watch to time the seizure, then flipped the light out to decrease stimuli.

In rushed other aids and a young, overly confident co-worker who flipped the light on, looked at me, and snapped disgustedly, seeing me simply standing nearby, "Did you get her vitals?"

Before I could speak, that chick had slapped a wrist cuff on Leese and was trying to force Leese's arm still in order to obtain a blood pressure.

"Turn the light off and get your hands off of her now! Please and thank you," I whispered between gritted teeth.

"Her blood pressure is two hundred and fourteen over one hundred and thirty-two," girl wonder professed, eyes wide, as she looked for me to join her in shock.

"Don't speak. Don't touch her. Decrease as much stimuli as possible. Simply observe and time the activity," I whispered more softly to an aid. "I'll be right back."

Motioning for girl wonder to follow, I stepped out into the hallway.

"The first thing one learns about seizure precautions is to ensure safety by getting anything away from them on which they might harm themselves. Second, decrease as much external stimuli as possible." I looked to see if she was even registering the input. If sarcastic eye rolling is a sign of registering, she was with me all the way! "The very last thing one should do is attempt to force an extremity to remain still during seizure activity, and the blood pressure cannot be accurate during muscle stiffness and twitching. You, in conclusion, placed Leese at risk of status epilepticus. Study up on seizure precautions and management. If you don't, do not enter the rooms of my patients again when I'm on duty, unless I call for you. Thank you."

Returning to the room, I saw that Leese was beginning to settle down, her eyes no longer darting. The darting then replaced with drowsy, droopy lids. I told the aid she could leave, and I left Leese to rest, then went to document a description of the seizure activity. A short while later I drew stat drug levels on Leese's seizure medications. The results were just as I'd suspected. Checked monthly, the levels had been running fine for over a year straight. Suddenly, Suzanne switched to our unit, and Leese had her first seizure in a very long time, as her drug levels had suddenly dropped.

Now, considering Suzanne signed that all medications had been given, we couldn't prove she hadn't given Leese her 2 p.m. seizure medication. However, I was still her evening nurse Monday through Friday; the weekend nurse had been in place for a long time. The only change had been Suzanne. And I had already proven, for a fact, that Suzanne would sign that a medication was given when it wasn't. Suzanne had *given* medications that I knew she had never touched. Suzanne had *given* medications that were not even in the building.

Similarly, the g-tube syringe is replaced in the wee hours of each morning by the night nurse. The clear, plastic, sealed packaging that contains the syringe is timed, dated, and initialed by that night nurse. The old syringe is discarded, and a new one is routinely placed, by the night nurse, for each new day. I'd already noticed that I was repeatedly opening the syringe for the first time when I administered Leese's five p.m. medications. I mean, I was breaking that seal. I had already wondered how Suzanne administered Leese's 2:00 p.m. seizure med via g-tube without ever opening the syringe. I'd already asked Suzanne how the packages remained sealed, and Suzanne had merely rolled her eyes. It's a mystifying miracle, as Susanne swore emphatically that she never missed giving a single dose.

"The syringes were never even opened, Suzanne." I pled for a sign of hope that accountability might lead to improvement. "The levels are near a third what they've been for over a year running."

"Well, I always gives my medicines." Suzanne shrugged, cocked her head to the side, smacked her gum, and walked away.

The fact that Suzanne lied, even when faced with all the proof, was what concerned me the most about her being a nurse. I could not fix it, so I wrote her up, as instructed by the cop-out, never-present director of nursing. But later, just as soon as I had the authority, I terminated Suzanne for countless medication errors and false documentation. I spread the proof across my desk until I ran out of space, dropped the remaining stack in the middle, handed her the termination papers to sign, and informed her she should feel free to write comments should she so desire. I didn't enjoy it. I hated every second of it. I do not like to hurt anyone's feelings. But these vulnerable people need our protection. Suzanne had long proven that she was going to cut whatever corners she needed to cut in order to clock out and go home on time. And I mean absolutely *whatever* corners she needed to cut. It mattered not to Suzanne. Getting off on time and finding herself a man were Suzanne's priorities.

Side note: Girl wonder here is Wynona, whom you will meet shortly. Some things are just so … mean, so unnecessary and cruel, that they stick with you forever. So, this is the one thing I'm going to share with you from memory. One night, at shift change, Wynona had just arrived, thus she was energetic and talkative, cutting up with the aids who'd just arrived for their shift as well. The two of us who had worked the two o'clock to ten o'clock shift, myself and Haley, were blocking the chatter out while quietly and diligently working to wrap up our documentation so we could clock out and go home. Suddenly however, Wynona's cackle pierced our focus-induced sound barrier. Glancing up at Wynona, I was horrified as the words she had spoken registered in my brain.

"What did you say?" I asked, seeking confirmation before I reacted. Haley, glanced over at me, then leaned back in her chair, crossed her arms and stared at Wynona, awaiting response.

Wynona, still cackling wildly with the aids, spun around cackling ever louder. Near squealing, she replied, "I said, I took care of us! We don't have to worry about being bothered by the ones who stay up late, or get up in the wee hours, drinking coffee every night. They might as well go to bed tonight because I dumped it!" Her voice shrill with excitement. "I dumped the coffee!" She added to ensure clarity and … admiration?

"You *dumped* it?" I asked incredulously. "You know we have no way of getting them coffee made now that the kitchen staff is gone. *That's* why they fill that big urn just before they leave every night. What does it matter to you if these people want to have coffee?"

"Because we want them to go to bed and go to sleep; get out of our hair," she glanced at the aids, cackled again.

"That's one of the absolute meanest things I've ever heard of anybody doing. That was just downright wicked. How would you feel if I dumped your bag of snacks that I'm fairly certain you have tonight, just like you do every night?"

"Aww girl! Don't touch my snacks!" She cackled again.

"That's how they feel about their coffee."

"That was a cackle-stopper," Haley glanced at me and winked.

Albert:

One afternoon I was helping the floor nurses process significant labs, just doing it to help out. I happened across Albert's TSH (thyroid function level, on which the doctor bases the dosage of his thyroid supplement).

Right away I noticed Albert's abnormal TSH level. A low TSH level means a high thyroid level. In short, if the body has plenty of thyroid, the TSH (thyroid stimulating hormone) will back off, so the TSH level is low. If the body is low on thyroid, the TSH (stimulator) kicks in, trying to get the body to produce more thyroid, so the TSH level is high.

Albert's TSH (stimulator) was really low, meaning his body had way too much thyroid.

Strangely, upon review of the results, I noticed that just three months prior, Albert's TSH had been super high, meaning his body was way low on thyroid.

Reviewing his records, I saw that Albert had been on the same dosage—75mcg—of thyroid supplement since 2017, two years his level remained within normal limits every check.

Then in April of 2019, suddenly his thyroid level was super low, his TSH super high. And of course, it appeared nobody had done any kind of review. Nobody had looked for the cause of the sudden change. The nurse had simply faxed the doctor the results, likely without even looking at them at all, and naturally, the doctor increased the thyroid supplement dosage, giving Albert more thyroid. The very next month, in May of 2019, his TSH level was super low, his thyroid level super high, after the recent increased dosage. No changes were made (likely because at that point, Doc had no clue *what* was going on), and the level was rechecked in August of 2019. It continued to be the same: high thyroid, low TSH. His level ran high until January of 2020.

This is where I came in, immediately curious, and reviewed Albert's records to see what had caused the sudden shift four months prior. Thyroid level matters! It affects the body in a multitude of pertinent ways!

Upon reviewing, as I said, I discovered that Albert had run smoothly since 2017, on the same dosage of 75mcg. Then, suddenly, in April of 2019, there was a huge change. 75mcg *suddenly* wasn't cutting it at all.

Why? I wondered. *There has to be a reason.*

As said, the very next month, following an increase in the thyroid dosage, based on the labs, Albert's level had swung to the other extreme.

Why? I wondered. *He apparently hadn't needed the increase. So, what the heck happened prior to the April level that made Albert so low on thyroid?*

The only possible explanation was that Albert hadn't received his thyroid medication.

Having already started the new year in 2020, the system wouldn't allow me to go back to 2019 to check medication administration records. However, I quickly realized, "It's just as well. I'm sure, given or not, the records will indicate given."

So I conducted a pharmacy review on Albert's thyroid supplement. A pharmacy review simply tells you if, when, and how often a given medication was filled and delivered. Ultimately, I determined the thyroid medication had not been filled for the month of March. In other words, Albert's thyroid level wasn't low because his body suddenly required a higher dosage. Albert's thyroid level was low, back in April of 2019, because for a full month he never received the medication. It was never filled. It was never in the facility to be administered for the entire month of March.

Ultimately, I had to get with the doctor, explain all of this, and get Albert's thyroid supplement dosage decreased back down. Albert's level has been fine ever since.

Albert had missed the medication for an entire month, and nobody noticed. Once I had my answer, I took it to the director. Predictably, she informed me later that everybody had signed that they had given it.

The director of nursing was "glad the state didn't catch that." That's it. That was her biggest concern. She obtained her sacred zero deficiency survey, which means absolutely nothing except that the state didn't find her dirt. 'Cause she no doubt had dirt. *They all have dirt.* She just swept it under the rug with the rest of it.

Upon looking, *call me curious,* I found that Albert, who was already skinny, had lost sixteen pounds during the three months he was taking the increased thyroid dosage he never even needed. Of course, that was swept under the rug, as well, with the help of the very system in place to catch significant weight change.

Nope, state didn't catch the related weight loss, either.

Harver:

Dalinda was a medication aid. I liked her. She was the type of person who did extra things during her downtime. Most medication aids sit on their behinds and do absolutely nothing between medication passes, as if there isn't a world of needs spinning out of control around them. It has always infuriated me and baffled me at the same time. Management is notorious for saying, "Nurses, help the aids. Answer call lights." As the nurses are already running in a thousand different directions. Yet in twenty-eight years I've never once heard any member of management instruct the medication aids to help anyone, except for the facilities in which I was part of management. I expected everyone to put forth the same effort and for that effort to be the very best they had. "Everybody has an off day now and then, but most days should be top notch." Anyway, Dalinda gave it heck. She was a good medication aid, had a good heart. So I was somewhat blown away recently when I overheard the charge nurse, Raven, giving Dalinda instruction. Raven sat at the desk, stretching her neck to yell to Dalinda over the high counter. "Hey, Dalinda, Harver's Furosemide is increased. He'll be taking four tablets now, instead of two, until his new tablets come in."

Kind of bent a bit at the hips, her torso leaning slightly forward, Dalinda's head arrived everywhere just a few seconds before her feet did. Her feet turned in as if her toes were kissing, Dalinda's torso also tended to bob with every step, the bob swaying the tail of her ever-present long sweater. Dalinda's smooth black wig suddenly popped up above the counter as she simultaneously propped her elbows on it. "Okay, now, tell me that again. You say Harver gone do what?"

I stood at the fax machine with a telling view of Dalinda's befuddlement.

Raven spun around in her chair, swinging her long, brownish-gray hair over her shoulder. "Okay," she said, prepping for clarity, "Harver was taking two"—she held up two fingers—"Furosemide tablets. Two ten milligram tablets to equal his ordered twenty milligrams, right?" Not waiting for, nor desiring, an answer, Raven continued, saying, "Now he's going to take four tablets." She held four fingers in the air. "Four ten milligram tablets to equal forty milligrams. Make sense?" She stared at Dalinda.

Dalinda stood and thought, her head cocked to the side, mouth gaping, gaze shifting to nothing as she processed, during which I stood at the fax machine, watching. *Harver hasn't been getting two tablets, has he, Dalinda? This is news to you, isn't it?*

"Okay." Dalinda had obviously made her decision to keep quiet. "So he gone get fo Furosemide tablets until the new ones get in." She held up four fingers. "Cuz he wuz getting two tablets?" She lowered two fingers, waving only two. I appeared to be the only one who noticed the "two tablets" comment was in question form.

Raven smiled victoriously, saying "Exactly!" before spinning back around to her paperwork.

I leaned on the counter, observing as Dalinda did precisely what I'd anticipated. She turned and bobbed back to her cart, sweater tail swaying. Unlocking her cart, she began sifting through blister packs of medications.

Just to satisfy my curiosity—confirm my gut feeling, so to speak—I strolled over, observing as Dalinda pulled out the blister pack she'd been searching for. Stepping to her side, my gut knotted as I watched Dalinda run her long, bony finger beneath the words on the instruction label. Stopping at "take two," her gaze again shifted to nothing as she processed once more.

Feeling Dalinda's inner struggle, I whispered, "Mistakes happen. But don't let them double it if you know he's only been getting half of what he was supposed to get." I smiled, then patted her shoulder.

Dalinda looked as if she'd seen a ghost, but she swiftly recovered. "Oh, he been gettin' two. So now he get fo." She held four slender fingers in the air.

One thing was for certain: Everybody could count on their fingers! One thing that was not so certain was how much Furosemide Harver had actually been receiving, which also made it unclear how much he actually needed. I finished what I'd been doing and sauntered back to my office while contemplating just how I might find the answer to the uncertainty.

Medication administration records are crap when it comes to determining what or how much was actually administered. Knowing this, I ran a pharmacy audit on the Furosemide.

Ultimately, it was clear that Harver had only been receiving one tablet as opposed to two. How did I know this? Simple. Harver was still on his first month's supply of sixty tablets, and he still had tablets remaining. If administered correctly, he'd have required a refill over two weeks prior. Another pickle. Dalinda hadn't meant to give an incorrect dosage. It was human error, which unfortunately continued for nearly seven weeks. However, the doubled dosage, if actually administered, was dangerous. So I had to do something to stop it. I decided to give Dalinda another chance to be accountable, to right the wrong and prevent a potential crisis.

"Hey, Dalinda. Just shooting straight, Harver has only been getting one Furosemide tablet, and we both know it." I shrugged, smiling. "Human error. It happens."

Her brow creased, and her black eyes frantically jumped from one place to another as her mind raced. She finally spoke, saying, "Naw, he been gettin' two." She raised two fingers into the air, smiling sweetly. "But I'm gone give 'im fo like Ms. Raven say to do."

"Okay." I was stumped, but then it hit me. "Tell you what. You hold off on giving Harver anything at all for now. Give me just ten little minutes"—yep, I held up both hands, spreading my fingers and thumbs dramatically and waved them in the air. "Ten, and I'll get back to you."

So I had to call the doctor and tell him about all the nasty little details and how I'd confirmed my suspicions. I asked him to hold off on the increase. Let us see how Harver was doing after he began receiving the correct dosage of two tablets.

Being one who truly hates to hurt anyone's feelings, I gave Dalinda one last chance to stand up. "Dalinda, the doctor discontinued the increased dosage. He wants the initial dosage of two tablets continued, and we'll monitor the effectiveness once he's actually receiving it before considering a change." I watched her face closely. "You understand?"

Dalinda stared.

"Make sense? No new order, after all. Okay?"

"So, two tablets now," Dalinda clarified. "Not one, not fo, but two." She raised two fingers into the air.

"Right," I raised two fingers into the air. "Two. It was never one." I curled the second finger, leaving one standing, allowed time for it to sink in. "Give Harver two"—I uncurled my finger—"tablets. *Two*. In fact, hand me the blister pack."

Dalinda unlocked her cart, sifted through, pulled out Harver's Furo-semide blister pack, and thrust it toward me, placing her hands on her hips when I took it from her. I then wrote *two tablets* with my red sharpie across the top of the pack.

"You want a label-change sticker?" Dalinda asked nicely.

I bit my tongue, then glanced up at Dalinda without moving my head. "No, ma'am. Thanks, but this isn't a change. It's always been two tablets." I raised two fingers into the air. "Dalinda, I think the world of you. And nobody's perfect; we all make mistakes. The thing that separates right from wrong when a mistake is made is ownership, account-ability. If a mistake is made, own it. Don't put someone in harm's way to cover your mistake. *That* is wrong."

Dalinda glanced downward, then raised her chin high. "Yes, ma'am. That's the truth."

I smiled, turned, and walked away. I found Raven and told her the new order was discontinued. I told her there was every reason to believe that Harver had only been receiving half his dose for the past seven weeks.

Harver's edema, mild lung congestion, and wet cough resolved once he started receiving the correct amount of diuretic.

Dalinda never said another word about it. Neither did I. Nor did any of the other med aids who had administered the incorrect dosage over the seven-week-long medication error.

Wynona:

Wynona was a young, snippy know-it-all. Actually, Wynona would make a fantastic nurse if it weren't for her attitude. Attitude can completely obliterate any good traits a person may have. You know? I feel certain that you do.

Wynona frequently boasted, in fact, every single time I worked with her. "I'm already finished. All I have left to do is to give my nine o'clock meds, and then I'm out of here," she'd add with her arms raised like a champion. "I've already got all my charting done!"

This was proclaimed every day around four p.m. So you tell me. She came in at two p.m. How has one given all of the four and five o'clock medications, checked everyone's pre-dinner blood sugars, given the insulin, reviewed all the labs, done all the treatments, assessed all the patients, intervened as indicated, followed up for effectiveness, managed all behaviors and documented everything... in two hours? How has one documented an evening that has yet to really even begin?

Thing is, Wynona wasn't a champion at all. Wynona was the norm. Her victorious cry was directed at me because I was almost notoriously late getting out. To this day, I do not understand how a nurse can actually *do* the job and get off on time on, not some, but undoubtedly the vast majority of days.

So anyway, when Wynona made her daily proclamation, I'd inevitably recall my first three days, during which Wynona *trained* me for, or *oriented* me to, the position. Fully cognizant that one gets faster as one learns the people, the personal preferences, and where things are, I wasn't surprised by Wynona's speed, and I didn't pay much attention, as passing medications is passing medications. The people and medications change, but the process is, or should be, the same everywhere you go. It was rather incidental that I noticed at all, but I did. I noticed.

As we made the rounds, passing medications, Wynona never once looked at the medication administration records. She'd already signed, in advance, that she'd administered all the medications. Wynona went solely by memory. This appears to be a popular concept in the world of medication administration. Now, I'll readily admit that after administering the same medications to the same people repeatedly, one innately memorizes them. But it's a dangerous practice to get into doing it by memory. Some medications may not be on the cart, and you may fail to notice. A medication may have new directions, and the nurse you relieved may have forgotten to tell you. A medication may have been discontinued, but the nurse failed to pull it from the cart and forgot to inform you. There are a host of reasons medications should be administered according to the administration record, signed for at the time of administration.

In any case, Wynona went entirely by memory. I hadn't noticed until I observed her prepping to administer a medication that had been discontinued. They had just discussed this in report, as I stood listening, a little over an hour before. Yet Wynona was putting the pill in the patient's medication cup.

"Isn't that discontinued?" I asked, genuinely thinking maybe I had misunderstood their conversation.

"Oh, yeah!" She cackled, plucking the pill from the cup and tossing it in the trash.

I began to pay attention, not to learn the job, but to learn Wynona. I noticed that Wynona skipped some of the patients on the four and five o'clock pass. So I asked if those patients were out on pass, in the hospital or some such.

"No, I give those people all their meds at dinner. The four o'clocks and the nine o'clocks," she replied as she pushed the cart down the hallway, intermittently chattering with random staff or residents. "Some of them like to get all their meds at one time so they can just go to bed whenever they're ready. So I give them out at dinner, all together." She shrugged.

You can bet I was paying close attention at dinner. I'll give her this: Wynona can multi-task! Her hands were opening drawers, punching pills, pouring liquids, and unlocking the narc box like the Tasmanian devil while she participated in and impressively followed ten different conversations at once. The only thing I never saw during this whirlwind was

Wynona looking at or touching the medication administration records. Not one time.

Sammy shuffled up to the cart mid-madness and asked for Tylenol. Wynona had it for him in a flash, not even stopping her "flow." I wondered for what, specifically, Sammy needed Tylenol. Did Sammy have an order for Tylenol? Was he allergic to Tylenol? Were we going to find out if it was effective in relieving whatever it was he took it for? Apparently, there was simply no need for any details.

Over the next thirty minutes, I observed multiple medication errors as two doses of medications, ordered four times a day, were administered together, meaning residents were getting one large dose rather than two properly spaced doses. Specifically, a seizure medication ordered every six hours, due at three and nine, was administered all at once, at six.

One poor woman was taking a heavy load of Lactulose, a stout laxative, to rid her body of ammonia. I watched as Wynona opened the bottle and poured the thick, sticky, clear liquid into an unmarked cup, meaning the cup had no measurement markings on it.

"Oh wow!" I blurted. "How much do they take?"

"Oh, girl!" Wynona cackled. "She takes ninety milliliters four times a day!" Shrugging, she added, "She wants the bedtime dose with this one," as she topped off the cup with the syrupy liquid.

My brain, as usual, kicked into gear. *Two doses would be one hundred and eighty milliliters, which would be six ounces, and you just topped off a four ounce cup and called it two doses*, I thought as I watched Wynona set the cup next to the woman. I watched as the woman quickly moved the cup from the reach of her tablemate, who had immediately attempted to grab it as Wynona turned away.

"Would you run this over to Dirk?" Wynona jerked me from my haze. "He's that guy in the red shirt." She pointed. "He's too lazy to come get his medicine. He'll sit right there and wait till morning if you don't take it to him." She cackled. "He wants you to bring it to him and set it right next to his plate." She rolled her eyes.

I was not touching that cup, nor was I going to set a cup of pills next to the plate of an individual who may well forget to take them, forget they're there, or leave them for the guy next to him, who appeared to consume anything he could find. No way. Not me.

"I can't do that. I'm sorry. I can so something else for you." I cringed. "But I have no clue what's in that cup, and I'd never just set medications down and walk away. Too many risks. I hope you understand," I said, sincerely apologetic.

She didn't. In retrospect, very few ever did, understand.

Important thing to take from this: Wynona is the norm. The corners may be different, but the corners are cut, and very few think things through sufficiently in order to determine if the corners cut may indeed lead one's steps down a dangerous path.

Once again, the needs, problems, vulnerabilities, weaknesses, and lives of human beings are the very foundation on which the long-term care industry is built, the very foundation on which it exists at all. There is an enormous difference between providing pertinent care for another human being and repairing a computer, selling a blouse, or landscaping. In the people business, few corners can be cut, safely.

Gable:

Eye drops are rather insignificant unless you are the person with the eye problem. Across the board, however, eye drops are, well, disregarded. If your loved one needs the eyedrops, you best be asking to check that bottle from time to time. Although, even that isn't foolproof.

I thought I was losing my mind, or at least my eyesight. I'd been transferred to a new unit after yet another staff reduction, and try as I might, I could not find Gable's eye drops. Gable was on contact isolation for pink eye. His poor, old, hazy brown eyes were crusted and itchy, and Gable wanted to get back out and sit in his rocking chair on the porch. The traffic was going unobserved, and that was driving Gable bonkers.

"Somebody gotta keep an eye on that traffic out there." He winked. "So I need my eyes, and I need to sit in that rocking chair so I can do my civic duty." He grinned, saluted, and then rubbed his left eye.

"Stop rubbing it, Gable." I chuckled. "You're only making it more irritated. Sit down. Let me get you a warm compress while I find your drops."

I searched high and low through that cart. I looked back at the administration log and saw that he'd already been receiving the drops twice a day for the past four days!

So where are they? I screamed to myself, purely frustrated.

Deciding somebody accidently took them home in their pocket, I called the pharmacy to get more drops sent right away. Gable's eyes were miserable.

"Well, they've been administering the drops for four days, so I guess you have filled them before," I rudely popped off to the pharmacist who had informed me that Gable had no such order and that they'd filled no such order.

"Ma'am, send us the order, and we'll fill it," the pharmacist said. "We obviously can't fill an order we don't have," he added sarcastically, which I deserved.

"I apologize, sir. I've been searching through that cart for over thirty minutes, which I don't have to spare. I took it out on you." I pleaded, saying, "Please forgive me and send those drops out ASAP. He's miserable, and I'm starting to think they've never been started at all."

"We'll get them out as soon as you get us the order."

I hurried to Gable's room just as soon as the eyedrops were delivered.

"Okay, dude, I got your drops," I announced as I sailed into Gable's room.

"Oh goodie!" He grinned. "Rocking chair? I'm a'comin' soon!" he proclaimed before tilting his head backward for the drops. "These gone fix my eyes, ma'am?"

"They should," I assured him. "They're good drops. Have they helped at all since you started them?"

Gable raised his head up, blinking his eyes, which then clouded with the milky fluid. "Well now, since I started 'em just this minute, ma'am, I don't rightly know jest yet." He chuckled.

"You haven't been getting drops in your eyes morning and night for the past few days?"

"No, ma'am. Was I sposed to?"

"Why didn't you tell me that when I told you I was looking for your drops?" I chuckled, handing Gable a Kleenex.

"I didn't know what you was talking about." He laughed. "I'm the old man who needs help cuz I don't know; you the helper cuz you do know." He shrugged.

I shook my head, laughed, patted his shoulder, and turned to leave.

"Ma'am?" Gable stopped me. "I am an old man, and I do needs help.

But I still got a head full of sense, and old don't mean stupid. Thank you for them there drops. I guess I never woulda got 'em iffen you hadn't started bein' my new nurse. I don't mean to burden you none, but would you kinda make sure I keeps gettin' 'em so I can get outta this room and back to the porch?"

"Consider it done. The community needs you." I winked.

Gable chuckled. "Mighty fine. We both be on the job."

Eye drops not needed can be dangerous.

Eye drops needed but not administered can be dangerous.

Eye drops matter.

Gable's eyes matter... Gable matters.

Olive:

Not a real pretty name, but what a beautiful, spicy lady. Somehow, Olive had dodged the aging stick repeatedly. She could still pass for sixty at eighty-four years old. Olive was my mentor.

Doris, the nurse, had asked me to see Olive because she was still coughing her head off, and her lungs still sounded bad.

I always start with reviewing the records, as those tell me the individual's history, status over the past few weeks, medications, etc. And then I assess the person to determine his or her status at that moment.

Upon reviewing Olive's records, I quickly recalled that she had recently completed an antibiotic for the same symptoms. Looking, I saw that the antibiotic was a good, broad-spectrum antibiotic and had been completed thirteen days prior. However, upon closer inspection, I noticed something strange.

The medication administration record (MAR) was contradictory. The medication aid on day shift was documenting that the medication was unavailable. The night nurse was documenting that the medication had been administered. Ultimately, the order was completed, thus there was no further related documentation on the MAR. The nurses did the required three-day follow-up in their notes, writing *No adverse reaction to completed Levaquin.* (Gotta love generic crap!) So I mentioned the previous antibiotic to Doris. She told me, "Yeah, I remember that. We were out of it in our stocked meds, so we had to wait to receive it from the pharmacy. Why do you ask?"

"Well, the medication aid documented consistently that the medication was unavailable. But one of the nurses on the night shift documented that the night dose was given consistently. The only other nurse involved during the five days also documented that the medication was unavailable." I looked up at Doris. "So, dang! Was it, or was it not?"

"Oh, all I can tell you is that the nurse who documented that she gave it probably didn't."

I called the pharmacy; the medication was never filled. This explained Olive's ongoing symptoms. I called the doctor, who reordered the original order, and we started over. By then Olive had a fever, and her lung effusion had consolidated to pneumonia.

I told the director of nursing and never heard a word about it again.

I did make sure the medication was received from the pharmacy and started. Olive got better. I guess it was all good in the end. But I have concerns when a nurse documents that a medication has been given when it's not even in the building. I mean, did it matter to her at all that the patient's infection would likely get worse instead of better? Did she ever actually administer any of the medications on her shift?

More false documentation.

Why had the nurses done follow-up on a medication never given, therefore never completed? How did they not know?

The medication aid who was documenting that the medication was unavailable was as outspoken as I am, and she told the nurse on duty each time she had to document that medication was unavailable. She told me the nurses kept telling her we had none in the backup medications, so we were waiting for pharmacy to deliver it. How long were they going to wait? Why didn't they have the pharmacy hot-shot it? Where is the … professionalism … the heart?

Jack:

Jack returned from the hospital the morning of my day off. I'd like to have seen him when he arrived. I'm fairly certain he was sporting his darkest sunshades, and said, "Jack is back!" in his Barry White-sound-alike way. He probably flashed a peace sign as he was rolled through the lobby. Jack is a firm believer that only the good die young, so he has made it his mission in life to be "bad to the bone".

Truth is, Jack is one of the best people I have ever met. Man shoots straight, holds nothing back, and is genuinely considerate of everyone. I heard him tell the nurse aid the day he first arrived, "I know you busy, and y'all ain't got nuff help. I hate that, too, but least for now that's just how it is. So I don't mind waitin' while you a'helpin' somebody else who needs help. But, little lady, don't let me find out my bladder done busted loose cause you on yo phone." His lips retained the 'o' shape as he paused, bent his head down, and peered up at her from beneath his gray, speckled, wooly brows. "This ain't my first ro-deh-o. I done seen all the clowns, and I know all the tricks."

As soon as the aid walked out of the room, Jack looked at me, relaxed, and said, "My mama ain't the only one who got eyes in the backuh her head." He roared.

Jack had been re-admitted to the hospital for an acute exacerbation of COPD (chronic obstructive pulmonary disease) and pneumonia, but Jack was back. I was told in a report that he'd come back on three more days of IV Cefepime, and we were in day one of follow-up. This follow-up should include, at minimum, answers to questions like these: Was there an adverse reaction? Was treatment effective? Is the problem resolved, or is further intervention indicated? But, notoriously, the vast majority of nurses documented *No adverse reaction* to virtually everything. From a multivitamin to a new heart medication, it was always the same thing, nothing else. They referenced nothing about effectiveness or even the rationale for the medication being ordered to begin with.

So Jack was back, and I hurried down the hallway to say hello before starting my rounds.

"Hey, hey, there's my little angel in disguise." Jack grinned. "Come on in and set me straight. I been lookin' forward to you fussin' at me 'bout my cigars some more." Raspy laughter rumbled from his throat.

"See there? It's slowly sinking in." I laughed. "Maybe by the time you see Jesus, you'll have stopped smoking those nasty things."

Looking horrifically shocked, Jack cried, "Jesus don't smoke cigars?"

I stared at him.

"Well then, I postpone my departure even further," he finished smugly. "How the hell are ya Cinderella?"

"I lost my slipper."

"Oh good!" His eyes popped open wide. "I think that's where your story gets good! You need a man to take care of you so you can stop workin' yourself to the bone."

"Jack."

"Okay." He raised both palms in the air, then flashed me a peace sign.

"The nurse take your IV site out today?"

"You know you always gone be the one to do things." Jack began again, saying, "I see how things go."

"Jack."

"Okay." He pouted like a lost puppy. "No, ma'am. I asked them to take it out two days ago. They ain't using it, anyway." He shrugged his massive shoulders. "But nobody has time. They say they gone take it out, but they never come back and do it."

"Well, two days ago they were using it, Mr. Impatient."

"I ain't had no IV nothin' since I left that hospital."

I didn't say a word as my mind began working in a fast motion.

"Uh oh." Jack pointed at me. "Somebody done me wrong, and my angel is 'bout to flutter them wings all over they head!" He laughed so hard I had to administer a breathing treatment. "Go get 'em!" He punched the air, still laughing, fogging his nebulizer mask.

"You do entertain yourself." I chuckled, shaking my head as I hurried out.

I discovered that Homer had re-admitted Jack, and per his never-failing sloppiness, Homer had never even ordered the IV antibiotic. I called the doctor, who wanted to add two more days now that three days had been missed, allowing time for opportunistic rebound. I told the doctor about Jack requiring a breathing treatment when he laughed, which wasn't Jack's norm. The doctor decided to redo the entire seven days. So I got it ordered, started a new IV site, gave the first dose, corrected the twenty-four-hour report, discontinued the old IV site, and grumbled to myself about Homer for the remainder of that shift.

Jack was silent as I started the new IV site after filling him in on the new orders. But later, when I disconnected the empty bag, Jack looked at me. "Hey." He hesitated, glancing toward the window, then back to me. "Thanks." He thrust his enormous fist out. I bumped it, winked, and left the room.

As I said, he shoots straight. He is the one who nicknamed the nurse "Homer." I just kept it because it was so perfectly perfect. Jack told Homer the next day, "I'm not one to hold a grudge, boy, so I'ma let this thing go. But this ain't no game you playin' here. This ain't no cartoon, Homer. This is the real deal. People pay for your mistakes with their bodies, their health, and their lives. If you can't walk the walk, keep steppin' right on out that door. Go paint houses. If it's ugly, it's just ugly. Nobody dies."

Homer made the mistake of laughing, thinking Jack was teasing.

"Boy, it takes a man to wear a man's shoes. If you can't fill 'em with a man's feet, step on out of 'em now. A man takes his responsibilities seriously. You keep that goofy, giggly outlook on this job you got here, and you gone kill somebody."

Homer requested to be allowed to switch patients with somebody else, complaining that Jack had threatened him. I stood behind Jack and told the director what went down and how, what Jack said and why. Jack was moved from Homer's care. Jack later proved to be correct in his ominous predictions about Homer. But it was swept under the rug along with the rest of Homer's dirt.

Trick or Treat

Rubert:

The first time I saw Rubert, I wanted to turn and run. Rubert looked very much like a serial killer disguised as a Duck Dynasty star as he slouched in his wheelchair, head bent, unmoving, staring intensely at the television.

In the few seconds it took me to cross the room, my imagination ran wild. My eyes swept over Rubert's thick tangle of kinky, salt-and-pepper hair hanging stiffly past his hunched shoulders; his scraggly beard splayed over his chest, tipping the curve of his rounded belly where his t-shirt stretched the tightest; and his beady brown eyes peering out beneath fuzzy, tufted brows. I thought I'd glimpsed nostrils, but I wasn't confident, and I sure as heck wasn't going to stare.

As I drew nearer, Rubert slowly peeled his eyes away from the television, shifting his gaze to mine, completely void of expression.

Yep. Serial killer for sure, I thought.

Rubert stuck his finger out robotically and turned slowly back to the TV, never making a sound. I introduced myself and checked his blood sugar, my mind reeling between sarcastic wit and sadistic fear.

"Enjoy your dinner. I'll come back after you eat and do your wound care." I smiled, turning to make a fast exit.

"You don't have to do it tonight if you don't want to," I heard someone say.

Okay, that voice cannot belong to that man, I thought. I turned slowly, almost expecting to see a ghost.

"They've been doing my leg every other night."

Oh wow! Grizzly has the voice of an angel! I grinned, blushing as I recalled my thoughts from just seconds before.

"They did my leg last night, so you can wait until tomorrow if you want. It's okay as long as it's for sure done tomorrow night. I really don't think it should go any longer than that."

"Well, no, Rubert, it shouldn't go that long. Your wound care is supposed to be done daily, so we'll do it right after dinner if that works for you?"

"Oh, yes, ma'am. That's fine with me." Rubert chuckled so heartily that it shook the belly fat peeping out from beneath his t-shirt. "I wish all the nurses would do it every night. Then maybe it would heal up, and I could go home to my dogs! I miss 'em real bad. Since Pam died, they're all I've got."

A serial killer, huh? I chastised myself.

It turned out that the Duck Dynasty cave man/serial killer was just a big ole Mamma's boy who was just then, at sixty-six years old, learning how to write checks and pay bills. His late wife, Pam, had always done all that kind of stuff. Rubert laughed, saying, "And ooooh, she would give me crap for it if she could see me today! Pam cut my hair every Saturday and made me shave every single day!" When Rubert later showed me a picture of himself with his late wife, Pam, I had to struggle to hide my surprise. I would not have recognized the man in the picture as the same man I was looking at that day.

After dinner, I went back to Rubert's room. I checked his blood sugar again, then went out to get the wound care supplies. When I walked back into his room, Rubert looked stunned.

"What?" I laughed. "I told you I was going to do your wound care!"

"Well, yeah, I know." He smiled as he shifted closer to the edge of the bed. "But I didn't really think you were going to do it since they did it yesterday! They all *say* they're gonna do it." His eyes sparkled as he literally giggled.

The mood had shifted so much that it felt much like Christmas morning. Rubert proceeded to instruct me on precisely where to put my supplies, what to do, and how to do it. I then proceeded to acknowledge Rubert's every word while I did as I saw fit.

Rubert was a severe diabetic, which had resulted in the recent amputation of his right leg, just below the knee. He still had staples, and the incision was intact, but what concerned me (other than the fact that he still had staples at that point) was the fact that he had a large open area on each side of, and beneath, the incision. Rubert informed me that these areas had developed a few days after he arrived, and they'd just kept getting bigger until he'd finally insisted wound care be done at least every other day.

"I mean, I didn't want to get nobody in trouble," he whispered. "But it was starting to smell, and that's when it got this yellow stuff in it. So I had to say something."

"Ya done good, Rubert. If you don't take care of you, who will, right?"

The next two evenings Rubert and I went through the same routine. He was exuberant as the wounds surrounding the incision rapidly improved in appearance. The yellow stuff was gone. As I was leaving his room that third evening, Rubert asked, "Can I get a shower tomorrow evening before we do my leg? I haven't had a shower since I went into the hospital, cuz I can't get this dressing wet."

I spun back around to face him, then stared, blinking, my mind scrambling for appropriate words. But before the words came, my thoughts tumbled right out of my mouth, "Rubert! You had surgery over four weeks ago!"

"I know." His fuzzy brows shot up.

"So you're telling me you haven't had a shower in almost five weeks?"

"Nope, well, yes," he giggled, "I've asked. I want a shower bad! I mean, I may not look like it, but I like to be clean!" He chuckled. "Heck, I'd like a haircut, but I can deal with that. I just want a shower!"

"I won't be here tomorrow, Rubert. I'm off. But I will put in the report that you have to have a shower. They need to take the dressing off, and you need some good soapy water running over those wounds, then rinsed off real good. Just gently pat your leg dry with a clean towel, and then have the nurse do the dressing after your shower. Wouldn't hurt to get a shave while you're in there, Grizzly."

Grizzly grinned like a six-year-old with a new bike. "Grizzly! I like that. I'm not gonna push my luck. I'll be happy if I can get the shower."

"Dude, we can take that dressing back off, and I'll get them to shower you right now."

"No, I can wait one more day. That wound care takes a while, and I'm kind of tired now. But thank you. Heck, now I look forward to tomorrow!"

I came back two days later, on Saturday, and Rubert still hadn't had a shower. Not only that, but the dressing I put on him on Wednesday was still there.

"What the heck, Grizzly?"

"I told 'em you said I needed a shower. They rolled their eyes, but they said they were gonna do it. They said they were gonna do my leg, too, but nobody did nothin'."

I went out to my computer to check things out. I found out that the nurse who had worked my two days off had written an order on Thursday to discontinue daily wound care per patient request. Then she had written a nurse note stating that the resident refused daily wound care. The same nurse had signed off for performing the wound care on Friday evening, and yet there I stood, looking at my initials and my date on my dressing - from the previous Wednesday—on Grizzly's stump.

After discontinuing the "order" the nurse had written, I wrote a clarification order to continue daily wound care, as ordered by the physician.

The nurse resigned, and word spread amongst the others that I was trouble. So Rubert's wound care improved significantly. In fact, it improved so much that I had to call the surgeon in order to obtain new wound care orders before Rubert's next appointment with him, because now that the wound was clean, it would heal much faster with a different dressing. Between the initial uproar, the new orders, and Rubert being a "routine fanatic" (instructing the nurses working my off days to do it as precisely as I did), I wasn't anywhere close to winning a popularity contest. But Rubert's leg was healing rapidly.

Meanwhile, Rubert was taking charge of his personal life. I walked in his room one day, and he was puffed up like a rooster.

"I just finished writing checks to pay all my bills. I've never written checks before!" His eyes were wide with excitement. "And I told Pam's mother she isn't allowed back in my house, because I found out she took all Pam's jewelry to her house. She said she took it to keep it safe, but it was safe at my house. I'm gonna get it back, too."

Rubert's smile faded, and he hung his head. "But she hauled Trudi off, my little dog. She was supposed to go by and feed them every day, let them out to potty. I think she got tired of it. She said they were making a mess in the house. But they never did before. She put Happy outside and hauled Trudi off."

"Is she going to feed Happy?"

Grizzly wiped tears from his eyes before looking up. "I called my neighbor. They have a dog, too. They went and got Happy, and they're keeping him for me. They said they'd bring him up to see me this weekend!"

"Oh Lord! You dog people!" I rolled my eyes dramatically.

Grizzly laughed. "So yeah, things are looking better! I'm getting a shower every Wednesday, and my leg is almost healed, thanks to you. I have my own checking account, and I'm paying my own bills!" He raised a hairy fist into the air.

"What do you mean by 'a shower every Wednesday'?"

"It's okay. I warsh up in the sink every day. I like to be clean. That one aid gives me a shower every Wednesday. She don't work on Monday or Friday, and them other aids don't do nothin' for me. But as long as I get one on Wednesdays, I can warsh myself at the sink on the other days. I'm gonna get to go home soon!"

I was headed out of Grizzly's room to address the shower thing when he called my name. I stopped and turned around.

"Hey, do you know anybody that wants to buy a truck? I'm selling mine. I don't need two vehicles no more. How much should I ask for it?"

Grizzly began giving me details on his nine-year-old Toyota quad cab, four-wheel drive pickup truck.

"I can't advise you on anything like that, Grizzly." I apologized. "First of all, I have no clue. Secondly, as your nurse, that's not my place. I hope you understand. Maybe ask your neighbor if you trust him, or ask the social worker if she can refer you to someone who can advise you."

A few days later I had been at work a little while when Grizzly gleefully rolled his wheelchair through the front door. He'd been to see his surgeon.

"Hey, hero! Doc was amazed at how good my leg looks! He asked me your name! And get this," he added breathlessly, "he took the staples out! He said he was getting concerned last time he saw me, but no more! That's a great report!"

"That is great! I think that calls for a celebration!"

"Like what?" His childlike expression was a total contradiction to his burly appearance.

"Leave that to me, nosy."

He giggled and rolled off down the hallway.

Later I called in an order to a local restaurant and had Grizzly a special dinner delivered. When I took it to his room, he was leaned over his bedside table, his glasses on, reading a piece of paper.

After drooling over his pending meal, he asked, "Can you sign as a witness on this truck title?"

"Not no, but heck no!" I laughed. "That would no doubt be crossing the ethical line. Besides, I think your witness signature must be notarized or something. Better ask somebody. But not me!"

The next day Grizzly was absolutely glowing. "I made my first business transaction without Pam!" he bragged. "I sold my truck!"

"I'm so proud of you!"

"Yep." He smirked. "Made six hunnerd dollars."

I struggled to hide my shock. "You sold your Toyota for six hundred dollars?"

"Yep." He grinned.

"Sold it, or you're selling it?" I asked coolly, hoping it wasn't too late.

"SOLD!" He smacked his hand on the table. "I signed the title today!"

"Oh! Well, I'm glad you're happy! Congratulations!" I hurried out, biting my lip.

The next afternoon, Rachel, the day nurse I was relieving, was running a bit behind. By the time I got a report, I was behind schedule, as well. Grabbing my things, I hurried down the skilled hall to assess my more critical patients before starting my first round.

Stepping out of Mrs. Stelford's room, I ran into Rachel, who was hurrying from Grizzly's room.

"See ya later, Rachel. Have a good evening!"

"You, too!" She smiled, then hurried off, yelling over her shoulder, "And sorry I was running late. I had to go to the bank at lunch, and it took longer than I thought it would."

My stomach knotted.

Later that evening Grizzly was still excited about his first independent business transaction in his "whole life". He added, "It was really sweet of Rachel to take the title down to the bank for me. I didn't even know that could be done!"

My stomach churned.

"But" Grizzly continued, "since I couldn't go to the bank, she called and found out how we could seal the deal. That's what she called it." He chuckled. "Anyway, she called to see how we could do it without me having to be there. She did all the work! Now she has a truck, and I have six hunnerd dollars!" He beamed. "Well, he added with exuberant pride, "I did have it! I put the six hundred dollars toward Pam's funeral expenses, so now I only owe three hunnerd."

I only owe three hunnerd, echoed in my ears.

Grizzly grinned like a hairy, overgrown kid. "I'm going home tomorrow! I get to be with Happy again. That's all I care about. My leg is healed, and Happy needs me. Heck, " he chuckled heartily, "I need Happy!"

Just knowing somebody took advantage of you makes me sad. Knowing who *took advantage of you… oh my… I need 'happy' too*, I thought as I hurried out.

Cal:

Cal was an enormous man with massive shoulders and huge, thick hands. His most outstanding feature, though, was his eyes, which were so chocolate brown that they were nearly black. More outstanding than the color though, was the size. Cal's eyes were so enormous, that they almost didn't fit on his face. Despite his head being as big as a basketball, Cal's eyes appeared to be at imminent risk of slipping right over the sides of his face and into his ears.

Cal was quiet and grumpy, so much so that his vocabulary was largely grunts. Cal could grunt with intonation in a way I'd never imagined possible.

I inadvertently met Cal while educating a nurse aid on proper response to call lights, during which Candy, the nurse admitting Cal, complimented him on his big, pretty eyes.

Cal stared at Candy for a few seconds, then grunted, his face void of expression.

Candy, thinking Cal hadn't heard her, chirpily repeated the compliment just a bit louder.

Cal stared. "Big eyes don't mean deaf ears."

Hesitantly, Candy chuckled.

Cal stared.

"Are you comfortable?" Candy grasped for neutral ground.

Cal stared.

The nurse aid chimed in, "You really do have some big, purty eyes, Mr. Cal."

Cal shifted said eyes to the aid and grunted. Then, beyond explanation, Cal shifted his gaze to me. "Guess you got an eye comment, too."

What I did have was Cal's number. Having an innate ability to feel others, I knew more about Cal by that point than Cal may have known about himself.

"Well, I didn't." I smiled sweetly. "But since you extended that lovely invitation, I'd feel rude if I had no comment at all. So I'm just curious. Are you afraid that if you smile your cheeks are gone push your eyes on over the edge?"

Cal stared, grunted. Then, to our amazement, that huge man roared with laughter. He laughed so hard that we had to raise the head of his bed so he could catch his breath. When he finally composed himself, he pointed a thick finger at me, nodded his head, and grunted.

I could tell. Cal and I were friends. Cal just didn't quite know what to think about it.

Candy started to remove the dressing on Cal's foot. He had a diabetic ulcer, and she needed to assess and then document a description of the wound. Cal grunted, pointed at me.

"You want her to do it?" Candy asked.

Cal grunted.

I washed my hands and gloved up. "Just because you're so drippy sweet." I rolled my eyes dramatically.

As I started removing Cal's dressing, he winced and grunted.

"You want pain medicine before your wound care, Cal?" I asked, feeling his pain as I gazed at the black, necrotic tissue covering his heel. "Looks like it might hurt."

Cal grunted.

"Candy, would you mind getting Cal some pain medicine? And make sure you put in the report to medicate thirty minutes before wound care."

Realizing I was late for a meeting, I blurted, "Cal, I've got to run. I'm sorry. I have a danged meeting to endure. I don't work on the unit, but Candy will fix you up. I'll tell her to let your pain medicine kick in before she cleans and dresses your foot."

Cal grunted.

A few weeks later, just after Easter weekend, Robert, Cal's oldest son, suddenly popped into my office. He introduced himself, and I motioned for him to sit.

Well, that apple not only fell far, but it rolled completely away from the tree! I thought as Robert smiled and shook my hand.

"How's Grumpy?" I grinned.

Robert sighed. "Only he knows. I've still not learned to speak grunt." He laughed. "But I think we have a problem, and that nurse up there won't give me any answers."

"So tell me about it. What's up?"

"I took Dad home for Easter."

I waited. Robert was silent as tears welled in his eyes. Handing him a Kleenex, I continued waiting.

After a few minutes Robert cleared his throat. "I'm sorry. I just never imagined. I feel guilty for bringing him here, but I don't know what to do. It took five men to get Dad into the shower. Three men had to stand in the shower and hold him up while the other two of us hurried to wash him. We don't have the equipment or the manpower to take care of Dad at home. It was Easter Sunday, so extra family and friends were there, or I wouldn't have even been able to clean Dad up. That's why I brought him here. He won't tell me what goes on, and that nurse just says Dad is difficult."

"Well, shoots, Robert, we can all be difficult! She shouldn't have said that. But forgive me. I'm not following. Did he have an accident while home? Why were you guys giving him a shower?"

"He stunk horribly! Body odor like I've never smelled before, like the monkey cage at the zoo!" His eyes wide as he explained. "The aids put him in the car for me when I picked him up, and I smelled him in the car pretty quickly. But when we had to hold him to stand him up and get him out of the car at home, we gagged. We gagged at my dad's body odor! And, ma'am, when we showered him, you could see the grime. We washed and rinsed him until the water ran clear, then wrapped his foot up in a clean towel until we could get him back to let the nurse put a bandage on it."

I struggled to swallow the lump in my throat.

"Ma'am, he's my dad. He hasn't always been like this. He gave up when my mother died. He's actually one of the funniest people in the world. Please help him. Help me help him."

Hunting down the Director of Nursing, Nixy, I reported all I'd been told and requested that she meet with Robert in my office. Nurses being very territorial, Nixy informed me she had the situation under control and that I could proceed with my duties.

Several weeks later I stayed late one evening and went upstairs to see Cal. After flipping the light switch on, I found his dinner tray sitting on the table next to his bed, untouched. Cal squinted in the light.

"Ya know," I started, "your eyes will get used to the light if you turn it on more often."

Cal grunted.

"You need to eat, especially the protein," I encouraged as I bent to straighten his blankets. "Protein is critical to healing."

Cal grunted, but the sound was different, and I was fairly certain Cal winced.

"You hurting?"

Nothing.

"You need pain medicine, Cal?"

Nothing.

"Robert must have gotten his delightful sense of humor from his mother."

Cal grunted, shifting his huge eyes my way. I struggled not to grin when I saw the corners of his mouth twitch.

"Well, he's a good man, your son. His mother did a good job with him."

Cal grunted.

"He has a good heart. Must've gotten that from his mother, too. And good-natured. Not a grumpy bone in that man's body."

Nothing.

Moving his tray to the overbed table, I continued, saying, "Takes a lot of energy to be grumpy, so you better eat up."

Cal turned his head toward the wall without a sound.

"He's witty, has a delightful sense of humor. I'm sure his mama would be proud of him! But I wonder… What would she say to you?" I persisted while setting up Cal's tray.

Cal grunted loudly, jerked his head back my direction, and burst into laughter.

"You just don't quit!" He laughed. "She'd tell me I'm an ornery old fool and kiss me on my cheek, and then I'd do any damned thing she asked of me and pretend I didn't like it. That boy did get her heart, but, by damn, he got that wit from his old dad!"

"Woo-hoo, Grumpy speaks!" I laughed. "Now then, you need pain medicine?"

"Well, my foot's rotting off. What do you think?"

"Oh, he's feisty, too! My kind of guy!" I winked. "Now, eat your dinner. And I'm not kissing you on your cheek, but I will get you that pain pill. We need to look at that heel."

When I walked back in, Grumpy was at least pushing food around on his plate. I gave him time to finish pushing, and time for his medicine to kick in, then returned to his room. I had to focus to keep my face from reflecting my emotions as I pulled Cal's blanket back and observed his drooping dressing, which was covered with greenish-black drainage. The stench enveloping my nostrils, I glanced up at Cal only to find his eyes closed in a grimace. Even medicated, it was clearly extremely painful for Cal as I removed his dressing. I stopped.

"You okay?"

Cal grunted.

I proceeded, amazed at how many layers were unraveling. When I finally pulled away the last of the filthy gauze, I glanced at Cal, grateful beyond words that his eyes were still closed. Quickly wiping my tears on my sleeve, I shoved the soiled gauze into a bag. Then, gently covering his leg with his sheet, I hurried to rewash my hands and regain my composure.

"Should I look at it?" Cal asked in a whisper edged with fear.

"Whatever you normally do is fine with me."

"Normally, nobody takes the dressing off. Every now and then one of them wraps some more stuff around it, over the old stuff. So I at least know there's still a foot there to wrap." He chuckled weakly. "I haven't seen it for a long time."

As he spoke, I began cleaning the wound, which was no longer a "heel wound," as it now covered his entire lower leg, going up to just a couple of inches below his knee. Hard, black tissue speckled with cracks oozing sticky, greenish-black drainage. I cleaned and dressed Cal's leg, then visited with him a while to distract him from what I knew in my heart that he knew in his.

Later I called Robert and told him his dad needed to go to the doctor as soon as possible. Robert had left town that morning on business for two weeks, so I encouraged him to call Nixy the next morning and insist that his dad be taken to his doctor as soon as the doctor could see him. I called Nixy and informed her of what I'd seen, then told her I'd notified Cal's son. Nixy was not happy with me, but I reminded her the family had to be notified.

"Next time let me do the notifying," Nixy popped off. "And we'll discuss this tomorrow. You had no business in Cal's room."

Wearily, I resisted all the things I so desperately wanted to say. The next morning, I called Cal's doctor's office, informing them of what I had seen. Within an hour I was called to the administrator's office and reprimanded for overstepping my boundaries. I was instructed to see to my facility and to stay out of the nursing facility unless my assistance was requested.

I smiled.

I'm not certain of the exact timeframe here, but I'll forever remember the call I received from Robert. Apparently, Cal was never taken to his appointment. Ultimately, Robert scheduled Cal an appointment and took him to the doctor himself. Robert told me that when the doctor lifted Cal's pant leg, something was moving under his dressing. The doctor had told the nurse to call the hospital immediately and arrange a direct admission. Cal had emergency, below-the-knee amputation performed that same day, after pictures were taken of his leg, the wound, and the flies infesting it—flies from all stages of the life cycle.

The next day I called Robert and asked if I could visit Cal in intensive care.

"Absolutely! He's asked to see you."

I then went to the administrator and resigned my position, effective immediately.

After hurrying to the hospital, I rushed to the ICU waiting area where I found Robert, his wife, and other family members. Robert stood and met me in the hallway, where he informed me that Cal had been rushed back in for a second surgery in which they planned to amputate more of Cal's leg. Robert told me Cal had sent a message to me, but he hadn't understood it. Maybe I would.

I laughed, wondering what on earth Grumpy had to say to me. "He grunted, right?"

Robert laughed. "No, he spoke in real words this time!"

"Oooooh, I feel special! Do tell!"

"I argued, but Dad said I had to say it just like he said it," Robert explained apologetically.

I laughed hard, rolling my eyes. "Oh Lord, please do!"

"He said to tell that short, mouthy nurse thank you for not stopping, not quitting. Yes! Tell the short, mouthy nurse thank you for not quitting. Tell her I'm fine and dandy. I'm going to get myself a kiss on my check."

"Thank you, Robert." I swallowed the lump and forced a convincing smile.

"I guess he thought he might play on some sympathy, sucker one of the nurses into kissing his check." Cal laughed. "And then he got even stranger. He asked me if I was aware that I had him to thank for my sparkling personality." Still laughing quietly, Robert shook his head. "Sparkling! Of all things. I think the infection has gone to Dad's head."

My eyes stung, but I maintained.

Cal went for that kiss that very day. Knowing him, he grunted at St. Peter as he passed through the pearly gates in search of his favorite kisser.

Much later, as the wheels of justice are slow, it was revealed in the records:

- Cal's "daily" wound care was actually done every six to eleven days.
- Cal received an average of one shower a month once he started getting showered at all.
- It was repeatedly documented that Cal refused his shower and his wound care, yet there was no documentation regarding interventions made to facilitate compliance.
- In fact, all of Cal's notes were regarding his being "grouchy," "noncompliant," and "difficult." There was nothing in his notes about medical issues, care, interventions, or his wound.

- Out of a potential 468 doses of pain medication, Cal received seven doses total, two of which I instigated. Both times I saw him, he was clearly in pain. Both times I saw him, he took a pain pill. It's not rocket science. It's humane.
- The corporation actually stood on the defense that leeches are still used for debridement in some cases, implying the flies weren't necessarily detrimental, after all. (Let's all close our eyes and simply overlook the fact that the flies put themselves in the wound due to filth, germs, and rotting flesh, which was caused by lack of showers and lack of wound care.)

Ms. Carolina:

Ms. Carolina was like a fresh spring breeze, always uplifting. She smelled like honeysuckle and was full of hope. If she had a way to go look, that woman could find living hope buried deep in the Titanic, all these years later. Most everybody called her "Mama." Her granddaughter worked at the facility as a nurse aid, and she called her "Mama," so after a short while most others called Ms. Carolina "Mama," as well. I didn't. I called her "Hope."

Hope wasn't my patient or resident. I happened to be on the hall one day, seeing to one of my patients, when I noticed her call light on. It was highly unusual, as Hope was one of those rare souls who seldom had a need or complaint. Spending her time reading or watching TV, Hope pretty much just took each day as it came. Hope was as patient as the floor and as trusting as a child. Knocking first, I entered her room and found Hope sitting in the recliner, filling every inch of it with her pleasantly portly self.

Beaming up at me with big, round, brown eyes, she asked, "May I have some ice water, please? I hate to be a bother. I wouldn't have pressed that light button, but I ain't had cold water all day. I'm sorry to bother yuh."

"Oh, good grief. You're the opposite of a bother, Hope," I chortled as I headed back out the door.

"This girl gonna get herself in trouble iffen it kills her." Hope laughed as I hurried back into her room carrying her jug filled with iced water. "I never seen such a blind determination to find trouble in my life." She chuckled, sending waves of ripples across her portly rolls.

"Oh Lawd, trouble finds me. I sure don't need to read a book about somebody looking for it." I leaned over to check Hope's wound vac. "I think that'd make me plumb resentful!" I laughed.

"Well, if trouble finding you so easy, you either in the wrong place or somebody thinkin' you the one can handle it." Hope chuckled, her gaze soft as cotton and sweet as cotton candy. "Mmm-hmm, I'm thinkin' you probably the one," she mumbled as she resumed reading, the quiet buzz of the wound vac the only sound in the room.

Sarcastic "trouble thoughts" were popping like popcorn in my head, and I stifled a giggle as I habitually checked the wound vac settings and functioning, glancing at the wound site to look for signs of infection. I saw none. However, I did notice that the date of the dressing was four weeks prior, just prior to Hope's admission to our facility.

"Everything's working properly, Ms. Hope. And use that button more often. Don't just sit in here waiting for somebody to come ask. I assure you that you will wait forever. Forever can take a long time if you're thirsty."

My mind reeling, I returned Hope's smile and hurried out the door, closing it behind me, knowing Hope preferred it that way.

Now, without getting too technical, allow me to briefly explain the wound vac. It's not appropriate for every wound, but for those it does work for, it has proven to be amazing in promoting and expediting healing. Great invention. In short, it's a sponge cut to fit the wound, and it's inserted into the wound bed. The site is then covered with plastic, and a tiny hole is cut in the center. Suctioning is then attached over the hole, which literally sucks or pulls oxygenated blood flow to the wound, thus promoting healing. However, it is beyond pertinent that the procedure be done strictly according to guidelines.

The facility had held an in-service on the wound vac prior to Hope's admission. I was completely surprised and overwhelmingly pleased to see this being done. Having worked with wound vacs previously, I was fully cognizant of the dangers related to improper use, though, I must add, I had never seen any related complications. The instructor's words resounded in my head as I sought out Matreece, the Director of Nursing.

"The dressing must be changed timely, or one runs an extremely high risk of the new tissue growing into and throughout the sponge." The instructor had continued to explain that timely meant per the doctor's orders. "It may be weekly, biweekly, or three times a week depending on the rate at which the wound is healing, but it's never less than once a week."

Matreece had newly been promoted from treatment nurse to director of nursing, and she was still covering the position of treatment nurse until a replacement could be hired and trained.

"That's none of your business," Matreece barked. "However, since you stuck your nose in *my* business, I haven't been able to get her into the wound care center yet, and the wound care center won't give me orders to change the dressing until they see her," she said with a sneer.

A no brainer for sure. They can't legally give orders on a patient they've never seen. I struggled to maintain a pleasant expression. "How about our medical directors?" I asked nicely. "They can give orders in absence of another avenue. And Carolina is at high risk of her new tissue growing into the sponge."

"I tell you what. I'm going to give you orders as your director," Matreece snarled. "You stay out of Carolina's room from this point forward. If you see her call light on, you go find her nurse or aid to answer it. I better not hear about you stepping one foot in that room."

"I apologize for any offense. None was intended," I offered quickly. "I'm just concerned."

Matreece smiled sweetly. "Oh, it's okay. I know you just didn't think before you spoke," she sang merrily as she walked away. Then she stopped and turned around. "But I meant what I said. Stay out."

Frustrated, I hunted Tara down. Tara was Hope's direct care nurse. I informed Tara of the status of the dressing and related concerns. Tara informed me she had expressed the same concerns herself and was met with a similar, though less harsh, response. Tara shrugged.

Not desiring to debate the Nurse Practice Act with Matreece, I simply hurried to the phone and called the medical director with whom I was most familiar. I got orders to change the dressing now, and weekly, utilizing the same settings until the patient could be seen at the wound care center. Simple. I entered the order into the system and proceeded with my duties on my unit. As much as I hated it, I avoided Hope's room, as instructed.

Two weeks later State was in the building again. I must add that this building seemed to be a frequent flyer for State visits. In any case, I was standing by the phone when it rang. No one answered by the third ring, so I picked up the receiver, glancing at the guy from State who stood just on the other side of the counter. My ears burned fast.

"This is Amanda with the wound care center," the voice on the phone announced before continuing without stopping for air. "We just saw Carolina, and her dressing hasn't been changed for five weeks! The doctor had to surgically remove the sponge from her arm. Because of your lack of care, the wound is now larger than it was when the wound vac was started in the first place. Thanks to you, she's starting over with an even bigger wound! The doctor instructed me to call you and inform you that if this wound isn't cared for properly from here forward, you will be hearing from him personally, and you will not like it. He wanted me to make certain that you understood this clearly. So, do you understand what I am saying?" she asked angrily.

"Yes, ma'am, I understand completely," I replied as I glanced again at the guy from State.

"Good. I'll let the doctor know." Amanda slammed the phone on the receiver, ending the call.

I was far from offended; I was angrier than Amanda could even imagine. As if it were a divine intervention, Matreece sailed into the nurses' station.

"Matreece? May I speak with you privately, please?"

"I don't have time for that right now. Speak to me right here if you must speak at all."

Stifling a grin, I began to relay Amanda's message.

"That's enough!" Matreece grabbed my sleeve, tugging me toward her office. Once inside, she continued to rant about my speaking of such things in front of State. I apparently overstepped my bounds in the first place by calling the medical director, she "should have terminated me right then." Blah, blah, blah. Matreece ended with, "Now get to work, and don't give me one more reason, or you're out of here."

A short while later I got word that Hope wanted to see me before she left. She hugged me tightly. "I been missin' you the past few weeks, but my granddaughter tole me you wasn't allowed to come in my room. I'm going home now. I won't stay here nigh nother minute. I wanted to thank you for trying to help me even though it got you in trouble. But I did tell ya you was probably the one can handle trouble." She chuckled.

I returned the hug. Having caught Hope's contagious chuckle, I walked out, chuckling myself, as a feeling grew in my gut.

Walking straight to the nurses' station, I checked Hope's records and found that the order I'd obtained and entered for weekly dressing changes had been struck out. My mind spinning, I then walked slowly to Matreece's office, then knocked on the door.

"What now?"

"I found that my order on Hope's dressing change had been struck out. So her dressing was still never changed," I said almost pleadingly, as I hoped she'd help make sense of it all.

"Her name is Carolina." Matreece then looked up at me. "And you best not mention that order to anyone else, ever, for any reason. Do you understand me?"

Maintaining eye contact, I smiled. "Yes, ma'am. I do indeed." I turned and, with a heavy heart, walked down the hallway, mentally penning my letter of resignation, knowing, without a doubt, that I had to mention that order again.

Kyle:

Kyle was a big ole boy, as lazy as a two-toed sloth and as useless as an empty bucket on a deserted island. His own mama had finally kicked him out of the house on his fortieth birthday. Kyle laughed, said, "She thought it would make me get a job."

The man himself admitted, "I've learned that if I don't do it, somebody else will. So I just wait until somebody else does things." He added with pride, "I'm a patient man."

This conversation started with Kyle asking me to hand him his remote control as I entered his room. "It's laying right there by your foot, Kyle." I chuckled, thinking he hadn't been able to find it.

"Oh, I know where it is," he drawled. "I was just waiting for someone to come in and hand it to me so I wouldn't have to go to all that trouble."

I stared, grinning. "Well, I guess you'll get it when you get tired of waiting. May I have a finger, please, sir? I need to check your blood sugar."

Kyle slowly pulled his arm from beneath his blanket, and the movement of the blanket wafted a foul odor to my nostrils.

"What's that smell, Kyle? You have food somewhere that needs to be thrown away?"

"Naw, I eat my food." Kyle sniggered. "I don't smell nothin'. I did the other day, but I don't smell nothin' now."

"Kyle, let me look at your tummy, please," I asked, recalling Kyle's newly placed g-tube.

"It ain't time for my medicine yet."

"No, but I've been off a few days, so I haven't seen your g-tube site. Please, sir?" I waited, not nearly as patiently as Kyle would.

Kyle looked at the television. "If you'll hand me my remote control."

"Never mind." I shook my head, rolled my eyes, and pulled the blanket back. The stench wafted so heavily that I had to wave my hand in front of my nose to catch a good breath. Glancing at the dressing, which was drenched with brownish-black drainage, I turned and grabbed extra gloves. "Good grief, Kyle! You can't smell that?"

"I guess I done got used to it." Kyle shrugged. "Nobody else has said nothin' about it when they give me my medicine," he added triumphantly. "Can't be that bad. I smell it a little bit now that you took that bandage off."

"Kyle, this is not your fault, but it is your body, your life. Pay attention to it," I pleaded as I began cleaning the site. Infection had broken skin down to the extent that the tube wiggled in the middle of an enormous hole, purulent drainage oozing out like a slithering snake. Finally, the drainage slowed sufficiently enough that I could dress the wound and call the surgeon.

Glancing at Kyle's oblivious face, I smiled at him. "Hey, dude, does your tummy hurt?"

"Only when you touch it."

"Does it hurt down here?" I asked, gently touching his lower abdomen.

"Yeah, when you touch it."

"Does it hurt here?" I asked, gently touching each side, then his upper abdomen.

"Yeah, but only when you touch it." He grinned. "I just don't touch it."

Handing Kyle his remote control, I tapped his nose with my finger. "There you go, my little sloth." I grinned. "So, has anybody changed that dressing while I've been off?" As suspected, Kyle was warm. He had a fever.

But Kyle was busy channel surfing.

"Kyle."

"Oh, what?" He was still looking at the television.

I grabbed the remote and asked him again.

"No." He grinned, reaching his hand out for the remote. "Nobody ever changed it but you."

I handed him the remote control. "I'll be back in a minute. I'm going to call your surgeon."

"The stoma is no longer there, Dr. Sill. It's just a large hole that smells like a dead animal, and it has copious purulent drainage," I rattled to the doctor. "His entire abdomen is tender to the touch, and the skin surrounding the site is gray, macerated. Surrounding that, the skin is warm to the touch. He has a fever, Doc. I don't know precisely what it is yet. I wanted to call you before I went back down to check his temp. But I felt his nose. He's warm."

"Send him to ER now," the doctor ordered. "Don't worry about the temp. They can get it there."

Kyle never came back. He was in ICU for several weeks, nearly dying twice, and then he moved from ICU to the stepdown unit for two more weeks. When he was well enough to leave the hospital, he chose to go elsewhere as opposed to returning to our facility.

The administrator called me into her office. "Dr. Sill called me." She frowned. "Kyle isn't coming back. Dr. Sill said Kyle told them you are the only one who ever changed his dressing."

I waited, not sure where she was going or where she wanted me to go.

"Is that true?"

"Oh." I shrugged. "I can't honestly say that nobody else *ever* changed it."

"You know, you pay attention to everything." She stared hard.

I stared back.

"You know Kyle nearly died twice, don't you?" she continued. "So I checked. Kyle's wound care was on the day nurse's duties, not nights."

I shrugged.

"You didn't know that?"

"Of course I knew." I shrugged. "It's everyone's responsibility to make sure needs are met. So, when I saw his wound care wasn't on my treatment record, I checked day shift's."

"So, why were you doing his wound care?"

I looked straight into her beady, black, caring eyes. "Because it needed to be done."

"Nurses have to date dressings."

"Yes, ma'am, we do."

"On the days you did Kyle's wound care, did the date reflect the dressing had been done that day?"

"No, ma'am."

"Could you see the date on the dressing you removed the day you sent him out to ER?"

"No, ma'am. It was soiled and bunched up. But I could see it was dated with a sharpie, and I always use a sharpie."

"So you likely removed the dressing you had put on the day before?"

"No, ma'am." I sighed. "I hadn't worked the day before."

"That's right." She feigned recent recollection. "You'd just come back from five days off." She stared hard once more.

"Yes, ma'am."

"So..." She leaned forward, propping her elbows on her desk. "Are you telling me you removed a dressing that was five days old?"

"No, ma'am. I'm telling you it is possible that I removed a dressing that was five days old."

"You don't seem shocked." Her brow creased, and she locked her eyes on mine. "Not even surprised. Personally, I was shocked."

"No, ma'am." I leaned forward. "This is something that occurs all the time, everywhere. This is no new thing. The only difference is that the dude spoke up. Otherwise, only he and I would know." I held my palm in the air. "Hold up a minute before you speak. I tell these nurses all the time. Maybe you've noticed I don't have a fan club despite my big heart and sparkling personality."

180

She laughed and nodded.

"These nurses are grown. It is my responsibility to my patients to address care issues with the nurses I find falling short. I do not hesitate, and I deal with my resulting lack of popularity. However, it is not my responsibility to supervise these nurses. I am a co-worker, not a supervisor. A nurse, not a reporter or investigator. So you need to speak to those you pay to supervise, investigate, and report."

What bothers me most is that this is far from rare. If a facility doesn't have a treatment nurse who performs the wound care, it's hit or miss, mostly miss. If they do have a treatment nurse, trust me, unless it's a major wound and/or pressure related, it's still hit or miss, but more hits than misses, at least.

Just two days ago a patient with necrotizing fasciitis, otherwise known as "flesh-eating disease," was completely skipped by the treatment nurse that day. The man had been through pure hell and was finally on his way back to health, wounds clean and healing. Then the treatment nurse decided to make him one of the corners she cut that day. The night nurse noted that the dressing was hanging loose, lightly soiled. The wound had a slight odor. Upon closer inspection, she noted that the date of the dressing change was the day before. She reported it, cleaned the wound, changed the dressing, and prevented a crisis. But his wound care never should have been skipped. What if the night nurse chose to ignore it? What if she hadn't noticed? What if…

Edith:

Edith was pleasantly plump, as tall as cotton, as sweet as candy, and as sharp as a tack, but Edith was as weak as a kitten after being hospitalized with a severe urinary tract infection.

"Who are you?" she asked when I sailed into her room. "I haven't seen you before."

"You're right." I smiled. "I guess today is just your lucky day. You get to put up with me."

Edith chuckled as I introduced myself.

"How long have you been coughing like that?" I asked, noticing that her cough sounded wet. I checked her legs for swelling, observing the tiny red bumps scattered over her legs. As if reading my mind, Edith scratched her tummy. "You got fleas?" I teased, placing my stethoscope over her heart. I noticed that the rash was also on her chest.

"I think I might," she chortled. "I feel like an old dog with fleas. I'm too worn out to wash with flea soap and too decrepit to reach all my itchy spots, so today my tail's not waggin'; it's draggin'!"

"Well, let me take a look, Rover." I winked.

After an assessment, I realized that Edith had tiny, red, raised bumps scattered all over her back, buttocks, chest, abdomen, arms, and legs. There were larger, softball-sized areas of intense redness on her back and abdomen.

Ultimately, I obtained some lab work and a chest x-ray, all of which indicated Edith had developed pneumonia and an acute exacerbation of congestive heart failure. This resulted in Edith being even weaker, and of course, she was short of breath, as well.

The doctor ordered an IV antibiotic for the pneumonia, an IV diuretic to reduce the fluid buildup resulting from congestive heart failure, and Benadryl tablets for the itching. I'd noticed the treatment nurse had already obtained an order for a topical ointment.

A short while later I went back to Edith's room to start an IV site. Clearing a spot on her overbed table was a challenge, but I managed to make enough space for my IV supplies. Edith was watching my every move.

"Don't move my Kleenex. I need those."

"I'll put everything back where I found it as soon as I'm done. I promise."

"You can take that coffee cup. I'm finished with it."

"Oh, thank you! You are too good to me." I chuckled.

"You know what I mean." Edith giggled. "Don't move my book!" She glanced up at me. "Okay, I'll hush now."

"No, you won't."

Edith grinned. "No, I probably won't!"

While scooting the last few items over, Edith asked, "What is that, anyway?"

"What?"

"In that little cup. The creamy stuff."

"I don't know." I shrugged, glancing at the little medicine cup holding the "creamy stuff." "It's your cup, your table. You tell me." I laughed, placing the tourniquet on Edith's arm. After getting the IV site started, I asked, "You really don't know what that is in the little cup?"

"Honey, I haven't a clue!" Edith chuckled, then shrugged.

"Okay." I laughed. "I'll play it safe, then, and throw it away."

The next day I checked to see if Edith's rash was improving. It wasn't. I called the doctor and asked if I could try a combination of ointments, thinking the rash may be two separate issues due to the difference in appearance between the tiny, raised, red bumps and the large, flat patches that were as red as stop signs. With the doctor's approval for my concoction, I headed to the treatment nurse's office to round up supplies.

Crystal, the existing treatment nurse, had recently resigned and was orienting Donay, the new treatment nurse. The two were busy talking when I knocked on the door, but they welcomed me inside.

"Sheryl said she came in at four in the morning to make sure she'd have time to get all the treatments done," Crystal exclaimed. "I wasn't going to do that. I just cut corners. I'm only going to work eight to five," she finished disgustedly.

I glanced at the two of them as I bent down to dig in a cabinet beside Donay.

"Me, too!" Donay laughed, kicking her head back dramatically "Imma cut corners, too, cuz I'm not *even* coming in at four in the morning." Her brows arched high as if to say, "Not this girl!"

"What are you mixing up there?" Crystal laughed as she watched me stir ointments together.

"A concoction for Edith's rash. It doesn't appear to be getting any better. Thanks, you two," I said as I hurried out the door, heading back across the building to Edith's room.

"Okay, Rover, stand up so I can reach your backside and kill those fleas." I snickered, helping Edith stand.

"Oh, thank you. I can't reach back there."

When I set my mixture on the overbed table, I noticed a tiny cup with white creamy stuff inside.

"I thought I threw that away yesterday."

"What, honey?"

"That cup, with the creamy stuff in it."

"What is that, anyway?"

"Edith." I laughed. "Where were you yesterday when you and I had this same conversation?"

"I was probably right here in this chair." Edith cackled. "But my brain was probably somewhere else entirely!"

I trashed the mysterious cup and made certain a coworker saw me do it. Linda laughed. "And why am I watching you throw it away?"

"Because I'm certain I threw it away yesterday, but there it was today." I shrugged. "This time I want a witness."

"What is it?"

"I have no clue. Edith has no clue."

The next day, when I was checking on Edith, I found yet another cup of white creamy stuff.

"Okay, Edith, think, love," I encouraged. "Who put this cup on your table? Because I have a witness who saw me throw it away yesterday." I laughed, half thinking I'd lost my mind entirely!

"Oh, honey." Edith chuckled. "I haven't a clue, truly!"

Ultimately, I sniffed the cup, noted a medicinal odor, and then went in search of the treatment nurse.

"Donay." I could not help laughing. "Do you have any idea what this is in this cup?!" I ran through a summary of the entire story.

"Ooooh! That's her triamcinolone cream!" Donay laughed. "I sit it there in the mornings—well, usually in the morning—and tell her to put it on her rash."

"She can't even reach half her rash, Donay. Her backside is covered." I shrugged. At least that explained why the rash wasn't resolving. "Donay, Edith doesn't even recall what it is or who put it there. She's not at risk of eating it, by any means; she's fully cognitive. But she has no clue what the medicine even is and she has a severe rash. Have you seen her abdomen, back, or her bottom?"

"No."

"They are thickly freckled with the rash and splotched with large, flat, vivid red, softball-sized patches. The lady is miserable." I sighed heavily. "Look, I didn't say anything, because no one was speaking to me, but that corner cutting thing, I get it. I do. Nurses have too much to do in too little time. But Donay, some corners can't be cut. Me? I'll stay over to get the job done. You? You want to cut corners? Risk your own fanny and cut documentation. Don't risk her fanny so you can go home on time. The problems of the nursing world are not her fault, nor are they any of your other patients' fault."

"I thought she was with it!" Donay exclaimed with eyes wide. "She seems all there!"

"She is 'with it' Donay." I reminded myself to be Christ-like. "She simply doesn't remember *it*. Most obvious...no, completely obvious is the fact that she can't even stand without assistance, much less reach her back, shoulders, or behind. How were you thinking she'd apply the cream by herself? Or had you decided her rash-covered backside could just magically resolve itself?"

"I'll start putting it on her."

"Thanks."

Realizing the weekend was fast approaching and knowing the real world, I called the doctor and got an order for a Medrol dose pack.

"Oh good." Edith chuckled when I filled her in on the solved mystery of the white creamy stuff and the upcoming steroid. "Maybe that will kill my fleas faster." Then, as an afterthought, she asked, "What white creamy stuff?" while scratching her upper arm ferociously.

"Rub it, Rover! Don't scratch. You're just spreading the fleas."

Edith cackled and scratched.

Elderly Elementary

If you are a gleeful participant in or a connoisseur of snacks, church, crafts, fingernail polishing, popcorn, singing, or bingo, you will find life in long-term care to be overflowing with delightful fun. You'll wake each morning full of joyful anticipation.

If you are not a said gleeful participant or connoisseur, you, like most, will find life in long-term care to be an endless, mind-numbing blur of nothingness. You'll wake each morning full of drudging acceptance that the new day will offer nothing different or more interesting than the one before it.

And if you're a member of the male gender…? I can tell you now that you should prepare to be bored into mindless oblivion.

I think ole Stew put it best when he spread his hands in the air, scrunched his brow, curled his lip, and said, "I don't want to string beads or make pretty things," his fingers wiggling in the air. "I'm not the bingo type," he added, raising his brows as if a label should be attached to those who might be. "Church is okay. I like to watch the others fall asleep." He chuckled "That is, if I can stay awake myself. But I don't understand why we don't ever do anything that grown men like to do." As an after-thought, Stew smirked and said, "They do things my grandkids did in kindergarten." He chuckled.

I couldn't argue with that a wink, especially considering I'd been in the office of several activity directors at several different facilities. Hobby Lobby is the only other place in which I have ever seen such a vast collection of glue, glitter, popsicle sticks, construction paper, finger paint, and other assorted crafty items.

In fact, when our church finally found a permanent Sunday school teacher for the four- and five year-olds they'd coerced me into teaching while they searched, I split my amassed craft supplies between the new teacher of the class and the activity director of the facility at which I was working.

I can hear the activity directors screaming "dementia" now, in addition to a host of other things. I can see their defensive expressions, their arms raised in dramatic shrugs. I get it. I do. I've lived and worked in the "real" world for many years. Some even enjoy the crafts. So get after it! Craft away! But dang, come up with some things the others like to do. Interesting things. Grown-up things. And, State, don't go knee-jerk reacting and pulling all the craft supplies. I shake my head in frustrated disbelief. It truly isn't rocket science. This shouldn't be so hard.

I've never asked what it is, but I'm aware that there is an existing budget for activities. That is perfectly understandable; we all live on a budget. But I wonder sometimes, in light of what I've consistently seen, what that budget might be.

For example, Christmas, the biggest holiday of the year. Corporate provides a little money for a dinner or a party. I say "a little" based on what I've seen produced by it. But the facility's administrative staff obviously feels the residents need, want, deserve, and should have a Christmas gift. With Christmas being "the time of giving," a time of loneliness for many who have no families, I wholly agree. However, it is not the multi-million-dollar corporation that gives their residents gifts. In every single facility at which I have been employed, it is the employees who give the residents gifts. The employees, many of whom make nine dollars an hour, are asked to purchase the residents' Christmas gifts. We either draw a name or sign a list, putting our name next to the resident for whom we plan to buy a gift. Either way, the outcome remains the same. The employees, who also get nothing in the way of a Christmas gift or bonus, are asked to buy at least one resident a gift. The activity director keeps a list of who is buying for whom to make sure everyone gets a gift. Then management hosts a party or dinner, with meager funds provided, and they pass out the gifts as if the devoted company lovingly selected and wrapped gifts just to put a smile on each face and to put Christmas joy in every heart.

Do not misunderstand. I usually select several names to buy for, as it brings me joy to bring joy to others. The point here is that these corporations are not in the computer software business; they are in the "people" business. They are in the business of providing a "home" for people who need it, for people who need assistance with medical care, health issues, and the activities of daily living. It's their home. It's a forever inpatient, move-in-and-live-here kind of thing for people who have no one else to provide these things for them. In essence, the corporation has stepped in and taken the role of the absent, unable, unwilling, or nonexistent loved one. Yet a Christmas gift for the people in their care didn't enter their minds, couldn't be taken from their allotted budget?

They are in the business of providing a safe home, yet they make no real provisions for *life*. Again, in essence, what they ultimately provide is a building in which said people sleep, receive medications, and eat three dictated meals a day.

One last example. How many elderly people do you know who like to sit on the porch, stroll around the yard in the early mornings or late evenings, watch the squirrels, or listen to the birds or the rain? How many of you recognize the importance of fresh air and sunshine? How many of you look forward to grilling outdoors, heading to the beach to soak up some rays, and hiking in the great outdoors? Yet, of the seven facilities in which I have been employed, only one provided any accommodations that allowed the residents to safely spend time outdoors. That one facility boasted a fenced-in area, which allowed for outdoor time while providing safety for those at risk of wandering. And yet that area was not only never used, but the fence was crumbling with decay, the bushes inside the fence were overgrown to the point of being homely trees, and there was absolutely no door to access this area from the inside.

We do not want our elderly thinking they "came here to die," and yet, if one truly thinks about it, once they step in that door, they do begin to die.

My poor child will be thrown completely for a loop one day if things don't change. To promote a healthy lifestyle, in addition to regular exercise, I've raised her on the motto, "Eat to live; don't live to eat." What's she going to do when she steps in the front door of long-term care and finds out I was wrong all these years, that people are indeed living to eat?

Folks should not be able to make a profit from sacrificing the happiness of others. I readily admit that people are a challenge. That includes you and me. And not one of us can make everybody happy all the time. But, if one chooses to go into business, to make a living by providing a safe home in which people can live, by dang, provide the means to *live*.

Living and existing are two entirely different things. Maybe corporate offices need to pull out their dictionaries.

Lastly, make a few random calls to facilities in your area, or across the country. Listen to the recorded message while you're on hold (you *will* be put on hold). Take notes on how wonderful life is in said facility, how much they care about and respect your loved one, and what measures they take to ensure quality of life for those in their care. It's the biggest bunch of bunk you may ever hear.

When it's my turn? Leave me at home. I may well not take my medicine. Who knows? I'd rather not take a bunch of medication to prolong a miserable existence, anyway. I may die and see Jesus sooner that way. I may well fall on my face and break a hip while trying to stand up to better see that little squirrel chasing the bird across my front lawn. But when I heal up, you better send my butt back home to live, even if I fall again.

If you do not offer me a home in which I can truly live, leave me in my home. If anybody forces me into yours? *You* better buy me a Christmas present! I will be watching. By the way, I like to go look at Christmas lights, so plan an outing for a change. Chop those bushes down and fix the fence. I plan to go outdoors. I plan to *live* until I die.

Happy Meal

Food is just about the only pleasure, pastime, hobby, or habit that older people can still enjoy. In every facility across the board, food is the main activity, the main concern, and the main complaint.

Vera:

Vera was *not* going to like what was for dinner, or breakfast, or lunch. And she was going to make the process of trying to please her just as difficult as she possibly could in her own, quietly disgusted, scowling way. Vera was grumpy. Vera was so grumpy that the facility had to separate Vera from her quiet, soft-spoken, gentle husband, Joe, whom I adored. In fact, I'd been working there for over a year before I ever even knew they were husband and wife. The two had proven they just could not get along in the same room. Vera once told me how very much she loved him, but then she said, "He's weak. I despise weakness." Truth is, underneath her tough exterior, Vera had a heart of gold. She just didn't feel the need to reveal it very often, or to very many people, or for very many reasons at all. But it was there.

Vera died one day while sitting at the table in the dining room. Her old ticker just stopped ticking. She'd been told years before that this is how she would likely leave this world, as her heart had stopped and restarted spontaneously many times before. Finally, Vera had signed DNR papers. She said, "I'm not in a hurry, but I'm ready to go home when the good Lord calls me. I don't want anyone restarting it for me. If He restarts it, who am I to argue? But I don't want some fool playing hero and dragging me back into this sad existence if I can be on my way to happy."

Unfortunately for Vera, she was resuscitated by her just-out-of-high-school nurse, quite by accident, before the nurse aide could find me to intervene. The young girl had panicked, then started rubbing and patting Vera's chest in an attempt to get her to start breathing.

Sadly, in the process of dying, Vera's body had eliminated itself of urine and feces. I'll forever remember that proud lady's expression when she came around and realized her circumstances. Vera being Vera, she simply resumed her scowl and didn't make a fuss. Disregarding the EMTs who'd just arrived, and the others who had helped me get her back to her room, she locked her hazel eyes on mine. Curling her arthritis-stiffened, knobby old finger, she motioned me closer and whispered in my ear, "Get them out of here now. I peed and shit all over myself, and instead of being with the Lord, some idiot drug me back, so I'm still here with the idiots, and now I have to live with this shit. Literal shit." Then she scowled at the floor, waiting for me to carry out her orders.

I cleared the room, then began gently cleaning Vera up in silence. She was exhausted and pale.

"I cannot believe my heart betrayed me by stopping in that damned dining room," she grumbled weakly but clearly as I cleaned. "Of all damned places. I'm never going back. I refuse to die in the same room in which that lousy kitchen tries to kill us every day by feeding us garbage."

Vera rolled over toward the wall when I had her cleaned and changed. I recognized my dismissal.

"Hey, you," I tried. "Nobody knows about this but us. Just remember that."

Without moving, Vera grumbled, "I guess I'm gonna have to kiss your ass a lot to keep your silence."

"Only once or twice a day. I won't take advantage."

"You're an angel."

"I can hear you rolling your eyes, you know."

"Oh, so you're an angel and a freak of nature."

I heard her chuckle quietly as I exited.

A couple hours later Vera's call light started beeping. I went down myself so I could see how she was doing.

"Hey, how you feeling?"

"I died, came back, shit myself, then took a nap. Busy evening. I'm hungry."

"The kitchen is closed, but I had them fix you a grilled cheese sandwich with some chips. You want me to warm your sandwich?"

"I want grapes. That's the only thing they haven't figured out how to screw up yet."

"Of course you want grapes, because I didn't get grapes." I stared at Vera, matching her scowl. "But you like grilled cheese. That's why I requested it. So don't give me any crap. You need to eat." I winked.

"That's why I don't despise you like all the others. You're strong."

"I love you, too, Vera. I'll go warm your sandwich."

A tiny smile flickered before Vera regained her scowl. I hugged her, feeling her lean her head against mine. Then she caught herself doing so and jerked it back up.

Four days later, on Friday evening, I was headed back up the hallway from Vera's room, having just answered her call light. She had predictably requested something else for dinner.

"But they asked you before dinner, and that is what you requested."

"Well, I didn't know they were going to screw that up, too. I do like lasagna when the lasagna is edible. This isn't."

So, I was headed back up the hallway, planning to call the kitchen and request tomato soup for Vera, when I heard somebody yell "Nurse!" Running toward the voice, I saw Meesha, the aid, standing in the door of Ms. Davis's room, frantically motioning for me to come, her eyes wide, her face as white as the moon.

I ran faster and found Ms. Davis lying on the floor, surprisingly calm, in an ever-growing puddle of blood, her left lower leg against the wall, bent grotesquely backward mid-shin, the bone protruding ominously from both halves. The leg appeared to be held together by only the posterior skin and muscle, which was now folded in the bend.

Forty-five minutes later, exhausted, I trekked back to Vera's room with a tray holding tomato soup and crackers.

"I'm sorry—" I began explaining as I entered her room.

"I've been waiting for an hour," Vera droned, interrupting.

"A poor lady just fell in her room, literally broke her leg in two," I continued as I set down the tray. "Bless her heart, I think she may well have been in shock. She had to have been in severe pain." I maneuvered Vera's overbed table in front of her.

Expressionless, Vera sat on the side of her bed. "Umph, I hate that for her. Can you get me some grapes?"

"No, the kitchen is closed, and you asked for soup. You got soup." I turned to walk out.

"It wouldn't have been closed if you hadn't taken so long."

"I'll put out a memo and post a sign in all the hallways that says, 'No falls during dinner so that the staff is free to run back and forth to the kitchen for Vera.'" I smirked.

"Be sure to sign it so they know to take it seriously."

"Anything for you, love."

"You should have already done it. Then you could have gotten grapes."

"I still wouldn't have gotten grapes. You didn't ask for grapes." I shrugged. "Eat your soup, Grumpy. I'll talk to the dietary manager tomorrow, see if I can arrange for them to provide a bag of grapes each week. We'll keep them in the resident fridge just for you."

"That's a good idea. Why didn't you think of that before now?" Vera coolly spooned a bite of soup into her mouth.

"I never had visions of throwing a cluster of grapes at you before now," I replied in a "Vera" tone.

Spewing tomato soup clear across the room, Vera exploded with laughter, falling backward onto her bed, literally rolling side to side.

Laughing with her, I turned to leave. I hurried back down the hallway, relishing the completely alien, never-before-heard sound of Vera's laughter echoing around me.

Mimosa:

Apparently, Mimosa's mother had grown up climbing a mimosa tree in their backyard, and that tree held her most treasured memories. Thus, she later named her only child after the tree.

Amazingly, Mimosa seemed to have embraced the name and was determined to live up to it. She wore her boxed blond hair as long and sweeping as the mimosa's branches. She applied blush, eyeshadow, and lipstick that almost perfectly matched the mimosa's pink, fluffy blooms, and she donned carefully selected clothing that was as bright as the sunshine beneath which the tree thrived.

Mimosa was largely responsible for the beautiful flower garden just outside the activity room, where she happily worked each morning. She always wore one of her brightly colored, flowing muumuus, along with her wide-brimmed straw hat, which had a neon green ribbon and a giant yellow sunflower. She nurtured those flowers as if they were her children, sitting amongst them each evening at sunset, sipping her doctor-approved-and-ordered glass of wine before bedtime.

Most outstanding about Mimosa was her attitude. The woman literally never said anything unpleasant and seemed eternally able to see the bright side of things. At least until the day her roommate was served dinner minus the meat.

Having chosen to have dinner in her room that evening, Mimosa stretched out, raised the head of her bed, and prepared to eat dinner while watching a movie. She later told me it was while she was unrolling her silverware that she heard the "Huh?" from the other side of the curtain that divided the room to create the illusion of privacy.

"She can hear me fart beneath my covers," Mimosa blurted. "How private is that?" Then, on second thought, she said, "Hell, I rubbed my nose this morning, and she asked me if I needed a Kleenex before I even realized my nose itched. Lord help us if our butts decide to itch! We got no place to scratch without flashing one another."

"Mimosa!"

"I know. I'm rambling. But that damned kitchen sent that woman a plate with watered-down brussels sprout, a soggy roll swimming in a puddle of water that was made by the tea while it sat there waiting to be delivered, a lump of mashed potatoes with no gravy, and the looks-pretty-tastes-shitty jello with fruit cocktail dumped into it. Not a speck of meat to be found! She wants a piece of this shoe leather, too!" Mimosa waved her chicken fried steak in the air. "And what's up with the gravy thing, anyway? Gravy ain't nothin' but flour and water cooked in grease, with some seasoning thrown in! That's cheap and easy! They like cheap!" She threw her hands into the air. "But we get rice and potatoes all the time without gravy. They dripped a stingy drop on this shoe leather, like the gravy was liquid gold, but they can't drip a drop on this lump of potatoes? This stuff needs all the help it can get to make it taste like food." Mimosa shoved her overbed table to the side, glancing toward her gaping roomie. "We'll eat our shoe leather together, thank you. We eat, sleep, and fart together in here, so I'll just wait."

Stifling a grin, I hurried out of the room just as the aid hurried in. "We don't have no more meat Ms. Sergeant. I'm sorry." I spun on my heels as I heard the aid announce this.

"The kitchen either didn't cook enough to go around or they keepin' some for themselves." She shrugged as I flew back into the room, my eyes on Mimosa. "You want a sandwich instead?"

Mimosa's sea green eyes widened, locking on mine as her left brow arched. "Well now, I guess that says it all," she all but whispered as she picked up her cell phone and looked away in dismissal.

I hurried to the kitchen, but the staff ultimately refused to prepare Ms. Sergeant a meal, offering soup or grilled cheese instead. Glancing around, I noticed the napkin-covered plates sitting on the side counter. Breaking all the rules, I barged through the door beside the serving line, lifted a napkin from a plate, and pointed at the thick, gravy-covered steak with its perfectly browned edges.

"We have already touched our plates, so they can't be served to anyone," Brenda, the cook, said, quickly adding, "And we've already cleaned up, so we can't cook more." She stared challengingly.

"The decision is yours." I shrugged. "All I can do is suggest you think about it before you decide."

"She want soup or grilled cheese?"

"Neither. She wants a meal." I turned, stomped out, called Cotton Patch, and ordered two chicken fried steak dinners with two extra bowls of gravy. I sent the aid to inform the ladies that dinner was coming.

Thirty minutes later I hurried into their room to serve the ladies dinner.

"Well, I'll be damned. Save your extra gravy, Sally! We've struck gold!" Mimosa cried as she reached out for a hug. "I'm sorry I took it out on you, little one. You didn't have to do all this."

"It's no big deal, and I didn't do it because you got upset. I knew you had a right to be upset, and I knew you'd calm down. I did this because you ladies are hungry." I laughed. "Personally, I love me some gravy! And I absolutely hate being hungry. Eat up. Fart. Do your thing." I grinned, winked, and hurried back to work.

I reported the kitchen staff the following day. I'd say more, but there is no more.

Mimosa's daughter spoke with the administrator on that Friday when she picked up Mimosa's laundry. He "addressed it with the dietary manager," so there's that.

Grizzly:

Grizzly was a big ole boy. Having lost his wife, thus having to become his own cook and housekeeper, Grizzly was somewhat enjoying the benefits of facility life. He'd watch the clock and literally prepare himself for each meal. He'd situate his wheelchair straight in front of the television, raising his overbed table to the perfect height, where it sat just above his enormous belly, and then he pulled it in close and locked down the chair and table. His elbows resting on the table, eyes glued to the television, he waited to be served.

Running late after checking blood sugars, I was standing at his side one evening as the aid slid his dinner tray onto his table before him. Ignoring my hand reaching for his, Grizzly grinned, grasped the plate cover with his pudgy hand, and lifted it, his eyes glowing the entire time.

I just about fell over as Grizzly's face scrunched, his chin dropped, and his hand froze midair as he stared at his plate. The plate cover still hovering, Grizzly turned his face to mine.

"What's that supposed to be?"

"Umm."

"That's not even a snack!"

"No."

"That's not even a good joke!"

"Nope."

"That's unbelievable!"

"Yeah."

"That's just wrong!"

"Yep."

"That's not going to work!"

I could stand no more. I laughed hysterically, pointing at Grizzly's plate cover, which was still hovering midair.

Replacing the cover over his plate, Grizzly chuckled. "I'm not even touching that," he said as he moved the entire tray to his bed and crossed his arms indignantly.

"I've simply got to have a reveal picture to show Stewart!" I cackled, snapping a picture of the tray with the cover on, and then I removed it and snapped a picture with the cover off, revealing the tiny sliver of cheese pizza, which was barely a speck of interruption against the stark whiteness of the otherwise empty dinner plate.

"That's really unbelievable!" Grizzly laughed heartily, his wide eyes watering beneath his fuzzy brow. "I mean…" He guffawed. "I've seen some incredible crap come out on those trays, but at least there is usually enough crap to fill me up! That's not enough for you, and you're not as big as a bug!"

"I know." I laughed. "That won't fill one tooth! Let me go get you enough to call a meal, dude. I'll be right back."

"We don't have enough to give him more," the server told me dryly.

"Well then, call Pizza Hut. But get that man some pizza." I stared, crossed my arms, leaned against the wall, and waited. "I'm not leaving this kitchen without it."

Suddenly, they had plenty. Looking back, I should have rounded the entire facility checking plates. My bad. Hope nobody went hungry.

Alvin and Odie:

Alvin was a soft-spoken, quiet man. He was skinny as a rail with legs so long that his knobby knees stuck up into the air as he skillfully wheeled himself about in his wheelchair. Alvin's beloved wife of sixty-three years lay in a bed down the hall from him, lost to the world as she silently wandered the Alzheimer maze. Unlike his beloved wife's room, which was decorated by hospice and was fully furnished like a bedroom in any comfortably nice home, Alvin's room was sparse. On his wall hung one lone picture of himself and his wife from years before. The two of them stood side by side in front of the home they'd built together using scrap material they'd scavenged over time from trash piles at construction sites. Alvin told me they'd moved in once they'd had one room completed, then added to the home as they'd found more building material. The two had lived in that same made-from-scratch home until Alvin could no longer take care of his wife by himself. Then he simply left the home as it was and moved with his beloved wife into the facility. "Till death do us part," he would say, shrugging, a distant look in his good eye. The other was scarred beyond vision after an accident with a nail gun.

On the far, far flip side, Odie was a loud, rambunctious, trench-coat-and-top-hat-wearing, cane-sporting jokester. He had gotten divorced from his fourth wife just nine years previous to the day I met him. I remember well because, Odie being Odie, when I was introduced as his new nurse, Odie grinned and shouted, "What a wonderful coincidence! I meet wife number five on the ninth anniversary of the very day I rid myself of wife number four!" He winked and tipped his hat. "So nice to meet you, pretty lady. My lucky day indeed."

Odie was a hot mess in the making! He always had a joke to tell, and he laughed the heartiest with every telling. The problem was, with Odie's progressing dementia, he frequently retold his jokes, forgetting completely that he'd already told the same joke to the same person, often on the same morning or afternoon, or even within the same hour. Odie was also a charmer. The man wore his trench coat and top hat with purpose, cocked his hat to perfection, and twirled his cane like a star in an old musical. Most unfortunately, though, Odie was a walking disaster. The man's behind was on the floor as often as his feet. He was much too busy laughing, joking, flirting, and twirling his cane to pay any attention to the hard fact that his balance was steadily abandoning him. Odie said his cane wasn't for body propping; it was for show stopping. He'd smirk, duck his chin, and peer at me from beneath the brim of his hat.

Odie and Alvin were both one of a kind, but from opposite ends of the spectrum. It goes to show that in some cases opposites do attract. In their case, the first attraction was food. Odie would talk to a fence post and not be at all concerned that the post didn't talk back. After all, the silence of the post only served to provide Odie more opportunity to talk. Initially, that's how it went with Alvin and Odie. Odie, always asking what time it was or when the next meal was, often hit Alvin up for the answers, as Alvin proved ever-available in his quiet solitude and predictable locations. Alvin gradually began requesting a sandwich for Odie every afternoon when he requested his own, and a fast friendship was in the making.

One day, after I saw the aid bring Alvin's full tray back out of his room, realizing I'd just seen Alvin sitting out on the porch, it dawned on me that, once I thought about it, Alvin's tray was always mostly untouched. He might eat the desert, but he never, ever touched the food. But as sure as dinner meant evening, evening meant Alvin would be requesting another sandwich. That particular day Alvin caught me in the hallway, so I told him I'd bring it to his room later, adding that I'd be sure to bring a carton of milk with it. Alvin loved milk! He grinned shyly, ducked his gawky white head, and rolled away.

Later that night I knocked on Alvin's door. Hearing his reply, I slipped in, placed his snack on a small table against an otherwise empty wall, and turned to face him.

"Thank you," he said quietly. "I hate to ask more of you, but could I borrow some scissors for just a minute?"

I reached into my pocket, handed Alvin my bandage scissors, and watched him place the scissors just below a hole in the leg of an old pair of gray sweatpants, then cut off the lower portion of the leg. Intrigued, I stood and silently observed as Alvin then tied a knot in the end of the cut piece, slipping the other end over his head, then rolling it into a cuff around his face.

"I make night caps out of my old pants to keep my head warm at night," he said quite seriously. "If my head is cold, I'm cold all over."

"That's because you don't eat, scrawny." I chuckled. "I see your trays. You don't eat a thing on them except maybe desert."

Alvin laughed and began telling me how his mother never cooked. They spent summers at the river, and the only thing he could ever recall his mother cooking was fish. Otherwise, they ate canned and boxed goods every day of their lives. Alvin's face glowed as he finished, saying, "Sardines and crackers with a cold glass of milk…still my favorite meal. I'd give up my nightcap for a can of sardines and some saltine crackers!" His bony shoulders shook with his quiet chuckles.

"Oh my, we could not have that!" I laughed as I turned to walk out, glancing once more at the knot sitting on the top center of his head. "Enjoy your snack, knot-head." I spent the next couple of weeks requesting that dietary send Alvin finger foods at mealtimes. I gave them examples, such as a sandwich and chips, a corndog, a hamburger, steak or chicken fingers, and fresh fruit. But it was to no avail. Surrendering, I bought Alvin a huge tool chest and filled it with canned and boxed foods, including, among a host of other items, a loaf of bread, a jar of peanut butter, a package of Chips Ahoy, six cans of sardines, and a box of saltine crackers. To ensure some actual nutrition, I added a basket of fresh fruit. I made certain to provide a padlock and key, which, once he got past his stunned silence, Alvin used to secure his treasure.

Alvin still requested his daily and nightly snacks, and he finally put a little weight on. I restocked his box from time to time, and Alvin refreshed my memory from time to time, saying, "Make sure you take that nice box home when I leave this world. That's a really nice box." He'd inevitably add, "Don't let somebody get it that will just tear it up." He'd then show me the key on the chain around his neck, tug on it, and finish with, "You know where it is."

Early one afternoon, while in Vera's room checking her blood pressure, I heard a commotion from the hallway. Poking my head out the door, I saw Odie pushing Alvin's wheelchair wildly down the hallway, looking much like an escapee from the loony bin, his eyes wide, his lips flapping nonstop, and his head in constant motion. Odie was moving so fast that the resulting breeze tousled his "Alfalfa" hair, which was sticking up from his thick mane of snowy white hair. Alvin, who clung to the arms of his wheelchair as if it might take flight any second, held his size-fifteen feet up off the floor, his knees pulled up to his chest, grinning like a schoolboy skipping class to go fishing.

As they grew rapidly closer, I heard Odie ask, "Chocolate Chip?" his head bobbing clumsily as his legs grew tired his feet grew heavy. But his grin kept getting bigger.

Alvin's replies were too soft to hear above the noise, but one could easily fill in the blanks using Odie's words and expressions.

"Heck yeah, I'm always hungry! Where'd you get a whole jar of peanut butter?" Odie exclaimed, a look of sheer disbelief consuming his face. "And a loaf of bread? A whole loaf?"

Predictably, Odie passed Alvin's room up as Alvin motioned for him to stop, pointing at his door.

"Oooh yeah, that's it right there." Odie chuckled and made a NASCAR turn with Alvin's chair. "Can I really make me a whole sandwich, not just a half? And you have jelly, too?"

Alvin reached one arm out to push the door open, knowing Odie paid no heed to his knees, but he held tight with his other hand as Odie banged his chair through the doorway, still at breakneck speed.

Seconds later Alvin's door closed behind them. I tiptoed over and eavesdropped, relishing the sound of the two rumbling through the box, chattering the entire time. Their words were muted, but their joy was crystal clear.

A short while later Odie bounded clumsily out Alvin's door, a sandwich in hand and a banana poking out of his pants pocket. Noticing me as he took a big bite, he said, in muffled peanut butter talk, "First whole sandwich I've had in years!" Licking a drip of grape jelly off his finger, he proceeded back up the hallway toward his room.

"Hold on to the side rail, Odie," I called out, still grinning to myself.

Odie chuckled, grabbing the rail just long enough to make it sticky before releasing it to hold his sandwich with both hands, shoveling it in his mouth faster. Looking like Alvin the chipmunk, he disappeared into his room, bumping into the door frame as he went.

In one smooth practiced motion, I shoved my cart against the wall and locked it, headed fast up the hallway to Odie's room. Just before I reached the open door, I heard the familiar crash, thud, profanity, chuckle.

"I'm glad I finished my sandwich before I fell!"

"Me too; no doubt!" I laughed. "But do you think you could stop licking your fingers long enough for me to help you up?"

"Don't worry bout getting me up! I'll just end up back down here," Odie shrugged, grinned, "Worry about getting me one of them magic boxes like Alvin's got!"

Laughing with him, I bent to offer Odie my hand.

Odie suddenly stopped, mid shift, his eyes wide as he locked them on mine then placed his bent old finger against his lips, "Did you know Alvin has a magic food box *and* a 'good fairy' that brings snacks to his room?"

Me:

I'm a snacker. I like me some snacks. And I want to be able to have a snack when I want one. I might not always want a snack at the same time. I might not want a snack at all. By golly, I might want more than one snack! I am undeniably a snack fan.

But I don't like graham crackers. I love peanut butter and jelly sandwiches! But do I want one every single night for the rest of my life? No. I can readily say, without hesitation, that I do not. Little Debbie oatmeal pies are something that one must have a taste for. And I don't. But, folks, if you move into a long-term care facility, you best be ready to eat one of those three things for a snack, or be prepared to go hongry! No, I did not say hungry. Hungry is an understatement. I said hongry!

At the first facility where I was employed after getting into long term care, I eventually battled with the kitchen—excuse me, the "dietary department." They ultimately hated me. It was the apples. The apples just finished off my patience. I could stand no more.

I ask you, who sends apples as a snack for a significantly elderly, denture-sporting population? That's much like dangling a big, juicy red apple on a string, just out of reach of a racked-up horse. Now, mind you, I said apples, not apple chunks or apple slices. The kitchen sent whole apples out for snacks. Big, shiny red ones. Real beauties! They sent them out on trays, knowing full well that we don't have knives at the nurses' stations, and of course, we'd be breaking every food handler law in existence, not to mention infection-control regulations, if we were to cut one up for some poor, hungry soul drooling for a delicious bite!

So they blamed me. *Me!* I had grown weary of the complaints about lack of variety in snacks. Now I completely understood said complaints. I had crucial nursing care to provide and not enough time to provide it, yet there I was, spending precious time getting chewed out because we never had anything but graham crackers or halved peanut butter sandwiches." I'm even going to throw this in: When it's my turn, don't give me half! I want the whole danged sandwich! I don't nibble. I eat!

In any case, I feel for these folks. I can easily stand in their shoes. And I don't like it. So I had requested variety. I suggested a little meat between the bread now and then. Maybe some unhealthy chips, like we all have at home. Or some cold cereal fortified with crap but loaded with tasty! You know, SNACKS! Oreos! You people ever hear of Oreos? And bring me a lil' glass of milk so I can dip 'em! Please and thank you!

I want snacks: good snacks, plenty of snacks, a choice of snacks, and, by golly, readily available snacks. And though I occasionally enjoy some fresh fruit, I like junk food, too. I'm grown. I got this! Who died and made you my mama?! And let's be honest. Graham Crackers and Little Debbie's are cheap! Yeah, I gotcha!

I'm not even going to do this chapter justice, as there is simply not enough time. But I am going to say this: Menu planners? We eat gravy on our rice down here in the south! We eat it on our potatoes, too! Sometimes we eat it on our biscuits! You don't have to. That's cool. But we do. Get it right before I get there!

I want snacks, and I want gravy. I do.

Sadly, I could go on forever. But the point is, no, you cannot please everybody. But you can stop cooking the vegetables to the point of mush. You can prepare enough to go around, and maybe even enough to have a bit of leftovers for those who want seconds. You can provide gravy for those who want it. You can sit those tea glasses on something, or fix them last, to prevent the inevitable puddle on the tray that soaks the bread and the single salt and pepper packets. For that matter, you could provide butter for a change. Some people like butter on their bread. You could staff sufficiently to prevent serving burned meat. I bet it is tough cooking for a hundred people. Hire that cook some stovetop help. And while I'm here, it's no added salt, not no salt. How's this for thinking? Send a little bucket of condiments for the aids to offer to the people. That way you don't waste any, so you take care of your budget, yet those who want them have them readily available. And the packets aren't too soaked to be used. Sometimes it's the little things that make the biggest difference.

I once smeared butter on a little man's dinner roll as I prepared to assist him with eating. The dude's normally vacant, dull eyes lit up when he bit that roll. Chewing happily, he asked, "Is this Thanksgiving?"

Before I leave this chapter, I have to add that many folks are on supplements due to weight loss caused by a host of things. Now, bear in mind that most people who need the supplements—not all, but most—are debilitated. It makes sense. Poor nutrition weakens the body. Maybe the weakness even induced the poor intake. Regardless, my point is that many have supplemental snacks ordered to facilitate adequate nutritional intake and prevent further weight loss. Many of these individuals are completely, or very nearly, helpless. Yet, the aids—*if* they take the snacks to the people at all—will set an unopened carton (just like the milk cartons in elementary school, the ones often difficult to open) or will lay sealed cellophane packages on the table next to a near comatose or physically disabled human being. Then they turn around and walk out, and somebody will eventually throw them away (I stress the word "eventually," as I've seen literal piles of snacks build up before somebody sweeps them off into drawers or a trash bag). This is happening everywhere, always and forever, while the administrative staff holds more meetings in an attempt to resolve the unexplainable, ongoing weight loss. They scratch their heads, bewildered that the high calorie snacks did nothing.

Your loved one is hungry and thirsty. And there is no doubt that you will be, too.

It's not all that hard. It's not. We just need to give a shit. We need some changes. We need you.

Crackers:

I almost forgot Crackers. After calling the kitchen three hundred out of three hundred and sixty-five days a year to request crackers for the man, one would think he'd have been the first person I mentioned.

In a nutshell, Crackers ate saltine crackers with everything, and I mean everything. Unless they were serving soup, or some other item with which most people eat crackers, I had to call the kitchen to request crackers for Crackers. On that note, even on the days they served crackers, they didn't normally serve enough crackers for Crackers, because on those days, he needed more, obviously to have more to eat with whatever it was crackers normally went with.

Now, initially, I ran to the kitchen to get the crackers, knowing they were all busy trying to get the meal out in a timely manner. However, after I requested, verbally and then in writing, that they simply send crackers for Crackers every evening meal and they still didn't send them, I let them bring the crackers to the unit themselves when I had to call for them.

Crackers sometimes pouted, sometimes grumbled, and sometimes cursed in frustrated anger, but he always wanted and waited for crackers.

No, I don't understand wanting crackers with everything. I cannot imagine wanting such a thing. But what I prefer is irrelevant in regard to Cracker's meal.

"I don't get it," the kitchen lady said every single day when I called over. "Why does he want crackers with everything?"

At first I expressed amazement and aggravation myself, chuckling with her, keeping things light, our working relationship cordial. Finally, though, I spouted, "You know? I don't get it, either. But then, I don't get why you don't just send the crackers any more than I get him wanting them. In fact, I get him wanting them more easily than I can wrap my head around the fact that you'd rather have this same conversation every day instead of just sending the danged crackers with his meal to begin with! I mean, at least he wants them to eat. Regardless of the fact that we wouldn't want them, he does at least have a reason for his actions. Please tell me, what is yours? Why won't you simply send them to start with?"

She hung up.

We continued the daily cracker chase. I kid you not. For two years I called the kitchen to request crackers nearly every single day I worked.

The difficulty of the simplest things add so needlessly to the difficulty of the difficult.

Many times the kitchen told me they were out of crackers. Then Crackers would call his overly devoted wife, and—bless her heart—she'd drive into town, get crackers, and bring the man a box. Then she, too, grumbled about the kitchen not sending crackers, and rightfully so!

Ultimately, I bought and kept a box of crackers on hand for the days the kitchen was "out." That was better than listening to Crackers grumble about not having crackers, and it was better than having his poor old wife drive all the way into town to bring him crackers.

One way or another, Crackers got his crackers, but getting Crackers his crackers just about made me crackers.

Dr. Seymore:

I once looked up and across the small dining room in which the "feeders" were being fed. I noticed a middle-aged man struggling to get a spoon to his mouth with at least a little food still on the spoon. His hands obviously not wanting to cooperate, I offered to assist the man. Tears immediately welling in his eyes, the man snapped, "NO!" as he turned his face to the wall.

After dinner, I asked one of the other nurses, "Who is the new gentleman in the wheelchair, the younger guy?"

"Oooh," Stacy replied, "that's Dr. Seymore. He had a massive stroke a few weeks ago. He's here for rehab, and he is not happy about it."

"Why doesn't he stay at home and do out-patient therapy?" I wondered aloud.

"He doesn't have anybody to help him at home, no family left at all. And, since he may never practice again, he is trying to save the expense of hired help."

I never offered to help the man again. I did take him an extra desert one evening after seeing him devour his first piece of cake.

"Thank you." He glanced up into my eyes. "The food is horrible. And I never imagined I would have to eat it. In thirty years of practice I never one time admitted one of my patients to a place like this. I've helped many families figure out alternatives. And yet... here I am in the very hell I worked so hard to keep them out of. Here I am with no alternatives. You can go now. Nothing you can do to help me." He looked back down at his cake and I took my que to exit.

Floor Masters

Maddie:

Maddie was ninety-nine years old. She was a towering four feet and ten inches, was black as a moonless night, and topped out at a hundred and three pounds, thirty of which were her pendulous breasts. All that, and the first thing you'd notice if you saw Maddie today would be her scrunched-up face. Maddie, completely blind, could not even see light. As her vision had faded, Maddie's determination to see as much as she could for as long as she could had proven to intensify and nearly petrify her scrunch. Her little face forever resembled someone who had just taken a bite of a sour pickle.

Thing is, though Maddie couldn't see to walk around safely, she still had the stamina of a teenager and the agility of a monkey. The latter was proven emphatically the evening I approached the nurses' station and found Maddie crawling nimbly across the counter before climbing as skillfully and slowly as a sloth down the other side.

Maddie was easy to love and hard to handle! If you turned your back for two minutes, you may well find Maddie feeling her way along a wall or counter, or you might find her down on all fours in a fast crawl, searching for the door. Maddie would say, "I need to get back home to them cows, and Lawd, the garden is prolly choked with weeds!"

Maddie simply did not have time to sit idle; she had things to do. She was a hardworking woman who had single-handedly raised eleven children on the meager wages she earned taking in laundry and sewing. She had a garden she plowed and planted, two cows she milked, the occasional pig that she slaughtered and processed, and a mess of hens and chickens, ruled by a rooster Maddie had named "Strut." Maddie would say, "Strut sho nuff thought he was a peacock."

Needless to say, Maddie was a high fall-risk, requiring diligent observation and creative intervention to keep her safe. Maddie wasn't my patient, but she required teamwork! Thus, I had placed her wheelchair next to me while I hurried through some documentation before my next round of the halls. Extremely conscientious regarding documentation, I was in the zone, head down, focused.

"Suuuuuuu-EE," Maddie suddenly squalled from her seat next to me! Startled, I jumped, and my arms flew up into the air, sending my pen sailing across the lobby.

"Maddie!" I laughed, slapping one hand over my racing heart. "What the heck was *that* for?"

Maddie, chin still jutted upward, explained candidly, "I'm a'callin' them cows back up. They done wandered off too far in that back field again. Come on home, Susie, and bring Bucket with ya now."

"Bucket?"

"Yeah." Maddie smacked her ever-pinched lips. "Got his head stuck in a bucket first day I brung 'im home. That's what bein' nosy got him. So's it was Nosey or Bucket, and them kids liked Bucket better. Seemed fittin' ta me."

"I like it, too!" I laughed "But, isn't 'suuuuuuu-EEE' how you call pigs?"

"Them cows started a'comin' ever time I called Bacon to slop, so that worked for everybody. Suit me jez fine. Saved me a'hollerin' two thangs steada one."

I have to add that all Maddie's hogs were named "Bacon." After all, she only had one hog at a time, and "bacon was what they were for". It made sense to me once she explained it.

Suddenly, Maddie began pushing herself up from her chair.

"Where you going, Maddie?"

"I gotta feed them chickens and make sure them cows come on home. I don't got no time ta jez sit here and yap. Always work ta do 'round heah."

"Well, hold on just a minute, and I'll help."

"Well, make it quick. Time don't slow down for nothin'. It sho don't."

Maddie sat quietly for a quick minute. Then she began reaching into an imaginary "sack," waving her arm out to her side as she tossed imaginary feed to imaginary chickens, softly clucking while she tossed.

I spent many a moment feeding chickens with one hand while writing nurse notes and doctors' orders with the other. The day we went from paper to computers, meaning I needed my chicken-feeding hand to type, I was momentarily stumped. Things worked out, though. Being blind, Maddie didn't notice. As long as I made the right sounds and comments, and as long as she felt my hand take feed from her sack every little while, it worked great. In fact, I felt really silly for not having realized sooner that I hadn't actually needed to go through the motions all along.

Late one Wednesday evening, Kerri, Melissa, and I were working hard and fast, trying to wrap up our documentation before shift change. Engrossed in necessarily detailed documentation of a particular resident's status, I blocked out the activity around me.

"I tell you what," Kerri huffed. "I'm just going to let her fall. I don't have time to keep distracting her or getting her back into her chair. I'd rather just do the extra paperwork for the fall than to keep jumping up and down, trying to keep her off the floor."

"I don't blame you," Melissa quipped from her corner of the station. "We don't have time to babysit Maddie. She needs one-on-one care! Maybe if she falls, they'll see that."

It took a second for their words to register in my conscious. I turned around and looked at the back of Kerri's head, then slid my gaze to the back of Melissa's. Both were busily at work while Maddie stood next to her wheelchair, both arms stretched out as she groped for a surface to follow. Kerri glanced over at Maddie, shrugged, and resumed typing.

I shoved my chair back to hurry over. As if on cue, Maddie stepped one foot forward, tripped on the blanket that had slid off her lap, and started a flailing descent to the floor. I made it to her just in time to keep her from hitting the floor. She landed on me instead…this time.

What about next time?

What if I'm not there and the others who *are* there feel the same way Kerri did?

I must add though: Kerri is a good person, a good nurse. Overload makes people do things, think things, and say things they wouldn't otherwise do, think, or say.

I would guess that if Kerri is reading this right now, she fully realizes just how wrong that was. But at the weary time…

And sadly, Kerri is far from the only nurse I've seen and heard doing and saying the very same things.

Harold:

Harold was an auto mechanic—a gifted auto mechanic—and was highly respected by many. NASCAR tried to recruit Harold! But Harold had two sons he loved with every ounce of his being.

Harold told me, "Thanks to their mama's drug habit, they ain't neither one of 'em whole. She was a selfish woman, and a liar. Told me she wasn't doing no drugs while she was pregnant. I ain't stupid, I watched her close. But I never seen her doing the stuff while she was carrying them boys. Oldest one looked normal, or I'd a never give 'er a chance to get pregnant by me a second time. We had the youngest, whose body was all messed up, before the oldest 'un got big enough for us to know his head was all messed up." Harold grinned ear to ear. "But together they make a whole, and they got hearts as pure as California gold!"

Harold ran the boys' mama off just as soon as his second son was born, and Harold saw the baby's deformities.

"On the very day the baby and his mama were discharged from the hospital, I told her to get out." Harold frowned. "I told that woman to get on home and get her things. Told her to be gone before I got home with the baby, and don't never come back. I haven't seen or heard from her since, and I don't regret that one tiny bit."

So Harold had declined an exciting position with NASCAR and kept his repair shop, adding an auto parts store to provide his sons a job they could handle. When I knew him, Harold literally ran that business from his bed. He spent most of his time on his cell phone. And every evening I'd find his two sons in his room, sitting on the couch, and Harold would be in his wheelchair, facing them and talking business.

Harold was proud of his sons, and he had confidence in them. They had proven themselves capable. But occasionally, Harold would have memory lapses or significant pain, which would inevitably cause him to call me to his room.

"Now, mind you, I ain't going nowhere. Lots of folks beat cancer, and I fully intend to be one of them folks, but sometimes I wonder what would happen to my boys if I didn't beat it. I will now, but what if? I mean, someday I'm gonna die. We all do. What will happen to my boys?"

Harold didn't expect an answer. He just wanted me to listen. So I did. Over what seemed to be no time at all, I listened ever-more frequently. One night, Harold talked much longer than usual. Maybe he sensed it, I don't know. But that night I said good night to my grown, demanding friend, and the next morning he was gone. His body still moved, his lungs still took in air and let it out again, but Harold was no more. Gone were the blue jeans he insisted his sons take to the cleaners to be starched. Gone were the button-up shirts that simply *had* to coordinate with his socks. Gone was the underwear that he had insisted be folded into a "square". My friend needed briefs. I discovered all this at once when I heard a loud crash, ran into Harold's room, and found this competent, intelligent man on the floor, pushing his cell phone around like a Hot Wheel on a toy racetrack.

"Harold? You okay, my friend?" I asked as I hurried to check him out.

Harold looked up at me with empty gray eyes, then glanced around the room before clumsily attempting to stand. Then he suddenly shook his head and looked me straight in the eye. "Well, don't just squat there like an idiot," he barked. "Help me up!"

His last coherent words, and the complete opposite of his character.

I gave him a hand, and he stood as easily and straight as you or me. Then he took one step toward the door and crumbled. Seeing his legs turn to jello mid-stride, I quickly stepped up behind him and bear hugged that six-foot, two-inch, dignified man to the floor, helping him to sit instead of fall onto the tile. He then bit my hand. I guess he thought I'd pulled him down. Who knows?

Thereafter, Harold required hands-on assistance for every aspect of life. His cell phone was forgotten, as were the papers he'd been waiting for his sons to bring him. But Harold seemed to still be driven; he simply didn't know his direction anymore. So he was constantly trying to get out of bed. And he could get out easily; he simply couldn't stand. Ultimately, Harold was in a Geri chair (a recliner on wheels) in hopes of keeping him safe. But Harold proved capable of crawling right out of that, as well. Keeping Harold safe was an ongoing battle, but we were determined to win, as Harold had won our hearts.

Then one night after Harold was tucked into bed and sound asleep, I instructed the aid to keep a close check on him.

"Oh, I know. I know all about Harold," she replied nicely.

Later I headed down the hall to start an IV and stopped to check on Harold on my way back. I thought it odd that his door was partially closed, as it was supposed to stay open for easy bed check. I found Harold asleep on the floor, a pillow tucked beneath his head and a blanket covering him.

When I found the aid sitting in the corner of the darkened dining room, on her cell phone, she said, "Well, he kept trying to get out of bed. I don't have time to check on him every five minutes. I figured that if he fell, I'd just leave him on the floor, where he'll be safe. He fell, so I left him there, but I made him comfortable. And he's safe. He can't fall now."

I called for help getting Harold back into bed and sent the aid home to think about what she might have done differently. Three days later, I arrived at work to find Harold with stiches across his brow. The nurse I was relieving said, "Harold kept climbing out of his chair, and I got tired of him fighting me, so I just let him fall. I had hoped that he'd see that it hurt and would stop trying to get out." She rolled her eyes, added, "But he's been trying to get out ever since he got back from ER. You deal with it! I'm going home!" She laughed.

The next day she denied every word. But Harold had stopped trying to climb out. Harold died, just before breakfast, with stiches across his brow.

Sara-Lee:

Sara-Lee was as sweet as maple syrup, and the lady purely amazed me! Being someone completely void of patience, I find myself in genuine awe when I encounter a being like Sara-Lee. At times I literally found myself unconsciously encouraging her to have some sort of need or want, maybe a little humanistic demand or two. But ultimately, she'd smile on, insisting, "No, darlin', I can't think of a thing," and I'd walk out, saying, "Okay, well, call me if you think of anything."

Sara-Lee had a broken hip, and a large surgical incision ran from just above her hip down to her mid-thigh. We were having a very difficult time controlling the bleeding. Strangely, the incision never burst open, despite bleeding so heavily that it saturated her bed linens and gown, forming a puddle at her side. This all came from a tiny opening between the sixth and seventh staples. Thus, we were keeping a pressure dressing on the site and repeatedly contacting the doctor and the orthopedic surgeon.

Additionally, we had to position Sara-Lee in bed so that there was no pressure to the areas around the incision, which could cause further bleeding. This meant Sara-Lee had to lie on her left side, rather awkwardly at times, to prevent constant pressure on bony prominences. Sara-Lee was a trooper throughout it all. The lady never once complained, never once used her call light. Sara-Lee simply lay in bed, waiting for whatever may or may not come next.

She had absolutely no recall about how her hip was broken, or even what she had done the day or the hour before, but Sara-Lee never forgot the face of her beloved daughter, Jaye-Lee. (Jaye-Lee was named after both her father and her mother). Jaye-Lee visited Sara-Lee every single day, never missing a beat.

I only meet patients if they have a problem, so often I'd be asked by the residents' roommates, "Who are you? Are you my new nurse, too?"

"No, I only see people who might be getting sick or have something going on that requires a closer look. That type of thing. So if I never see you, it's a good thing!" I'd laugh.

I once had a jolly gentleman retort, "Well, in that case, I think I have a fever!" His grin was as wide as the Grand Canyon.

Anyway, Jaye-Lee walked into Sara-Lee's room one afternoon, and there I stood, bent over her mom, applying a pressure bandage. Of course, Jaye-Lee was curious as to who I was, so I began explaining my position and purpose. By the time we finished talking, Jaye-Lee had filled me in on Sara-Lee's journey up to that minute. Jaye-Lee was a delightful person, full of life and warm as sunshine.

Apparently, Sara-Lee had fallen at home, resulting in hospitalization to surgically repair a broken hip. Sara-Lee had then been transferred to another nursing/rehabilitation facility for therapy and incision care.

"Everything was going fine." Jaye-Lee smiled. "Then I walked into Mama's room one day, about mid-morning, and began chatting with Mama like always. But Mama's roommate, who seldom said anything at all, interrupted. She asked me if Mama had hurt herself when she fell," Jaye-Lee continued calmly. "I was about to ask her roommate what she was talking about, but the nurse hurried in and began explaining that Mama had fallen out of bed some time during the night. The aid had found Mama asleep on the floor when she'd brought Mama's breakfast tray in."

My expression remained unchanged as my mind began to click.

"The nurse said Mama just smiled at her when she checked her for injuries. Mama wasn't upset or uncomfortable in any way. She said Mama had been asleep in bed when she'd disconnected Mama's last IV at about eleven-thirty the night before. Then she laughed and said Mama had pulled the blanket down on top of her and never called for help." Jaye-Lee shrugged. "But I asked for an x-ray to make sure Mama's hip was all right, and by the end of that day, Mama was sent back to the hospital for a second surgery. Now she's here."

Jaye-Lee's face saddened ever so briefly. I could feel Jaye-Lee forcing herself to be positive. Smiling brightly once more, glancing lovingly at her mother (and obviously her best friend), Jaye-Lee continued, saying, "I just want Mama to get strong enough to come home. She was walking fine before she fell. Now she just doesn't seem able to bear weight on that leg anymore. I just hope therapy can help Mama get strong enough to stand so I can move her from the bed to a chair, or from the chair to the toilet. I'll do anything for her that she needs. I just can't lift her."

Her gaze fixed on Sara-Lee, who smiled glowingly back at her daughter, Jaye-Lee finished emphatically, "If I have to hire someone to help me, Mama's coming home when that incision is healed."

Sara-Lee cocked her old head to the side, smirked at Jaye-Lee, and proclaimed just as emphatically, "Sweetheart, I'm going to stand for you." She chuckled. "You may well have to remind me to stand, maybe even a few times. You might even have to remind me 'how' to stand someday soon, but I'll stand, sweetheart, every time, just for you. Never you fear."

Jaye-Lee grinned through the tears that had suddenly welled in her eyes, got up, and took the few steps from her chair to her mama's bedside. Hugging her mama, she said, "I know you will, because you love me as much as I love you."

Then, in unison, the two ladies said, "I can do all things through Christ, who strengthens me!"

Both laughed, pinched one another playfully, and said, again in unison, "You owe me a coke."

Jaye-Lee turned her head and looked back at me, her eyes wide with delighted wonder.

"I know," I whispered, smiling huge. Sara-Lee's sudden burst of cognition was purely amazing.

"I love you, Appleseed." Sara-Lee reached her age-spot-speckled hand and patted Jaye-Lee's cheek.

I felt her overwhelming love and joy as I watched Jaye-Lee choke with emotion.

"I'll buy both of you a coke if you stop the mushy stuff so I don't stand here and bawl like a baby." I stepped over, my arms stretched wide. "Come on. Group hug!"

The next morning I walked into Sara-Lee's room to check her pressure dressing. Physical therapy was there with her, trying to coax Sara-Lee into standing so they could transfer her from her bed to her wheelchair. Sara-Lee was trying—she always cooperated—but each time she attempted to use her right leg, she would wince and give up. Todd, the therapist, gently encouraged another try. I asked if Sara-Lee had been given pain medication, and Todd assured me he had ensured the nurse had given a dose thirty minutes before starting therapy.

"Alrighty then!" I grinned. "I can do all things."

"Through Christ, who strengthens me," Sara-Lee finished quietly, peering up at me with loving hazel eyes and a honey-sweet smile.

"So…" I smirked at her, knowingly. "Stand for Appleseed."

Sara-Lee's face lit up! Her eyes sparkled like ripples on the surface of a clear mountain spring in the light of her sunshiny smile, which spread swiftly from ear to ear. Still staring at me as if I were the seventh wonder of the world, Sara-Lee grasped her walker with both hands. Todd silently stood to grip the gait belt around Sara-Lee's waist.

Hazel eyes locked on mine, and Sara-Lee's expression transformed to a picture of sheer determination. Grimacing with the strain, she slowly shoved herself up, lifting her bottom from the bed. Once off the mattress, she hesitated briefly, her face wadded with pain.

Still holding her gaze, I stood behind Todd, nodding my head slowly.

"Stand for Appleseed."

Her face at once resolute, Sara-Lee nodded once, then shoved with every ounce of strength she could muster, and Todd helped lift her the remainder of the way into a standing position. Sara-Lee stood, trembling, for a full sixty seconds before tiring out, her posture starting to crumple. Todd, holding tight, helped Sara-Lee slowly lower her bottom back down onto the bed.

"Appleseed" continued to work miracles for therapy until Sara-Lee was healed up and strong enough to go home. Every time, of course, it was as if it were the very first time she'd heard anyone use that lifelong term of endearment, which, to Sara-Lee's limited recollection, no one was privy to except her and Jaye-Lee.

Jaye-Lee told me that when she was a small child, each time she had eaten an apple, she had planted the seeds in their yard. She had told her mama she was going to grow an apple tree. Thus, she became Appleseed.

Sara-Lee will never walk again, but she could stand safely with assistance, so Sara-Lee was going home. Jaye-Lee had a surprise for her mama. She'd paid a landscaper to plant an apple tree outside Sara-Lee's bedroom window. Maybe Sara-Lee will get to see it produce some day; maybe not. But Jaye-Lee will. I'm fairly certain that tree will live long and prosper under Jaye-Lee's tender, loving care.

So, a happy ending for Sara-Lee. But the thing is, she should never have fallen that second time in the facility. Sara-Lee had no recall, but she was completely cooperative and amazingly content. Thus, she never even attempted to get out of bed unless instructed to do so. She was far from needy or demanding. Sara-Lee probably rolled out of bed due to poor positioning. I say "probably" simply because I wasn't there.

My questions would be:

Why? Why did Sara-Lee fall out of bed?

When/what time did she "fall"?

How is it that the nurse's last report was at 11:30 the night before?

How is it that Sara-Lee wasn't found on the floor until breakfast time? I mean, what about the night aid's every-two-hour rounds? Incontinent care? Turning and repositioning? Why hadn't the oncoming day shift aid seen Sara-Lee until she was bringing breakfast in?

Had no one entered Sara-Lee's room from 11:30 p.m. to breakfast time the following morning?

Did no one hear the inevitable thud when Sara-Lee hit the floor?

Otto:

Otto was as pudgy as the Pillsbury Doughboy and slower than a crippled turtle. Otto even spoke slowly, and to make matters worse, he included every minute detail, never, ever cutting to the chase. Me being me, I'd often have to mentally chastise myself to keep from spouting, "Come on, dude! *Out* with it already!" But Otto was a sweetheart, so if he needed to take a full three minutes to say, "I need some ice," so be it.

In fact, allow me to demonstrate:

How I would ask for ice: "I need some ice, please." Or, "May I have some ice, please?"

How Otto asked for ice: "Hey, sugar, I don't mean to bother you. I know you're busy. I see you running all over the place. Would you hand me that Kleenex, please? Thank you, sweetie. I don't think you ever have a minute to rest. I hate to add anything to your load. But I haven't gotten any ice since this morning. Scoot that trash can a little closer to my chair, would you? Thank you. I think it was this morning." He'd rub his big, bald head and shrug. "Anyway, that little girl with the big braids— the one that talks real fast; she has them two little boys—she brought me some ice. Oh goodness, I think that was this morning. Regardless of when it was, it's all melted now. She didn't fill it to the top. I don't like that much ice all at one time. So, anyway, my water isn't cold anymore. I'm thinking a little ice. Not too much. Now, don't fill it to the top, but a little ice would be right nice. When you get a minute, I mean. I can wait until you come back this way. I know you're busy. I'm not in a big hurry for it. Or you can just tell that other girl, the tall, quiet one. I don't think she has any children. I don't know. She might. I don't recall her ever mentioning any. Nonetheless, she's pretty good about bringing me stuff when I need it. She knows just how much ice I like. However you decide to do it is fine with me. I don't want to be any trouble. I just need a little ice. Not too much now. Can you see to that for me?"

I would nod, smile, and hurry away as every neuron in my brain fired sparks out my ears to prevent self-implosion.

But no doubt about it, Otto was indeed a sweetheart. Not a mean bone in his body. And Otto absolutely adored his wife, who shared his room with him until she divorced him at seventy-eight years old so she could go home and live with her son. They'd been married for sixteen years, and

Otto was lost without her. It broke my heart. It was none of my business, though, and I don't know the facts. We all need to remember that. We don't know the whole story, and there are always three sides to every story. In this case, there was Otto's side, Mary's side, and the truth. Regardless, Otto was alone, grieving, and he fell during the night while trying to get to the bathroom.

I arrived to work that afternoon, and Otto filled me in. I'm going to summarize his story for you.

"I didn't hurt nothin', but it was cold on that floor! It was even colder because I peed all over myself when I fell." Otto rolled his eyes, smacking his pudgy hand to his forehead. "Maybe I shouldn't drink so much water, after all. I lay there peeing on myself all night long. I couldn't reach my call light, and I'm too fat to move myself around. Maybe I need to go on a diet. I had no idea I'd gotten so big. I'm *fat*! I couldn't even roll over! I was like a big, blubbery whale." His belly rolled with his chuckles. "And it seemed like the harder I tried not to pee, the more I needed to pee. I concentrated and tried to hold it, but my bladder didn't like that plan. It had a plan of its own." He winked." Naturally, I didn't sleep a bit, and I guess nobody heard me holler. So, I just lay there, peeing and waiting for morning."

"You're not fat, Otto; you're fluffy." I smiled. "Let's clip your call light to your clothes at bedtime from now on. Most importantly, at least at night, please call for assistance to the bathroom. I know you can get there by yourself. This was just an accident. But to be on the safe side, what would it hurt to call for help before you try to get up, just in case?"

That night I asked Cynthia, the aid, if she knew anything about Otto's fall the night before.

Immediately defensive but polite, Cynthia explained, "We don't ever go in there at night. Otto goes to the bathroom by himself, and he changes his own pull-up. We don't do no incontinent care on Otto. So there ain't no reason for us to go in there unlesson he uses his call light, and he never used it." She shrugged.

"So you guys don't make rounds on everybody at night?"

"Naw, girl. We just make rounds on the ones who need they brief changed."

Seeing my blank stare as I processed all the implications, Cynthia took her leave.

The night nurse, who I affectionately nicknamed "Care Bear," was a good one. She was an older lady with a slight case of paranoia, which, from my perspective, served her patients well. Care Bear checked on everybody. So naturally, I was glad to see her back, as her alternate had been on duty the night before. Her alternate was one of those typical "I'm gone do as little as I can" nurses. It was amazing just how little she could manage to do. Anyway, I informed Care Bear of what Cynthia had told me, and predictably, Care Bear called the aids to the station and informed them, point blank, that everyone had to be checked on every two hours regardless of their continence status. Go Care Bear!

Otto didn't break anything in the fall. But that night on the floor, combined with losing his beloved Mary, seemed to rob Otto of his spirit. He began a fast decline. Within a month Otto had requested hospice services, and a week or so later, he got out of bed for the last time. When he lay back down that afternoon, he just never allowed anyone to get him up again. I missed his long, drawn-out conversations. Otto was still the sweetheart he'd always been, but he had suddenly mastered the ability to summarize. I found myself wishing he hadn't.

One evening Otto told me, "I miss my Mary so much it hurts. It really hurts, right here." He patted his old hand over his shrinking belly. "I realized that night, while I was lying on the floor like a beached whale, that I was no good for her anymore, anyway. A grown man laid out on the floor in his own urine, too old and fat to get himself up. I'm so thankful she wasn't here to see that."

"Oh, come on, my friend! Your bladder was full! Everybody in this place is here because they need assistance. It happens to most people as they age. You had an accident. Accidents happen. We are the ones who fell short. We are the ones who should hang our heads in shame, not you. Put this thing in perspective. And I don't know what happened with you and Ms. Mary, but I know she loves you. She needs assistance, too. She gets that. In fact, she would think less of us, my friend, not of you. And you're not a whale. You're a delightful dolphin who happens to be a blessing to all of us in the sea, so start eating, please and thank you."

Otto laughed heartily. "A dolphin, huh? Well, that may be because I squawk and chatter a lot."

"You did! I'd like to hear you squawking and chattering again. And I want to see you eating, for that matter." I scowled playfully.

"I'm planning to do just that, little mermaid. I promise." He winked.

The next afternoon I was standing at Otto's bedside, assessing his vital signs, when he opened his recently-clouded brown eyes. "I keep my promises. I'm going to dinner." He grinned weakly, reached for my hand, and squeezed it.

I knew. I felt peace emanating from my old friend for the first time in weeks. "Put in a good word for me?"

"I already did." His eyes were suddenly sparkling as he lowered his lids, never opening them again...well, not in the earthly realm. I got to hold his hand as he took his final breath less than an hour later. Oh, and what an honor that was. I stood there, chuckling through happy tears as I imagined the loving but exasperated expression on God's face as Otto described his journey to heaven, Otto telling his story with all its backroads and byways. Otto telling Otto's adventure in his uniquely detail-laden, time-consuming, around-the-world-and-back kind of way.

Jannie:

Jan became "Jannie" when she met Chuck seventeen years prior. Chuck loved to talk, and Jannie seemed to love to listen to Chuck talk, especially when he talked of how they met and married. Jannie was twelve years Chuck's junior, and from the way they both told it, Chuck had lots of ladies. Jannie smoked cigarettes when they met, but Chuck said he finally told her, "If you'll quit those cigarettes, I'll marry you." Smugly, he added, "She knew she'd be the luckiest lady alive to marry me, so she quit right that minute, never touched another one." He smirked.

"Yep, I got lucky, and you hit the jackpot." Jannie winked, drawing Chuck's gaze to her own, transforming his face into the very picture of a love letter written and sealed in his heart. A moment so raw and tender, I instantly felt as if I were invading their privacy. I instinctively sat perfectly still, holding my breath, so as not to reveal my presence and stop the flow of unspoken words.

I heard the story the first day I met the two of them. And I heard it a hundred more times during Chuck's never-failing daily visits, which inevitably involved him wheeling Jannie all over the facility and grounds.

During one such venture, I stepped outside to find Jannie and administer her medications.

Following the sidewalk, I immediately felt I'd stepped unknowingly into another moment meant only for two as I heard Chuck's deep voice sing, "I got you, babe," as he pushed Jannie's chair.

In perfect time and key, with a huge, mischievous grin, Jannie leaned her head back to look Chuck in the eye. "I got you, babe," they sang in practiced unison, and then Chuck leaned down, wrapped his arms around Jannie's shoulders, and cradled the back of her head against his chest as she hugged his arms, pressing them tightly against her heart.

Suffering the effects of end-stage liver failure, Jannie's abdomen swelled up with fluid to such an extent that she often looked nine months pregnant, with quadruplets. Her abdomen would get tight and painful until she'd go to outpatient at the local hospital, where they'd drain the fluid off in a procedure referred to as paracentesis. At a pace far too rapid, Jannie was requiring the procedure more and more frequently.

"Just two months ago she could go as long as three or four months between drains. When she came here, she was going about every three weeks," Chuck told me, handing me the paperwork from outpatient. "They say there is no point draining her anymore, but they'll do it every other week for now as part of pain management." He rubbed his hand through his already mussed hair. "*If* we want them to, they said." He looked away. "*If* we *want*."

A while later, while assessing her neighbor across the hall, I heard Chuck and Jannie arguing again. Jannie's mental status was changing with the increased levels of toxins building in her blood, as her liver failed to eliminate them. Confusion made her boldly express thoughts and feelings that she had born in silence for years.

Chuck loved his wife—that was undeniable—but Jannie's confusion had opened the box in which she'd packed the memories of their lives together. Slowly, often bitterly, she pulled them out, one by one, waving them like flags, exposing Chuck as a walking contradiction, while Chuck struggled, sometimes angrily, to stuff them back into the box as fast as Jannie pulled them out.

Moments later Chuck opened Jannie's door and motioned for help. Jannie was hurting badly.

Standing beside Jannie's bed, waiting for her to swallow the pain medication, I winced as Jannie peered around me at Chuck, saying, "She's my best friend, Chuck, or she was. I'm not stupid."

Chuck readily interrupted with, "You are the love of my life, Jannie."

Jannie raised her round, eggplant-colored eyes to mine, wadded her face in a disgusted smirk, and said, "He's right." She spread her palms in the air, saying, "He loves me fiercely. The problem is that he loves every other woman he sees, too." Her laughter pealed and then ceased just as quickly as it had begun. "I'm so *thirsty*." She tried to smack her dry, cracked lips.

"You want some cold water?"

"No! Heck no! It tastes like…water." Jannie scowled severely.

"Want me to see if I can find you a popsicle?"

Jannie gasped, her eyes wide, "A popsicle?! Oh boy, that sounds soooo *good*!" She ran her hands over the enormous mound her belly made beneath the blanket, grimaced, and then looked up, smiling radiantly. "Yes! I want a popsicle!" She grinned like a kid ready for his prize after getting a shot.

"I'll go get you some right now." Chuck popped up and was out the door before I could turn around. Twenty minutes later Jannie was relishing every lick of her "green" popsicle while Chuck sat on the side of her bed, grinning, as he held the popsicle to her lips.

"I got you, babe," he sang to her as I passed the open doorway.

Later that night the falls started. Jannie's belly was so big that when she tried to roll over, the momentum of her belly's weight pulled her on over the side of the bed, onto the floor. I heard her confused grunt, followed by a moan she forgot as quickly as it occurred. Giggling, she looked up at me. "My bed threw me out."

Unable to resist a chuckle, I got down beside her and checked her for injuries before gathering help. It took all five of us, plus an aid borrowed from another unit, to safely maneuver and lift Jannie's dead weight from the narrow space between the window and her bed. Afterward, we moved her bed farther from the window, placed fall mats on each side, and lowered her bed to the floor just in case.

Jannie fell several more times, as the state would not allow the use of siderails. They were, and still are, considered a "restraint," and should a facility and family choose to use them, of course, there is a massive amount of extra paperwork involved, and there would an unspoken mark against the facility, as it affected the numbers.

Ultimately, I discovered that the million pillows Chuck brought for Jannie should have been a sign. I learned through loving but often frustrating trial and error that if I positioned Jannie on her left side; cozied a pillow against her abdomen; placed a pillow between her legs, with her right knee propped up; draped her right arm over the pillow at her abdomen; and positioned another pillow between her face and the edge of the bed, Jannie would snuggle in, hug the pillow close, and sleep soundly. She was far too weak to move and build enough momentum to pull her over the pillows. The only requirement was that someone needed to ensure that the pillows remained in place anytime she fell asleep. Jannie wasn't interested in attempting to get out of bed at all by that point. Thus, sleep was the risk, and Jannie was sleeping more and more.

When awake, Jannie was calling my name, as it was "Popsicle time." Between popsicles and pillows, Jannie kept me hopping. "Orange," she would say, her eyes bright, before I hurried back down the hallway to the freezer.

"She wasn't my friend. I know that now. That's so good, so cold and tasty." Jannie licked her lips, holding the popsicle at a precarious angle. "I thought she was. She came over to see me all the time. But she has never come to see me here." She gazed toward the window. "I smelled her on his shirt yesterday. I've smelled that perfume for years. I know that smell."

I just listened, unable to think of a single word to say.

"He can't be alone. He just can't." She glanced at her popsicle, sucked the juice dripping on her hand, and shifted her gaze to me, focused. "That's why he married me. Oh, but it was good, him and I. So I don't want him to be alone. But he could wait until I'm gone. Damned fool." She chuckled, then licked her drippy popsicle.

"Good grief, let me wipe you down, drippy." I stood, stepped out for a cloth, and ran smack into Chuck, who stood just outside the door.

Ignoring his hand, which was wiping tears from his eyes, I held my finger in the air, indicating he should wait. Grabbing a cloth, I took it back to him. "Wet this with some warm water and wipe my sticky friend down while you talk, please, sir."

"My pleasure," he replied, his gaze a thousand miles away as he plastered a smile on his face and hurried in.

"Ya know?" Jannie asked during her red popsicle at bedtime that night. "She gets Chuck, but he loves me. I get Jesus, and He loves me, too."

I held the popsicle to her lips, and we giggled as she bit a big chunk. "Well, all that and a red popsicle with me? Looks like you win, my friend." I grinned and wiped her chin with a readied cloth.

Jannie died two days later. I returned to work, and the nurse filled me in. She'd just checked on Jannie a short while before, when she'd given her a pain pill. She went back about thirty minutes later to see if the pain pill had helped, and had found her dead in her bed. It apparently looked as if she'd just fallen asleep.

However, the aid later told me Jannie had died on the floor, half on, half off the fall mat next to her bed, her pillows scattered over the floor on the other side of it.

Shakira, the aid, told me, "I'm sorry. I know I promised you I'd keep them pillas right, but I was down the hall cleanin' up Ms. Jones. She done shit all over everything, and it took me a while. I feel real bad about Ms. Jan."

"All you can do is all you can do. Don't feel bad. It's not your fault." I hugged my sincerely distraught friend. "The system is broken. Those who allow it to go on as it is are the ones at fault here," I reassured her before I hurried to run a copy of the related nurse notes, which detailed Jannie's quiet passing while lying in bed. I took the copy and headed over to the administrator's office, mentally prepping for yet another futile debate, another round of emphatic denial.

The thing is, I get it. I understand the facility's firm declination to utilize a "restraint." I fully understand the state's somewhat outdated perspective. What I don't get is why somebody hasn't revised the system so that someone in Jannie's circumstances could easily, readily, and immediately be provided the protection that she needed in the form of simple siderails. I feel certain that one with an IQ of four could distinguish the difference between a restraint and protection. And, dear Lord, don't add a mountain of *nonexistent-time-consuming* paperwork and a stigma in order for one to be provided that protection. It simply isn't rocket science. We are an intelligent people, aren't we?

We should be able to come up with a workable solution, shouldn't we?

I think, first, we must acknowledge that a problem exists and that a solution is needed, don't we?

Chloe:

Thirty-seven years old. Slowly and painfully dying from cancer of the vulva, secondary to cancer of the cervix, which was the result of having contracted genital herpes years before. The cancer had resulted in Chloe's suffering a huge, gaping, draining wound that made urinating and defecating excruciatingly pain. The wound meant it was even more crucial that incontinent care be done quickly and thoroughly. Thus, Chloe used her call light frequently during all waking hours.

In addition to the cancer, Chloe had bumpy red patches covered with white scales scattered over her torso and extremities, most severely to her scalp, elbows, knees, and lower back. This was due to an exacerbation of psoriasis. Despite all, Chloe was determined to live life to the best of her ability until it ended. She read books and interacted with friends and family on her cell phone during all waking hours. She tried to take as little pain medication as possible during the day so that she could stay awake. Not having had an easy life, Chloe was a bit rough around the edges. But her heart was good, and she was openly grateful for all care received and any act of kindness.

Covering an extra shift one night, I slipped in to check on Chloe in the wee hours. Exhaustion and the pain medication she took at night resulted in deep sleep. Therefore, Chloe wasn't often awake to utilize her call light and relied solely on staff to ensure her needs were met.

Knowing the aid woke her at least every two hours for incontinent care, I slipped in quietly, using only my flashlight, merely checking to make sure Chloe was resting comfortably.

However, upon approaching Chloe's bedside, my foot suddenly slipped, then both feet slid out from beneath me, landing my behind smack on the floor. My eyes wide, grunting from the pain, I reached my hands down to push myself up, realized I sat in a puddle. Very carefully,

I pushed myself up, stepped over to the door and flipped on the light. Seeing urine dripping from Chloe's bed I was horrified! *Urine! I slipped and fell in urine!* My face twisted with disgust, I rushed to Chloe's bathroom to wash as much of me as possible.

Hurrying out to get help, I found the aid sitting in front of the nurses' desk, on her cell phone. Describing what I'd just seen, I asked when Chloe had last been cleaned and changed.

The aid responded, and I quote, "She ain't been cleaned at all." She sneered. "And she ain't gonna be by *me*. I ain't touchin' that nasty bitch!"

"You're terminated. Get your things and leave, now." I struggled to control my rage as I headed to laundry to dig through the unclaimed clothing items for a pair of dry pants to get me through the remainder of my shift.

That same aid was at work the next night. The assistant director of nursing had determined, without a word to or from me, that it was "a wrongful termination." She did, however, assign the aid to a different unit so that the aid wouldn't be responsible for Chloe's care.

Forever Sixteen

I'm a fully-grown woman with a fully-grown child, yet one of my favorite things to do is to go to a park and swing. In fact, one day I hope to have a huge, park-sized swing all to myself, ready and available every day in my own backyard. I absolutely love to swing. You should try it. There's just something about the wind in my face as I push harder to swing even higher. And the flip of my tummy as I feel my weight lift slightly from the seat as the swing hesitates midair, then changes direction. Thrilling! Freeing! Exhilarating!

We grow older on the outside, but we are forever young *inside*.

Shirley and Grace:

Shirley and Grace had been roommates for several years. They seemed to adapt well to one another. Both had their own room, as both ignored the other's presence almost entirely. But, hey, it worked well for them. Neither of them seemed to want the other to know, but they watched out for one another, each reporting if the other seemed sick or uncomfortable, always in a secretive manner. Otherwise, neither of them seemed to care one hoot if the other was present or not…except for that one day.

Grace snored. Grace not only snored, but she also frequently snorted while snoring. And after years of listening to Grace snort and snore, Shirley had reached her limit. She turned up her television to drown Grace out.

Grace woke up. "Turn that down," she fussed.

Shirley ignored her.

Grace pushed her call light button. Burna, the aid, went in to find out what was needed, and Grace told her to turn Shirley's television down so she could nap. Burna later told me that she had asked Shirley to turn down her television, but Shirley just stared at her like she hadn't said a thing!

Burna said, "I done been in there five times and didn't get nowhere with it. So's I just decided I wasn't going back in there. Let them handle them." She shrugged.

That's about where I came in.

I was sitting at the desk, reviewing lab results, when I noticed the call bell beeping incessantly. Somebody's television was about to blow the roof off, and nobody was doing a danged thing about either problem. Pushing up from the desk, I headed fast down the hallway to answer the call light, which appeared to be Shirley and Grace's room, and I quickly realized the blaring television was coming from there, as well.

Rounding the door into their room, I found Grace sitting up on the side of the bed with her elbows on her knobby, glow-in-the-dark white knees, her hands over her ears. Shirley was leaned back on her bed, the remote control in her hand aimed at the television.

Grace's dusty white curls bounced wildly as she proceeded to yell, "Tell that crazy old woman to turn that TV down so I can take my nap!"

I looked at Shirley, who remained unmoving, reclined against her pillows, staring at me with hooded black eyes.

"See?" Grace shouted. "She's crazy as an old bat!"

Shirley grinned but still didn't move a muscle; she just stared intently at the television as if completely engrossed in the show.

"You need to send her somewhere," Grace shouted. "She's lost her mind, if she ever had one!"

Shirley grinned.

I stifled my grin.

"Ms. Shirley, would you please turn your television down so Ms. Grace can nap?" I yelled, ever so nicely, over the noise.

"Yeah, you old bat!" Grace chimed in. "Turn it down!"

Shirley grinned.

"Ms. Grace, no more insults, please, ma'am." I sighed. "Ms. Shirley, please turn your television down? We can hear it all the way down the hall."

Shirley glanced over at me, guilt flashing briefly across her face.

"Did you hear the nurse, you old bat?" Grace shrieked.

As sure as I'm breathing, Shirley turned that television up even louder, ducked her chin, and stared at it ever more intensely.

"That's it! She's bonkers!" Grace cried, flinging herself down on the bed and pulling the blanket up over her head."

I bit my lip, hard, to keep from grinning.

Shirley glanced over at the lump on Grace's bed, looked up at me, and grinned victoriously, just like a spoiled child.

"Okay, Shirley, turn it down, please."

"I'm watching this, and I don't hear too good." Shirley spoke for the first time, that mischievous grin still plastered across her face.

"Ms. Shirley, you hear just fine, and we both know it." I smirked at her. "More importantly, that's the Spanish channel, and you don't understand a lick of Spanish. We both know that, too." I winked.

Shirley's grin literally sunk into a pout that was poochier than any two-year-old's I'd ever seen.

"I *know* you are not pouting!" I laughed.

Shirley stared at me for a second, then grinned and cackled as she pressed the volume button, turning the television down.

Ms. Grace popped her little head out from beneath the blanket, and Ms. Shirley stopped her mid-pop.

"Don't you say a word, you goofy old bird with your lawn mower nose, or I'll turn it back up even louder and keep it that way till you die and go to snore the angels right out of heaven!"

Grace stared at Shirley. Shirley stared at Grace. I looked back and forth between Shirley and Grace. Then Grace snickered, Shirley roared, and I threw my hands in the air and walked out, shaking my head and allowing myself to grin once out of sight.

Golden Girls:

Sybil and Rue were nearly inseparable by day. They were the very best of friends, but they had proven incompatible as roommates. Thus, they were separated only by night. Both were attractive older ladies. Both had married well and were accustomed to living well. Both were busybodies. Both were bossy. Both were artificially sweet. Both were wheelchair-bound, and both were hypochondriacs. They often shared symptoms with one another, literally concocting a variety of illnesses.

Sybil and Rue ate every meal together. They spent their days rolling about the facility together. And, together once more, they spent the majority of their waking hours poking their slightly elevated noses into everybody else's business, wanted or not. I can still see the tops of their poofy gray heads gliding smoothly past the nurses' station as they expertly propelled their wheelchairs with their feet, en route to stir some crap.

Lastly, both had doting daughters who could not see their mothers realistically even if Van Gough himself had painted them a portrait. Both mothers and both daughters tended to get on my very last nerve. For this, I cannot apologize, as only a saint could bear the mothers and daughters without severe frustration. And I am no saint.

For that matter, that is one thing for which I must give my family full credit, and I do not pass kudos out all willy-nilly; I give them to no one undeserving. But my family is realistic. When my mother was in the hospital, being a royal pain in the nurses' behinds about how she took her medication at home? We readily told her, "Well, Mother, you aren't at home right now, so let it go. Take your medicine when they bring it to you, hush about it, and when you get back home, proceed with your schedule." When that proved to have only a temporary effect, we told her we wouldn't visit or bring her dog to visit again if she didn't shut her flapping lips about her desired specifics and just dive in and do her therapy. That worked. Side note: The woman had undergone emergency brain surgery, couldn't speak clearly, and couldn't swallow effectively, but, by dang, she could still flap them lips!

Sybil and Rue needed kids who demanded the same realism from their mothers, as opposed to kids who encouraged their mothers' dissatisfaction and somewhat ridiculous habits, preferences and demands.

All that said, both Sybil and Rue had a delightful side as well. Their delightful sides simply weren't their dominant sides.

Rue and Sybil adopted Ms. Isabella, a tiny little woman with advanced Alzheimer's disease. Isabella was four-feet, eight-inches of spit and sparkle, and strangely, she "loved" my voice and face. In fact, it proved to come in right handy. Isabella was as lost as a newborn kitten with no mama. Sunup to sundown, Isabella oscillated between a sweet, glittery southern belle and a tiny dragon lady who demanded we call her daughter or take her home immediately. In between the southern belle and the dragon lady, she would randomly become a little girl crying because her baby (doll) was hungry, cold, sick, or upset. Sadly, Isabella spent the vast majority of her time either demanding or crying. But as I said, strangely, she loved my voice and face. All I had to do was get her to look directly at me (which wasn't always easy) and say, "I love you." She would stop whatever she was doing, smile radiantly, put her cool old palm on my cheek, and say with gusto, "Ooooh, and I *love* you, *too*! And I love that *voice*! And that pretty little face." Needless to say, there was a lot of "I love you" goin' on around there!

Anyway, Sybil and Rue adopted Isabella, against everyone's wishes except their own and, of course, their daughters'. I was especially dismayed, as I fed Isabella dinner most nights. Otherwise, Isabella would most often sit and demand or cry instead of eating. After being off work for a few days, I returned to find that Rue and Sybil had moved Isabella to their table. To make the situation even more delightful for me, Rue's daughter, Shelby, lived nearby, so she frequently joined the two of them for dinner. Shelby was one of those people who covered her nosiness with friendly banter while soaking up every word, listening closely for bits and pieces that might tip her off about what to ask the next guy. Shelby wanted to sound informed so that *next guy* would speak freely, ultimately giving her the lowdown she so craved.

Even worse, Shelby was obsessed with her mother's care, to the point of being ridiculous. She once threw herself a literal hissy fit because she found out her mother's saline nasal spray had been discontinued. About three months prior, Shelby had gone out of town. Before leaving, she had directed us to call a specific friend of hers if anything came up during her absence. Well, the friend had forgotten to tell Shelby that the nurse had called to inform her Rue's nasal spray had been discontinued due to lack of use. Shelby found out when she took Rue to see the doctor and the doctor reviewed Rue's current medication list. Almost predictably, Rue up and developed allergies due to her nose being all dried out.

You tell me. What can one do with *that* mentality? I just resumed the nasal spray, which Rue forgot all about after about four days, never asking for it again.

So that was the mentality I dealt with the entire time I fed Isabella. In-between scanning the dining room and commenting on those of whom they disapproved for various reasons, Rue and/or Sybil, and even Shelby, would encourage Isabella to eat her carrots, saying they were good for her. This encouragement never failed to alert Isabella to the fact that she was eating, completely spoiling my laborious efforts to distract Isabella and keep her eating. I'd have to stop, wait a few minutes, and then strike up a conversation about some other random topic so I could resume poking food into Isabella's mouth. I suppose the Golden Girls and their not-so-mini 'mini-me' were just too self-absorbed to notice the added challenge they created for me in getting Isabella fed sufficiently.

One evening I had had my fill of the three ladies' encouragement. Mid-meal, just after Sybil told Isabella to eat her chicken because it was good protein," I moved us. I stood and said, "You're going to have to excuse us, ladies. Come on, Isabella, this isn't our table."

"Oh, okay," Isabella sang. "Well, where is our table?" She giggled, squeezing her beloved baby doll closer to her chest in anticipation of the pending move.

"Over there. Follow me. I've got your plate."

All three ladies chimed in like a bunch of magpies. I just smiled, thanked them for their kindness in sharing their table, and led Isabella to another.

After dinner, I couldn't spot Isabella's aid, so I helped her change into her pajamas so she could go to bed. I must add here that Isabella was well loved, and she had also married well, in addition to being born into money. Thus, Isabella had more diamonds on her fingers, wrists, and ears than I have hairs on my head. Additionally, and this was more my point, Isabella had a host of pajamas! It appeared that once she wore a set one time, they were replaced, as all of them looked brand new. But with her being four-feet, eight-inches, it was rather like dressing a doll, so choosing from the variety of spiffy PJs was fun! Isabella looked absolutely adorable in her tiny, powder blue PJs, which were scattered with miniature white daisies. I just *had* to hug her!

Isabella handed me her "baby," told me how to hold her right, folded back a pile of soft, fresh-smelling comforters, and climbed her tiny self into bed. I placed her "baby" next to her and pulled the covers up to their chins. Folks, it was a mental polaroid moment that I will forever carry with me!

After turning out her light, I walked out, grinning ear to ear, only to run slap into the Golden Girls. Both Rue and Sybil smiled up at me like rays of morning sunshine.

"Is Isabella in bed?" Sybil inquired with a sugary sweet—or shall I say sweet and low—smile.

"Yes, ma'm." I tried to walk on by.

"Wait a minute," Rue insisted. "Did you help her change into night clothes or leave her in her day clothes?"

I turned back around, stared, reminded myself these ladies also needed love, and chastised myself for my thoughts.

"Yes, ma'am, we changed her clothes."

"Who is we?"

"Isabella and I, of course." I smiled. "Now, I've got to get busy. You ladies have a good evening."

"Excuse me." Sybil smiled with Rue-matching sincerity. "But why were you helping Isabella instead of the aid? Isn't that the aid's job?"

Biting my tongue, I replied pleasantly, "Oh, Ms. Sybil, I don't think Isabella cares one hoot who helps her into her PJs, so long as it's done when she's ready. Now, I'll see you ladies later." I hurried away, pretending not to hear Rue yell "wait" again.

When I turned the corner, I saw Rue rolling into Isabella's room, Sybil right behind her. Both ladies' feet were propelling them in a smooth, practiced glide, their elbows propped on the arms of their chairs, hands clasped, torsos leaning forward with their heads and necks perched forward like a couple of twin hens. Because Isabella was a high fall-risk, I didn't want her getting out of bed without our knowing it. So, I watched to ensure that the twin hens rolled right back out before proceeding down the other hallway. Both ladies caught sight of me watching.

An hour or so later, Rue rolled up to my medication cart, smiling so sweetly that a honeybee would have been right at home on her ruby red lips. "I know you're upset with me, but may I have a headache pill, please?"

"Sure, you can," I agreed merrily. "And my goodness, why would I be upset with you?"

"Well, because we went into Isabella's room to make sure she was in her pajamas, and you saw us. We were just making sure." She smiled again. "You understand." She nodded.

"Oh yes, ma'am. That I do. I understand completely." I smiled back, stifling a chuckle as I handed Rue a tiny cup with two Tylenol.

Rue looked at me as if she weren't quite certain of my exact meaning, but she maintained her smile, thanked me, and rolled off toward her room. I heard her stop to speak to Sybil. "I got myself a Tylenol to help me sleep. You should go get you one."

As sure as the sun rises, Sybil rolled up about two minutes later.

"I know you're busy, but would you mind getting me a Tylenol to help me sleep?" She, too, was dripping honey.

Yes, I was mischievous.

"Tylenol isn't a sleep aid, Ms. Sybil." I avoided eye contact so I wouldn't smile. "If you're having trouble sleeping, I can talk to your doctor for you," I offered lovingly.

"No, I don't want a sleep aid," she dripped. "I want a Tylenol, please."

"Ms. Sybil, are you feeling okay?"

"Why, I feel fine. Thank you." She smiled big, batting her blue eyes.

"What do you need the Tylenol for, then, sweet lady?" I asked with a matching smile.

"Because I want one." Her voice was almost shrill.

"Yes, ma'am, I understand that. I'm simply trying to find out where you hurt so I can make a note and follow up to make sure the Tylenol was effective. That's all." I shrugged.

"Missy? Rue got a Tylenol, so I want a Tylenol!" Sybil snapped. "If she gets a Tylenol, I should get one, too!" Then, quickly regaining her self-control, she added, "I would appreciate it so much." She clasped her hands and lay them in her lap, suddenly revealing her halo.

"Coming up." I smiled, handing her a tiny cup with two Tylenol. She, too, swallowed them and handed me the cup with the remaining water. Then off she rolled toward her room as I turned the other way and rolled my eyes, laughing quietly to release the built up...love, which felt more like extreme annoyance right at that moment.

We're all kids until the day we part from this world. They say that as we age, we become more exaggerated versions of ourselves, more "fully realized." I say that if that's the case, look out, world! I probably won't demand anything just because someone else got it, but I'm going to be a handful! That, I can promise. In fact, while discussing my preferences just this morning, specifically regarding my later years, my daughter said, "Oh Lord, you *aging* is not going to be fun."

"Oh, I beg to differ." I laughed. "I plan to have a ball!"

The Twilight Trio:

"Who's going to take us out to smoke?" Sila (pronounced Silla) asked in her "I'm about to go off if you don't take us quick" tone.

Both floor nurses were working diligently on their rounds and a load of admissions. Nurse aids were scattered down the hallways, helping people, or they were scattered to the winds, helping themselves. But I knew well that the smokers were not one bit concerned about the possible excess of the nurses' workloads, nor were they worried about the priority level of what the nurses were doing at the moment. Smoke time was an unbending, undelayable, and undeniable *priority*.

Zola, Sila's nurse, glanced up from her paperwork, frantically scanning the hallways for an aid as frustration and desperation washed over her face. "Gimme just a few minutes, Ms. Sila, and I'll find somebody to take y'all out." She sighed.

Always so polite, and a darn good little nurse, I thought to myself before speaking.

"I got this, Zola," I offered. "I'll just sit away from the smoke. It won't kill me to take them out one time, will it?" I grinned.

"Oh, thank you, girl! I didn't know who I was gonna get to go, but I was gonna get somebody, or…well, you know." Zola cast a wide-eyed, sideways glance at Sila, who was tapping her foot irritably, her mood escalating rapidly.

Lorene sat quietly and waited. Both she and Sila were full-blooded Indian. But Lorene? Lorene couldn't deny her Indian heritage even if she was goofy enough to try. All the lady needed was feathers, and she could have starred in a cowboys and Indians remake. I told her so one day. Having lost one leg to diabetes, Lorene replied, quick as spit, "Better put me on a horse in every scene unless you want to cowboy up my wheelchair, or, in my case, I guess it would be Indian up." She'd laughed. Lorene was easy.

Sila? Sila was purely delightful and cute as a button provided every-thing was going precisely as she desired, anticipated, expected, and often demanded. As soon as it wasn't? Her Indian heritage came charging down the warpath! One could see it in her eyes, hear it in her voice, and almost smell the smoke from her fire. As a matter of fact, Sila had a traditional Cherokee name: "Atsila," meaning fire, which suited her perfectly.

"Head on down the hall, ladies. I'll meet you at the door," I called over my shoulder as I went to gather the ladies' lockboxes, knowing each kept their own key. I grabbed Carmela's while I was at it, fully aware that she'd come waddling down the hallway with her walker any minute. Carmela, like me, was always late everywhere she went, but also like me, she was consistent. In my humble, frequently voiced opinion, that very consistency is indicative of our reliability. The world simply has a habit of rushing the day, making it appear that we are late.

During every other designated smoke time throughout the day, there would be a fairly large group gathered at the end of the hall. However, at the last break of the day, it was only the twilight trio, as I'd come to think of the three.

Whirling around the counter of the nurses' station, I trotted off down the hallway to open the end door for Sila and Lorene. After backing them down the ramp in their wheelchairs, one at a time, I handed them their lockboxes.

"There comes Carmy," Lorene announced quietly.

I glanced up, and there she was, illuminated by the light, waddling toward us down the hallway. Hurrying up the ramp, I met Carmella at the door, then walked her down and took her out to the covered smoking area while she chattered nonstop about all the things going on in her world. Carmella had somehow gotten it in her head, when I first started working there, that I was a doctor. Having grown weary of correcting and explaining, I simply became "the doctor" where Carmella was concerned.

"Look at'chu," she exclaimed, her accent still thick with Spanish. "The doc-tor taking us out to smoke!" She beamed as she waddled on.

"Gives me an excuse to play hooky from work for a little while." I nudged her amiably with my elbow, and she giggled delightedly.

Carmella sat on the picnic bench, facing the other ladies, and I made sure everyone was lit up. Then I made my way over to the far picnic table, away from the impending cloud of acrid smoke. Climbing up to sit on the table, I pulled my cell phone out of my pocket to kill time. Sitting atop the table, my elbows on my knees, I played on my phone, occasionally glancing up toward the shadows to ensure nobody was in flames or about to hit the ground for some bizarre reason. One never knows in the world of the independently dependent.

A small raucous of laughter caught my attention. Looking up, though I couldn't see faces or details, I could easily tell which shadow was who. Lorene sat with her back to me, the three of them forming a small triangle. Had Lorene turned her head, I could have easily seen her face illuminated by the guard light just behind me, but they weren't paying me any attention whatsoever.

The picture of the three shadows, just three girls laughing in the twilight, captured my gaze, touching my heart. Their voices were muffled, but their laughter carried far through the stilled quiet of the night.

I watched as Lorene leaned forward in her chair, Sila's arm suddenly flailing in full animation of something unheard as Carmella threw her head back with a burst of laughter.

"We should!" I heard Sila exclaim.

The shadows' heads nodded vigorously.

"Ahhh, yes! No doubt abou-that!" Carmella exclaimed.

Their voices muffled once again, but Sila continued talking in full animation about *something* the three clearly found engrossing.

"I'm telling you, we *should!*" Sila's voice rang out loud and crystal clear.

"We aren't bothering anybody," Lorene added more softly than Sila but crystal clear! "And we are perfectly safe out here," she finished, spreading her arms out to her sides in demonstration of the "here."

"And nobody is burning themselves up with their cigar-ette," Carmella chimed in. "That's what they always say." She chuckled as if the very idea were purely ridiculous.

The shadows pealed with laughter.

Thrusting herself forward again, Sila insisted, "Some of them aids are younger than my grandchildren!"

"Don't flatter yourself, old woman," Lorene chortled. "They're younger than your great-grandchildren."

I thought I might have to do CPR the shadows laughed so hard.

Catching her breath once more, Lorene announced, "We should band together and rebel! Roll right up to that front office and demand our freedom to come out and smoke anytime we want to!" She raised her fist into the air.

"We're not kids!" Sila threw her fist into the air.

"Yes, adults! No shildren!" Carmella's tiny fist shot up into the air as well.

"We grown! We got this!" I shouted from my seat on the picnic table, thrusting my fist into the air as each of them had done.

All three shadows turned my way, once again exploding into laughter. I thought for a hot minute that little roly-poly Carmella might tumble right on over the edge of that bench as she leaned sideways to brace herself with her free hand while she roared.

"Tha doc-tor is something else!" She laughed, shaking her head.

A few seconds later Lorene reached down to unlock her wheelchair, and Sila and Carmy recognized the familiar sign that it was time to go inside.

I pushed Sila and Lorene back up the ramp in their wheelchairs, one at a time, assisting each just inside the door, then turned back to assist Carmella.

As I headed back down the ramp, she gazed up at me with enormous chocolate-brown eyes that sparkled mischievously as another smile spread across her face, its very plumpness smoothing the wrinkles of time from her olive skin.

Smiling myself, I fell in behind her at the bottom of the ramp. Grasping the handles of her walker, Carmella began waddling up, chattering incessantly, her ever-voluminous, thick Spanish accent challenging the silence of the moon with every waddle.

Instinct had me spreading my hands out protectively behind her as I slowly followed, frequently glancing down at her tiny red tennis shoes to check her gait. My gaze then returned to the back of her little head. Her cropped brown hair, still rich with the darkness of youth, denying her years, bounced in unison with her ever-dramatic chatter.

My heart suddenly overflowing with genuine love and affection, I impulsively reached down and tickled Carmella's ribcage, immediately spreading my arms again.

Carmella squealed and wiggled, threw her head back, her face to the sky, and giggled like a teenage girl. I, too, raised my face as the magical sound of her laughter tinkled musically through the twilight, causing the blanket of stars to twinkle ever more brightly against the velvet black of the night sky.

Forcing myself from my reverie, I helped Carmella through the doorway. Then, side by side, we proceeded up the hallway.

"Pssssst."

Carmella giggled. "Wha wus *that?*" she asked, glancing at me.

"I don't know." I laughed. "Doctors don't know *everything*. Let's find out!"

"Les do! But shhhhh." She placed a tiny finger to her lips. "People are sleeping," she reminded me in a thundering whisper.

I couldn't help smiling at the irony.

"Psssssst," we heard again, louder this time, and from somewhere behind us.

Turning my head, I saw Lorene peeping one eye around the doorframe of her room, her wheelchair and leg barely visible as she motioned for us to come.

"Come on, Carmella. It's Lorene," I whispered conspiratorially.

"Oh good! Lez go see what she wants," Carmy whispered in reply.

I followed Carmella's waddle, and we entered Lorene's room only to find Mary, Lorene's roommate, and Sila with her, waiting for us amidst a pile of deliciously carby snacks and sodas.

"Whaz all this?" Carmella asked excitedly.

"We're having a slumber party," Sila announced. "And nobody can stop us."

"Come on in! Y'all can sit on my bed." Lorene smiled.

Deciding to forget diagnoses and simply let them relish the moment, I sat down and asked for the Reese's Cup I had spied at the edge of the pile.

The nurses might just have to give a bit more insulin than usual come morning, I thought, my heart warm as I glanced about the room, seeing girls with gray hair and wrinkles laughing and talking, eyes wide with pure delight.

After all, what is life, really, without slumber parties? I thought, reaching for a soda.

"She said he held her hand in church last week." Sila grinned around the bobby pin between her teeth as she pulled back her braids, then began pinning them atop her usually hot little head.

"Wait." I raised a finger into the air. "I missed that! Who held whose hand? Do tell!" I giggled, ripping into my Reese's.

While driving home later, it struck me that the shadows were truly… ageless. The wrinkles, gray hair, and handicaps were all cloaked in the darkness, leaving nothing but the delightful spirits within, the pearls inside the shells. We should see the shadows more often.

The Prom King:

Gilmer had big, puppy-dog brown eyes and long, sweeping eyelashes. Even at eighty-two, age had only etched lines into his still handsome face, and the ladies noticed. Oh, I could tell you some stories about the ladies! Maybe I will someday. *But for now, poor ole Gilmer: lost as a goose, old-fashioned to his core, still devoted to his late wife, and yet … still in high demand with the ladies.* Bless his heart. I mean that as sincerely as one can possibly mean anything. Gilmer could *not* escape the ladies, and Gilmer had *not* a *clue* as to what the heck the ladies wanted.

Gilmer leaned politely forward in his wheelchair so he could better hear whichever lady was giving him attention at the moment, his brow creasing as he struggled to understand what she was trying to communicate. Ultimately, I watched his brows raise in acceptance of, and maybe even preference for, blissful ignorance. He'd smile nicely at the lady, then glance over at me and shrug.

One evening Marcel got a wild hair. In her demented state, she decided she wanted Gilmer to be her man, in every sense of the word. I ran across the situation while checking the pre-dinner blood sugars. Hearing a tussle of bumping and banging behind me, I turned around and observed Marcel clumsily crashing her wheelchair through Gilmer's doorway, intent on reaching his side.

I closed and locked my cart, hurrying to make sure all was well. But all was far from well. I knocked, which is something Marcel had demonstrated no interest in doing, and walked in. Gilmer was sitting in his recliner, his brown eyes as big as half dollars, his mouth gaping! Glancing up, he realized it was me, and relief flooded his face.

I stifled a giggle. "Ms. Marcel, this is Gilmer's room. Your room is down the other hallway. Come with me, and I'll show you where it is."

"Well, I know whose room this is. That's why I'm in here." Marcel proclaimed the obvious.

"Yes, ma'am, well, Gilmer wants to be alone in his room... by himself, I think." I glanced at Gilmer, who now looked more confused than ever.

"I want to be alone in his room with him," Marcel announced. "So you may go now." She wheeled herself closer to Gilmer's knees. "We need privacy."

Gilmer looked up at me, purely panic-stricken, nearly falling as he tried to scramble up from that recliner.

"Whoa!" I hurried over to stop him. "Sit back down. It's okay!" I could not help laughing.

I cannot give you the details of what Marcel proceeded to announce she wanted, but I can tell you that, without a doubt, I had no choice but to take her chair and assist her out of Gilmer's room quickly and in a hurry, as Gilmer sat oscillating between horror and confusion.

I did not want to tell Marcel's daughter what she'd said, but her daughter insisted. When I told her, she gasped, then shrieked with laughter. "Mother would lay down and die of humiliation if she knew she'd said such things out loud."

Regardless of it all, I am here to tell you that I spent the remainder of the evening saving Gilmer. I had to push his wheelchair with one hand and pull my cart with the other all evening. Marcel was a determined woman. At one point I had to wheel Gilmer down one hallway to lead Marcel, cut through the dining room before she could see us, and then hurry back up another hallway to throw Marcel off the path. Gilmer would look at me with wide eyes and shrug, clueless one minute, wise to Marcel the next, then back to clueless, as his recall and comprehension were as rare, brief, and/or about as effective as an August breeze.

Long story short, Marcel's daughter had to take Marcel home. Marcel never got over her...desires, and her daughter was concerned about placing Marcel anywhere. So she took her home and hired help.

Phyllis was thrilled to find that her competition was gone. She took Marcel's spot in the Gilmer chase. Phyllis was fully ambulatory, even more determined, and so much more successful. It's strange. Minds that cannot recall pertinent things—even minds that digress to the point that effective use of simple words becomes near impossible—still remember desires without fail, even when the mind no longer recalls how to properly manage said desires. More on Phyllis and poor ole Gilmer in a later chapter. I promise. I will add this, though: Phyllis and Gilmer won Prom King and Queen at the Senior Citizens Prom, which is held at a different facility each year. Phyllis preened over it for months. She hung the picture of them that she'd cut from the local newspaper on the lobby wall. Poor Gilmer could not recall that he'd ever even attended the prom, except those moments when Phyllis pushed his wheelchair to the lobby and pointed their picture out to remind him that he was, no doubt, her man. "We're a couple." I heard Phyllis say, "After all, the proof is in the picture."

Puzzling Puzzle:

"I want it back!" Mozell stated emphatically. "I worked hard on that puzzle. I bought it and put it together for my daughter, Shezell. I was going to shellac it and frame it for her birthday, and I just insist that you find out who took it. I'm just not going to let this thing go, I promise you that." She crossed her pudgier than pudgy arms, lifting her chins defiantly.

"Mozell, I have no clue who would have done such a thing," Jackie implored from the other side of her desk. "But please know I am truly sorry, and I'm going to do everything I can to find it for you."

Mozell huffed, "You certainly better," then backed her wheelchair out into the front lobby, glaring at me as she rolled off down the hallway.

Jackie, the administrator, looked at me helplessly. "Who would do such a thing?"

"I have no clue." I shook my head and stepped into her office, still struggling to stifle a giggle after hearing "Shezell." "She's been working on that thing for over a month!" I grinned. "For Shezell. She was going to shellac it for Shezell. Shazam!" I could contain myself no longer, and my laughter pealed through the lobby and likely down each hallway.

"Stop it!" Jackie grinned, slapping her hand over her mouth.

Two days later Mr. Trey demanded, "I want to see somebody right this minute about my slippers! They were there next to my bed when I laid down for my nap. I wake up? No slippers! I can't get out of bed without my slippers!" He jutted his whiskered chin and closed his golden-brown eyes to emphasize his adamancy.

Before Luke reached the desk to call Jackie down to the unit, Hazel stomped up. That lady was ninety-one years old and could still do the splits on the therapist's mat. The therapist had to help her up, but she got down in a full split all by herself.

"Somebody took my little squirrel! I just know it was that aid. She was always talkin' about how purty it is. I want it back!"

Now, mind you, we all talked about how pretty Hazel's squirrel was, because if you didn't mention it, Hazel was offended. The first time I met Hazel, I started walking back out of her room when she suddenly shouted, "I guess you didn't notice my beautiful little squirrel! You sure didn't say anything about it!"

I had turned, quickly scanning the room until I spotted the object of my unintended offense: a tiny pink ceramic squirrel with emerald eyes, ruby lips, and a cubic zirconia bedazzled tail. How I missed the gawdy little creature was what amazed me!

At that point we had a missing puzzle, slippers, and a squirrel within just three days. *Strange*, I thought.

The next day Mr. Trey still refused to get out of bed. Shoes would not do. He was not getting out of his bed until he had his slippers. Jackie surrendered to the madness by going out and buying him a new pair.

"They aren't like my slippers," Mr. Trey grumbled. "But since you haven't found the robber yet, I'll wear the ugly things."

The following Monday, the unit was in an uproar, the nurses exasperated.

"Five more patients have things missing, including Joan's phone," Jen whispered. "They all want locks put on their doors."

"Well, locks aren't allowed. It's a safety issue," Jackie said to no one in particular.

Her palms in the air, Jen replied, "Hey, don't tell me. Tell them!" She pointed at the activity room, where a large group of residents were gathered.

Jackie and I tiptoed to the open doorway.

"So I think we all need to work together here," we heard little Ms. Nicole say. "Do any of you have anything valuable in your room?"

"All my stuff is valuable!" normally sweet Gabe professed irritably.

Nicole (aka Nikki) grinned. "We know, Gabe. Of course, it is. All of it. But do any of you have anything in your room that cost a lot of money? Or anything that means something special to you?" Gabe wasn't at all offended. Everybody loved little Nikki and her enormous, vivid, hazel eyes; plump, rosy cheeks; contagious smile; and inexhaustible energy.

"I have a diamond tennis bracelet that I keep in my bedside drawer," Ada said anxiously. "On my goodness, if anything happens to it, I'll just lay right down and die!"

Interrupting, Joseph proclaimed, "I've got some high-dollar baseball cards hidden under my socks. I'll whup somebody's backside if those come up missing."

Jackie stepped into the room, encouraging everyone to take anything valuable to the office immediately so that it could be locked up and protected while we solved the mystery.

Nobody budged. They all insisted that they wanted to keep their things right where they were.

Jackie begged, explained, and reasoned for half an hour, but still no one budged. In fact, Mr. Raynard, who rarely spoke at all to anyone for any reason, said, "Why don't you stop asking us to lock our things away and start finding the thief who's taking them? Lock them away." He finished in more of a grumbling mumble.

As slippery as soap, the thief struck again and again. By the end of that week, the thief had taken every single item that had been mentioned in the group, and then some. The person even took Odis's favorite book about trains. Odis loved him some trains! Odis was hot!

But that was our first break. Odis's book was the only large item that had been taken, and it would be difficult to hide. However, try as we might, we could not find that book or any of the other missing items.

Our second break was in fact a clue, but we missed it at the time. We went an entire five days and nights without a thing coming up missing! We'd almost convinced ourselves that everyone had simply misplaced their missing items, that they'd show up eventually, until Becky reminded us that Mozell would never have disassembled her puzzle. So we were back to square one.

Taking every precaution possible, Jackie called an all-staff meeting, informed staff of the situation, and asked them to be on the lookout for the missing items.

Everybody's nerves were on edge by that point, even my own.

Later that evening the facility sweetheart returned from a pass with her daughter. I helped Nikki settle back in, appreciating the pleasant distraction.

"Nikki, why do you have all these things piled on your bedside table?" I laughed. "You can't even use the table!"

I hung Nikki's clothes while she busily unpacked her personal care items and put them in the bathroom.

Thinking we were finished, I suggested we head for the dining room, but Nikki began fixing everything really quickly, taking random hangers from the closet and turning the clothing items around so that, once completed, all of her clothing and hangers hung facing the same direction.

"Oh, okay, miss OCD." I chuckled as I followed Nikki from her room, then walked with her to the dining room, where she joined her friends and tablemates. Everyone smiled, delighted to see her coming, as she hurried across the large room.

Back in my office I dug into paperwork. A mental image of Nikki's cluttered bedside table repeatedly popped into my head, followed by a mental replay of her "fixing" her closet. Eventually, I realized what was niggling me was that one simply contradicted the other. Finally, too restless to focus on my paperwork, I stood and ultimately found myself standing in Nikki's doorway, staring at the clutter on her bedside table. I then noticed that the table sat a bit lopsided, which stuck out like a sore thumb next to her meticulously made bed, so I walked over to straighten it.

"Dang, it's heavy." I shoved and heard something thump the wall. Glancing behind the table to make sure I hadn't knocked anything off, I saw the book *Trains and More Trains* leaning against the wall.

"No way!" My hand flew to my mouth as I hurried out of the room, leaving the book and table right where they were. I went straight to my office to think.

A short while later Nikki passed my open doorway as she returned from the dining room.

"Hey, little OCD Queen, want me to help you clean off that table?"

Nikki stopped, turned back, and stepped into my office, her eyes filling with tears as she hurried in, slamming the door behind her. "May I talk to you for a minute?"

"Whoa there, it's okay!" I laughed. "Here, sit down and talk." I pulled a chair close and patted the seat.

"I took them, all the things!" Nikki cried, tears rolling down her cheeks.

Handing her a Kleenex, I watched her expression transform from genuinely distressed to just as genuinely determined.

"Some of them act like they're already dead! I just wanted to give them their fight back. I thought they'd get feisty and hunt their things down. I sure would! But they're just grumbling, and Trey wasn't even going to get out of bed!" Frustrated, she threw her hands in the air.

"Nikki, how could you destroy Mozell's puzzle? She worked so hard on that thing!"

"Oh! I know!" Her eyes grew wide. "That was an accident! I had gone in to check her progress. Oh my, she did a good job! It was beautiful. But then a loud noise in the hallway startled me. I jumped and knocked the card table over, and the puzzle slid off the table into a million pieces. I didn't know what else to do, so I scooped up the pieces and hurried back to my room. I was going to put it back together for her, but I can't figure out how to do it without anyone catching me. Please help me!" Her eyes filled with tears again.

After mulling this over, it made sense. Except for Hazel's squirrel, every other item had been taken from an individual who seemed to have just given up, making no effort to live or enjoy life.

As if reading my mind, Nikki spouted, "Oh yeah, Hazel's squirrel. That one was just because Hazel is so arrogant about the tacky little thing. I know, I know, it doesn't make it right. But, truth is, I was heading back to my room one night and remembered how she'd treated poor old

Henry at dinner. Next thing you know, I was stuffing that ugly squirrel in my drawer with the other things. Maybe I didn't have such a great idea, after all." She looked at the floor.

"Ya think?"

Nikki didn't look up.

"Okay, I'll talk to Jackie, and tomorrow we'll hold a unit meeting. You be thinking of what you want to say and how you're going to say it."

Nikki hugged me, long and tight. "Thank you for helping me even though I did a dumb thing," she whispered into my shoulder. "Okay, a reeeeally dumb thing." She snickered as she bobbled out.

The next day after lunch, I had the aids gather everyone who wasn't bed-bound into the activity room. Nikki straight up told them what she'd done and why. She looked at Hazel and said, "Except for your squirrel. I took that to teach you how it feels for somebody to be mean to you, like you were mean to Henry that day in the dining room. But I was wrong"—this appeared to take great effort—"and I apologize. I was wrong, but you're meaner than a rattlesnake, old woman! Okay." She sighed dramatically. "I'm sorry." Then she rolled her eyes again, grunting in pure exasperation. "But it's the truth. Mean as a rattlesnake! Own it!"

The room erupted with laughter! Had I closed my eyes, I'd have easily been back to the junior high school cafeteria, when Raymond Jeffrey randomly jumped up onto the table and mooned the principal! His buddy Steve jumped back wildly and pointed at Raymond's butt, yelling, "Dookie smear!" The cafeteria went wild with laughter, just as the activity room was right that minute.

Ole "Rattlesnake" finally stopped laughing long enough to skip over and hug Henry before sticking her tongue out at Nikki. Hazel grinned smugly, retrieved her precious squirrel from the table of stolen goods, and went over to show it off to the new guy, Sam, who appeared to be purely delighted that he'd found a place where everybody was still breathing. He was obviously less enthused about Hazel's beloved squirrel. She insisted he hold it, so he did. "Look how beautiful it is," Hazel demanded. "You can say so. We all know it's beautiful," she gloated.

Sam stared intently at the squirrel, then whispered almost reverently, "Ooooooh my, I owe my last wife an apology. I told her she was the tackiest decorator ever born. I got a feeling you top her." He chuckled as he handed Hazel her squirrel, then looked up at her. "I bet your husband died on purpose."

Old Habits Die Hard:

Remember "Crackers"? Crackers is Clinton, and Clinton was a perv. No two ways about it. He was a "good ole boy," the type my brother would call "a bubba." He was a truck-driving, beer-drinking, tail-chasing "Bubba" back in his day. Clinton had eight sons, whom we can only hope didn't pick up their daddy's philandering ways. As you know from his previous story, Clinton also had a wife, a devoted one.

As I talked with Clinton again about keeping his hands off the female staff, he said, "Well, they shouldn't dress like that. They're asking for it."

"Asking for what?"

"To be grabbed, of course!"

"Of course. So how should *they* dress?"

"Well, with their blouses up to here." He drew a line across the base of his neck with his pudgy old finger. "That way they're breasts aren't hanging all out, making us want to touch them, of course." He demonstrated massive breasts with his hands.

"Making you. Of course." I smiled. "That's about the most ridiculous, immature, antiquated, chauvinistic, and downright ignorant excuse for 'reasoning' that I've heard in a long time, my friend." I chuckled. "Keep your hands off the staff. Period. Please and thank you." I looked him in the eye, smiled, walked out of his room.

The office handled it the same as always. They held another meeting with Clinton. I rolled my eyes. I felt certain it was handled most professionally and ineffectively. But you know, dementia, natural desires, rights, and census entered the clouded, though clear, picture.

One crazy afternoon, with everything imaginable going on and going wrong, Clinton took full advantage of the chaos. I caught him sitting in his wheelchair, cozied up next to Ms. Flora, who, at any other time, he'd have had nothing to do with. His left hand was on the arm of her chair, just an inch away from her right breast. His face told *all* as he peered around to make certain no one was looking. Then his eyes met mine where I stood watching from behind the nurses' station. His chin dropped, his eyes popped open wide, and his face turned ten shades of red as he jerked his hand back, fast as lightning; so fast that he bumped himself in the chin.

I laughed, shook my head, and pointed for him to remove himself from Flora's side. Honestly, Flora would probably have liked it. She, too, talked of sex quite often. She missed "all the good stuff" she "used to enjoy." Flora wanted to "go dancing" and "bring home a man" as much as Clinton wanted to grab some boobs. But Flora's daughter and Clinton's wife wouldn't have liked it at all. Clinton slumped away, glaring sideways at me as he passed, then disappeared down the hallway, going back toward his room. One thing was for certain: If I hadn't caught him, and Flora hadn't liked it, Clinton would have thought he'd stuck his old hand right into a hornet's nest! I can picture it now. Flora's legs may have completely failed her, but her arms still worked mighty fine.

The phone ringing incessantly, admissions arriving, behind on my first round, I was drowning. The world of nursing consumed me, and yet I still picked up on...something. Something was persistently niggling me as I spun in a thousand different directions, doing a thousand different things for a thousand different people all at once. Suddenly unable to deny it any longer, I stopped amidst the madness. Turning in a slow circle, I gazed around, and there it was. The niggling became a knowing.

There, lurking in the shadows behind the row of wheelchairs to the side, where my defenseless angels were sitting, I saw the top of an old white head as it peered over a narrow shoulder. A large, sleeved arm reaching stealthily around a tiny, half-bare arm, and a large, old hand spread out like a vulture's claw about to grab dinner.

"Freeze!" I yelled.

The old fart literally ducked his head and hid, his hand slithering backward like a snake. He hid from me like a child caught in the cookie jar, ducking behind the counter.

I just stood and waited him out, knowing his arthritis and bad temper would flare long before my patience gave out. And I was right.

His head rose up in the shadows, and his facial expression was flashing between anger, guilt, frustration, and indignance.

I watched as he backed his wheelchair out, methodically turned it toward the lobby, rolled himself past me with his chin set high, and proceeded to his room. Then I followed and found him sitting in his chair facing the door, fully aware that this was far from over.

"Clinton, what on earth were you trying to do out there today?"

"You know exactly what I was trying to do, and I'd have done it if you would just do your job and stop watching what I'm doing," he said indignantly.

"I'm well aware of that. That is the problem and the very reason I watch you. So what, pray tell, is little Ms. Alice wearing that *made* you want to grab her breasts? I mean, her top comes up to her neck. That seems to destroy your theory of that being the *cause* of your behavior, right?"

I waited, but he just sat staring at me in silence.

"So, do you realize how completely defenseless she is? Of course you do. Do you realize what her family would do to you should they ever find out that you even attempted such a thing? That little lady is a prim and proper retired librarian. She was married faithfully to the same man for sixty-two years, and you will respect her. You took it way too far this time, my friend."

Clinton interrupted angrily, saying, "Well, my wife isn't healthy enough to be interested anymore. I mean, I don't want to make her feel bad about it, but I still have desires."

"So how would you feel if some old dude groped your wife?"

His face turned fire-engine red. "That's different!"

"I'm not even going to stand here and try to reason with you." I laughed. "You are completely unreasonable. You best remember that even old men go to prison. I don't like you right this minute, but I love you, and I'd hate to see your stupidity land you in prison for the rest of your life. I'm going to say this, just between you and me."

He cocked his head, fear having peaked his interest.

"Your 'desires' are between you and your wife. I suggest you speak with her about that, because one more time, Clinton, and I'm speaking to her."

Clinton blew a proverbial fuse. I briefly worried about his possibly having a stroke from being angry, or scared, or, more likely, both. Then I decided that was between Clinton and the good Lord.

I stood there and listened to him rant about how I better not say a word to his wife, that it was none of my business. According to him, he wasn't hurting anybody, boobs were supposed to be grabbed, it was natural for a man to want to touch breasts, and his wife didn't deserve to have to hear that kind of thing, as it would hurt her.

"You finished?"

"Yes!" he barked.

"Good. That's a bunch of bunk, except for one thing."

"What's that?"

"You're right. Your wife doesn't deserve to have to hear that kind of thing. In fact, she doesn't deserve to have a husband who would do that kind of thing. So be the man she thinks you are. Regardless, you're lucky I'm not singing like a canary right this minute. What you almost did was molestation. I best not see you anywhere near these ladies, or even hear that you might have been. Do not make the mistake of thinking that I'm kidding. I'm not. And I think you know me well enough by now to know that. Do not put these defenseless ladies in harm's way. There is no second chance here. Not only will I tell your wife, Clinton, but I'll also tell the authorities." I turned and walked out.

Clinton was a different man. Finally, a "meeting" had proven effective. In fact, Clinton went out of his way to keep a distance from every female resident in the building. Not a word was ever spoken about the incident again.

Strangely, I did get a random thank-you gift from Clinton's wife, though she wouldn't tell me what she was thanking me for. All she said was, "For putting up with Clinton and being my friend."

One evening I went to Clinton's room to assess him. I'd noticed him coughing during dinner, and it was a hard, persistent, wet-sounding cough. I wanted to listen to his lung sounds. I knocked on his door and walked in. He was sitting on the side of his bed, and motioned for me to sit, so I sat on the chair next to his bed.

"How you feeling?"

"Not so good." He coughed as he spoke.

His forehead felt warm, so I checked his temperature. He had a fever of 100.9.

"Let me listen to your lungs. That cough sounds bad." I reached my stethoscope around and placed it against Clinton's back. After listening to every lobe, I started to sit back down to inform Clinton of what I'd heard. Before my behind hit the seat, Clinton reached his hand out toward my chest.

"What on earth do you think you're doing?" I cried, dodging his hand and shaking my head. "I told you to keep your hands to yourself."

"I just wanted to touch that listening thing there around your neck, that's all." Clinton grinned like a devilish child. "You didn't say I couldn't touch you; you said the staff and the ladies."

"Good grief, even feverish and sick, you're still a perv." I laughed. "Dude, keep your hands to yourself. Don't touch any female besides your wife. You hear me?"

"Yeah." He pouted. "You just killed a sick old man's last hope."

"Oh my, a drama king." I rolled my eyes. "Let me go call the doctor and get you well."

"You said not to touch the defenseless ladies," he hollered behind me. "You're far from defenseless. You're tough as nails." He chuckled... coughed.

I could have fun going on forever about this topic, but for the sake of time, I won't.

My point is that our elderly are just kids with wrinkles. Just the same as we are just kids with kids. We all reach an age when we are "us," and though our bodies age and our minds learn more, we remain "us."

Our elderly are still very much alive. They simply need someone to help them *live* again.

Helping Hands

Lewis:

Lewis arrived about at eight-thirty in the evening on Thursday, looking a bit weary that his next stop had turned out to be yet another facility instead of home. He was a quiet man who was recovering from a bad case of pneumonia, which still appeared to be a bit difficult for him to accept, but he settled in and did his therapy to regain his strength, never complaining.

I was asked to take a look at Lewis, as his family had reported in his care plan meeting that morning that his blood pressure had been running high.

His family *reported?* I thought. *Absolutely, I'll check him out now.*

The first thing I did, quite naturally, was look at his blood pressure record and medications. Lewis had been with us at that point for fourteen days. He'd started out with 126/74. That was so good that if he could have bottled it, he could have sold it like hotcakes. But the second day it started to rise, and by the fourth day Lewis was running toward stroke level with 181/90. Before his family spoke up, his blood pressure had gotten as high as 182/110.

Now, in my humble opinion, it's far from rocket science. Think on this:

Lewis's family had to mention it for anybody to consider it at all. (That's just wrong. The nurse should have caught it. What if Lewis had no family? Many do not. And how did the family know? Who told the family but no one else?)

- All Lewis's blood pressure readings were first thing in the morning, taken by the medication aid before he got his medications. (This tells me that the nurse used the medication aid's reading for her notes. Thus, she never actually assessed the guy, and she knew the extreme highs yet never followed up to ensure the blood pressure had come down.)

— Hurrying down the hall to see Lewis, I checked his blood pressure and heart rate. His blood pressure, at eleven-eighteen in the morning, three to four hours after his medication, was 156/94. I talked with Lewis, who clearly informed me about his blood pressure history and how he had taken his medications at home. He denied having chest pain and headaches but said he had been experiencing "some dizziness here and there".

Lewis was a sweet, easy-going guy, but I could see the edge of desperation on his face. I could hear the edge of frustration in his tone when he said, "I've been telling the nurses all of this."

"Lewis, I'm sorry. I really don't know what else to say." I reached out to shake his hand. "But I'm going to change your medications to the way you took them at home right now, and we probably need to talk to your doctor so we get an increase in your Norvasc or something similar, at least for the time being."

Ultimately, his doctor agreed and doubled Lewis's Norvasc. I changed his medicine regimen so that he took one of his blood pressure medications in the morning and one in the evening, which was how he'd taken them at home. I informed Lewis and his family that his elevated blood pressure might resolve once his life began returning to normal, so it would need to be monitored closely. I added an order for the nurse to check Lewis's blood pressure every six hours for fourteen days, making certain his blood pressure would be monitored and addressed, as changes could occur.

Little did I know.

The next day, Wanda, Lewis's nurse for the day, waddled over to me and ceremoniously, with an enormous smile on her pot-stirring face, said, "Therapy said Lewis's blood pressure is low today. I don't know why you got his medicine increased. His blood pressure been fine every day. I checked it myself, and it's low."

"Well, Wanda, when I checked it yesterday, a few hours after his meds, it was still a little high for comfort, and he had the remainder of the day and night for it to go back up even more," I explained. "Additionally, according to the documented record of readings, which, by the way, indicates only the aid has been taking Lewis's blood pressure, it's been at stroke level ten out of fourteen days. Furthermore, Lewis's family expressed concerns in his care plan meeting regarding his persistently elevated blood pressure, and Lewis told me that he's been telling the nurses he's having dizzy spells, and his blood pressure meds aren't being given right."

"Oh." Her eyes popped open, and her full lips smashed together as she snapped her mouth shut.

"You nurses need to monitor it closely, Wanda. It may well come down as he gets closer to knowing he's going home."

Icing on the sugarless cake, Wanda never said a word, but Lewis had been told that very morning that he was going to be discharged home the following day, on Saturday. Having been constantly called all over the facility, it was late that evening before I had time to think more on Lewis. Therapy was long gone. So Monday morning, as soon as I arrived, I sought out a therapist to get further details on Lewis's blood pressure. Dee, the therapist, informed me Lewis had been discharged on Saturday. Dee further informed me that she'd read the nurse notes. One note stated that Lewis's blood pressure was low at 97/54, and the very next note said *discharged home.* "Yeah," Dee said, shaking her head. "Discharged home. Nothing more. And that man is active. He's up doing things all the time, cooks for himself and everything."

"Crap! He's at high risk of dropping to the floor! I've got to call him now! Thanks, Dee!" I hurried to the phone to call Lewis. But Lewis didn't answer. Lewis was back in the hospital with a broken hip and a torn rotator cuff, which had resulted from a fall at home, secondary to hypotension.

Etta:

I passed Etta in the hallway just yesterday as she sat in her wheelchair, waiting to go outside to smoke a cigarette. Etta was wearing a powder-pink, rooftop-sleeved t-shirt that read, *I'm not listening because I don't care.*

"Etta, I love that t-shirt!" I laughed. "And it's perfectly pink!"

"Yeah." Etta chuckled quietly. "My boyfriend gave it to me for my birthday. He said I should just roll my eyes and point at it when them aids tell me I can do something for myself and won't help me to the bathroom."

My mind flashed back to about a month before, when Etta's son and daughter-in-law stood and peered over the high counter of the nurses' station at Etta's nurse, expressing concern that Etta was always told she didn't need help and could do for herself. Etta's son, Denny, let his wife, Kelly, do the talking. No surprise there, right?

Kelly said, "Etta has multiple sclerosis, and sometimes she can do for herself, but sometimes she can't. That's the only reason she's here."

In fact, I overheard Kelly discussing this with several different nurses on several different occasions, and on the most recent occasion, Kelly had said, "If it doesn't get better, we'll take her out of here." That stuck with me, as I had thought, *Bless your hearts. It's the same everywhere.*

Etta jerked me from my daze.

"I get all the help I need now!" She kicked her head back and laughed. "I just tell them I'm gonna tell you if they give me any problems!"

"I'm not at all sure what that says about me, Etta." I laughed and shrugged. "But as long as you get your help!"

"Says you care," Etta mumbled.

"Okay, yeah, let's leave it at that." I chuckled as I hurried on my way.

Charlotte:

"She don't want to get a shower. She said no, and I can't make her," Jessie said again.

"Jessie, you have to try. Be creative. I can almost promise you that if I go down there and put forth a little effort, be a little creative, I can persuade Charlotte to take her shower. But that's your job. You aids suggest a shower, probably making it sound like the worst thing imaginable, then run to the nurse spouting that the resident refuses. If you think about it, that rather indicates you can't do your job." I smiled mischievously, hoping I'd pressed the right button.

Jessie rolled her eyes and stomped away, resurfacing a short while later with Ms. Charlotte in her wheelchair, headed to the shower. Ms. Charlotte stared at me with eyes the color of old pennies, and just as dull. She never said a word.

A short while later Jessie rolled Ms. Charlotte out the shower room door, her wet hair plastered against her head, water dripping from her bangs onto her enormous smile.

"You smell good enough to bite, Ms. Charlotte!" I grinned.

"I feel good enough to bite back." She smirked as Jessie pushed her off toward her room.

A few days later I walked into work mid-buzz. Cell phones were flashing as the news spread at the speed of light.

"Girl! She gone get herself in trouble one of these days!" Crystal exclaimed, thrusting her cell phone in front of my face.

"Yeah, taking pictures of yourself goofing off at work and posting them on Facebook isn't exactly a bright idea." I chuckled as I glanced at Jessie's "glamour shot" selfie, which she'd taken in the shower room. "She isn't the sharpest tack in the wall, that's for sure."

"Look closer." Crystal thrust the phone back in my face.

Grunting, as I had much to do, I took her phone, scanned the picture, handed her phone back, then grabbed it again as my mind registered what I had seen.

"Oh my! Ms. Charlotte! That's Ms. Charlotte!" My hand flew to my mouth as I stared at the screen, as I stared at Ms. Charlotte sitting naked in the background, soaping her arm, her head turned so that her profile was as clear as the sky on a crispy Fall day. Her right breast peeked out beneath her raised, soapy arm, and her large buttocks squashed against and bulged over the seat on the shower chair.

I thrust Crystal's phone back into her hand, immediately feeling overwhelming mortification for Charlotte.

"She will just die!" I cried.

"Oh, they already made Jessie delete the post," Crystal assured me, as if all was well and she weren't showing me her copy of the picture as we spoke, as if others weren't showing others their copies of the picture.

My mind raced back in time. As if it were that very afternoon, I recalled Logan, Zeek's grandson, stirring a hornet's nest in the office.

Logan came to the facility three days a week to get his grandfather in the shower. Zeek never spoke to anyone, and Logan was the only person Zeek would listen to. Logan always came by between four and four-thirty p.m. That day, like all the others, Logan left the facility after walking Zeek into the shower room, seeing to it that Zeek was allowing the aid to help him undress.

Yet Zeek was later discovered on the shower room floor at eight-twenty p.m. The medication aid had gone in to give Zeek his bedtime medications and had noticed his dinner tray sitting untouched on his table in his room. So she started looking for him and found him lying on the shower floor, cold water raining down over him.

Due to severe pain, Zeek was rushed to the emergency room, where they found he'd broken his hip. After his surgery, Zeek returned to the facility. I hadn't been working the evening he fell, but I was there the evening he returned from the hospital. I was present when he saw Jessie, pointed his old finger, and said, "You tha one."

Logan told Zeek that the aid had reported that Zeek had gone back into the shower by himself. She'd found him turning the water on, and when she called his name, he'd turned his head, slipped, and fell.

Zeek told Logan, "Bullshit. She left, never came back. The water got cold and I was freezing, so I tried to get out of that big chair they sit us on, and I fell."

"Zeek has dementia. His recall is completely unreliable," the director of nursing had said.

"He can't remember what he had for breakfast," the administrator had chimed in.

"Hmm." I had looked from one to the other. "He remembers it was cold. He remembers the shower chair is big. And he still, to this day, remembers Jessie is 'the one.' Not to mention the fact that he never touched his dinner that night. Why not? I guess he forgot to eat."

"The records show he ate one hundred percent," the director had proclaimed.

"The medication aid saw his tray! He never touched it!"

"I looked. I saw the records. He ate one hundred percent." The administrator smiled patronizingly. "And the notes say Jessie saw him turn the water on, slip, and fall."

"So the man whose grandson has to come coax him into the shower, in order for him to get one at all, just up and pranced into the shower room to get a shower all by himself? Not."

Zeek spoke one other time, when he saw Jessie later that evening. Zeek looked at Jessie, clicked his tongue, nodded his head, and said, "You tha one. You won't get my narrow ass back in there again."

Logan moved Zeek home and hired a caregiver he couldn't afford. He said he'd hired an attorney he couldn't afford for a fight he couldn't afford to lose. Logan has this idea that our elderly deserve our love and respect. Logan thinks that since his grandfather was in the facility because he needed assistance, that assistance should have been provided. Logan thinks people should be honest and stand accountable. "They're fighting back though." Logan shook his head. "And fighting hard."

While the same aid is taking glamour shot selfies in the same shower room, I thought disgustedly. *With an innocent, vulnerable elderly woman sitting naked and wet behind her, unattended, in the same shower chair that Zeek fell out of.*

Of course, upon asking, I was told they couldn't draw attention to Jessie's actions, or the facility would look bad. "People would link it to the facility. You know how it goes," the director said, shaking her head. "I'm going to hold an in-service for the staff so we can talk about HIPPA again, stress that no pictures are to be taken in the facility because a resident, or resident information, might accidentally be captured in the picture." She rolled her eyes. "Always something."

"Well, count your blessings. At least it wasn't a picture of you naked and vulnerable that Jessie posted on Facebook." I smiled.

"I can't imagine!" she cried, eyes wide, as she stood and hurried out of her office to run copies for her upcoming in-service.

Oma:

I held her hand and told her my name as the nurse performed the procedure. The human spirit and mind being the miraculous mysteries that they are, Oma suddenly perked up, pale blue eyes shining brightly.

She asked me, "Do you know my first name?"

"I do indeed." I chuckled. "Oma!"

Oma smiled. "What am I doing here? How long have I been here?" She squeezed my hand tighter, as if not willing to release it until she had the answers she needed. "Did my family bring me here?"

"You're here to get well and strong again. You've been here since the day before yesterday." I squeezed her hand tighter. "And yes, all twelve of your family members brought you, and they have been here nearly twenty-four seven!" I smiled. "I'm glad to see you're awake, even if you did wait until bedtime to get perky!"

Oma smiled big, running her free hand through her thin but fluffed gray hair.

"I'll check on you in a bit," I assured her. "I'm going to call and let Ralph know you're perky. Your family loves you more than biscuits and gravy!"

Oma laughed quietly but sincerely. "That's a lot of love! Those boys could happily eat biscuits and gravy every day of their lives."

Earlier that day, Oma's nurse, Raina, had asked me to take a look at Oma and talk with the family.

"Her family is upset because she is sleeping so long and hard. They think therapy left her up in her chair too long," Raina explained. "I checked her vital signs, and they're all good. I don't know what they want." She shrugged. "I just can't make them happy."

I had rounded the doorway into Oma's room only to find it chock-full of family! I introduced myself.

Ralph, Oma's eldest son, introduced each of them.

I laughed, saying, "I'll remember Oma's name until the day I die. I remember all those I have the opportunity to love. It just sticks." I shrugged. "But I won't remember any of your names by the time I get halfway back up that hallway."

Everyone laughed, and Ralph said, "Well, Mama's is the name that counts." He then proceeded to quite efficiently detail Oma's journey from the first sign of illness at home several months prior, through two hospitalizations, and up to that very moment.

They were all smiling when I left the room, as I had assured them that Oma had just become my priority and reassured them that, for the moment, Oma was simply resting well, and therefore there was no reason for immediate concern. I asked them to give me the afternoon to take a look at things. A short while later Oma's room was empty, and she slept peacefully on as I assessed her, then began reviewing her records. During said review, I discovered that labs had been drawn the day before.

Oma had been admitted to us on three different intravenous antibiotics for a urinary tract infection (UTI). This, no doubt, indicated a severe UTI. I then focused on the labs, noting her white blood cell count (marker for infection) was higher than it had been upon her discharge from the hospital to us, which had been just a few days before. And all her kidney function levels were significantly off.

Moreover, I found an order from back on January fifteenth, per Oma's nephrologist (kidney doctor), for a renal ultrasound, bloodwork, discontinuation of two different medications, an order to change her fluid pill administration, and an order for a urinalysis. Much of this hadn't been done as of that day, February eighteenth, which was over a month later. Oma was still receiving one of the discontinued medications and she had never had the renal ultrasound or urinalysis. So, I kicked into high gear getting the renal ultrasound done and discontinuing the ongoing medication.

At five-thirty p.m., the ultrasound tech arrived. She was finishing up as I walked into Oma's room to draw some blood for testing. The tech informed me, "Her bladder is distended," as she pushed her machine out the door. (This meaning Oma's bladder was overfilled with urine that wouldn't drain naturally.)

Raina popped in at just that moment and said she was about to place a foley catheter (to drain the urine from Oma's bladder).

Three hours later, at eight-thirty p.m., I had all my test and lab results, noting that the white blood cell count was even higher than the mobile lab results had indicated. I'd noticed wet lung sounds and a mildly irregular heart rate upon assessment, in addition to swelling and fluid retention all over, even in her face, so I had drawn a BNP (related to the heart). Oma's BNP was eight times the maximum normal. The renal ultrasound revealed bilateral hydronephrosis (Meaning a kidney swells due to urine failing to properly drain from the kidney, which, if left untreated, can lead to kidney failure. It most often involves only one kidney, but in Oma's case it was both.) And Oma's white blood cell count was 14.26, well above the normal range of 4.8 – 10.8.

I was about to call the doctor, then realized I needed to know the amount of urine that had drained after placement of the foley catheter. I went in search of Tommy, the nurse who had relieved Raina, to find out what Raina had told her in report, as she had documented nothing related in Oma's records.

"Hey, Tommy, how much urine drained from Ms. Oma's bladder when the foley cath was inserted?"

"I haven't done it yet." Blah, blah, blah. Tommy rattled at the speed of light, her short brown hair bouncing with every syllable.

"*Wait!*" I stuck my palm in the air. "She hasn't been cath'ed yet? Her bladder is still distended?"

Tommy batted her eyes, cocking her head to the side. "I haven't had time yet. I'll do it when I get around there to her."

"But she's got to be in pain by now! That was three hours ago, and her bladder was already distended then!" I struggled not to yell. Raina should have done it immediately. Tommy was a veteran nurse but was new at the facility. Therefore, she was understandably still as slow as a slug. However, she should have known the catheter procedure couldn't wait. Both nurses were dead wrong. Quietly, I explained, "That's a priority, Tommy. That can't wait," as I turned and hurried away.

The other two nurses on duty assisted, and we placed the catheter. Oma moaned quietly when I palpated her firmly distended bladder, then moaned again as I continued holding her hand and used my free hand to massage her bladder externally, facilitating the bladder emptying after the foley was in place. Over one thousand milliliters of urine drained immediately. We had to empty the drainage bag into a container as it filled, because it wouldn't hold it all. That's at least over a quart of urine. A healthy human bladder can hold between 400-500 milliliters of urine, or about two cups, before reaching capacity. Oma was holding over double that amount. Additionally, that's a lot of urine for someone whose kidneys work great. But remember, Oma's kidneys were swollen with urine due to not draining properly themselves. This strongly indicated that Oma had not urinated for a significantly extended time frame, yet no one had noticed.

Once her bladder was empty, thus her discomfort resolved, Oma smiled. When I asked, she said she felt much better. I had introduced myself as soon as I saw her eyes open so she wouldn't be afraid. After we were finished and had Oma covered back up, she repeated my name and asked if I knew her first name. It seemed to comfort her that I did. She smiled again and started asking questions.

A few minutes later I'd informed Oma's primary care doctor of all the results, and I told him about the severely belated renal ultrasound the nephrologist had ordered back in January. I told him I'd already faxed all results to the nephrologist's office. The doctor wanted the results of the US faxed to his office, as well, but he said, "Based on what you tell me, we needed that UA a month ago!" He then gave orders to repeat the urinalysis and culture, telling me to refer Oma to an infectious disease specialist due to her white blood cell count elevating further while on three IV antibiotics. I entered the orders into the system, wrote it on the report, completed a referral sheet for an infectious disease appointment to be scheduled ASAP, and then went to find Tommy again so I could update her on the new orders and rationale.

"Hey, Tommy."

Tommy interrupted me, sticking her pointer finger into the air like a tiny flag. "I'm about to go do that foley right now," she assured me.

"Tommy, it's eleven-thirty-five at night. We placed that foley three hours ago, just as soon as I found out it hadn't been done three hours before that," I droned wearily. "Now, hear me. The doctor just ordered a repeat UA with C&S related to persistently elevating WBCs, despite treatment and bilateral hydronephrosis. The UA her nephrologist ordered a month ago was never done. So make sure you get a urine specimen and have it picked up by the lab in the morning. It is critical. And the doctor referred Oma to infectious disease, as well. I completed the appointment sheet and put it in the book to be scheduled. I don't want to call the family this late, so call them before you leave in the morning and update them on the new orders, please." Shaking my head, I reflexively added as an afterthought, "Really? Six hours later you're going to do it 'right now'?" and walked away.

Finally, after midnight, and a sixteen-plus-hour day, I checked in on Oma, who was wide awake, comfortable, and pleased I'd stopped in to see her. Then I called February eighteenth done and drug myself home to bed.

On February nineteenth I moved on to the next residents I had been asked to see for various issues. It wasn't until February twenty-sixth that I heard anything further about Oma. I heard Oma had died. I was stunned. Me being me, I dug in, went back through her records. This is a brief summary of what I found:

11/25: Oma was admitted to the hospital after a fall at home. A renal ultrasound was done that day for acute kidney failure and chronic kidney disease. The renal ultrasound was negative, meaning no problems were found. White blood cell (WBC) count was within normal limits, so no other infection was present. But urinary tract infection (UTI) was confirmed via urinalysis with blood, 4+ bacteria and white blood cells in the urine, in addition to other abnormalities. Per hospital records, no culture was done on the urine, and no antibiotic was started.

11/29: Oma was discharged from the hospital *to us* with this admission diagnosis identified on the admission nursing assessment: "falls and failure to thrive." And orders were given for Oma to follow up with her nephrologist (kidney specialist) in one week. Oma was alert, oriented, participated in therapy, and frequently went out on pass with her family. Oma was kickin' it! (Naturally, the admission was slammed, so nobody had reviewed Oma's records. Thus, nobody at our facility knew Oma had an untreated UTI. And the admitting nurse failed to ponder the rationale for the diagnosis of "falls and failure to thrive" with a completely unrelated referral to a Nephrologist.

12/2: Serum (blood) white blood cell count was 7.2 (within normal limits). Oma was hanging despite the untreated UTI, though it still lurked.

12/22: Oma's primary care doctor started her on diclofenac for arthritis pain, which has potential to cause kidney issues, and Oma's kidneys were already compromised with chronic kidney disease.

1/15: Oma saw her nephrologist and received orders (related to "acute kidney injury", per blood work results) to discontinue both Vitamin D3 and the recently ordered diclofenac, to adjust fluid pill administration, to obtain a renal ultrasound, and to do more blood work and a urinalysis. Raina, the nurse receiving the orders, overlooked the urinalysis, the renal ultrasound, and the discontinuation of the Vitamin D3. (None of these three things were done.)

1/16: As said, Raina did obtain the ordered labs. The white blood cell count was up from the previous 7.2 to 12.1 (now well within abnormal). The night nurse faxed the results to the primary care doctor instead of the nephrologist, who'd ordered the labs.

Per the records, there is no indication that her primary care doctor ever saw the lab results, and they were never sent to the nephrologist.

1/25: We discharged Oma home with home health services, as she had "progressed very well, and her status improved." (WBCs still up and with no related treatment; a UTI found 11/25, still untreated; no renal ultrasound done; no urinalysis done; and still taking the discontinued Vitamin D3.) Oma was discharged due to her medicare days ending, thus therapy completed.

1/29: Oma was readmitted to us from home with "general weakness and unsteady gait." (not surprising with an untreated infection, or infections)

1/30: Oma was admitted to hospital with acute febrile illness, UTI, acute kidney injury, and urine and blood cultures positive for E coli (stout bacteria), indicating that the bacteria that was likely the cause of the untreated UTI (from 11/25) was now in her bloodstream.

2/14: Oma was readmitted to us from the hospital with metabolic encephalopathy and UTI. On three different IV antibiotics due to the severity of her infection.

2/18: I was asked to take a look at Oma, as per the story above, and WBCs were now 14.26, per my blood draw processed at the hospital lab, which was higher than the level of 8.4 on discharge from same hospital on 2/14. Her WBC level had nearly doubled in just four days, clearly indicative that the infection was worsening despite the three different IV antibiotics. Her bladder was distended, and we inserted a foley catheter, which immediately drained over a liter of cloudy yellow urine. And at this point I discovered and discontinued the ongoing Vitamin D3. I discovered and order the missed renal ultrasound, which revealed bilateral hydronephrosis, and I received an order to repeat the urinalysis that was never done, with a culture, and refer to infectious disease. I then stepped back out, as I was not the resident's nurse. I was asked to help determine the problem and get a plan of action in motion. That, I did. I then moved on to other people with other issues and left Oma in the hands of the nurses and the assistant director of nursing.

2/19: Nurse documented that Oma was drinking fluids. No reference to urinary catheter. No description or amount of urine output. *Urinalysis was not done.*

2/20: Nurse documented urine yellow. No reference to amount or resident's status otherwise. *Urinalysis was still not done.* At 8:12 p.m., nurse documented that resident was admitted to hospice for muscle weakness.

2/21: Hospice revoked, per family request. Resident remained unresponsive. No reference to urine or output all day. *Urinalysis still not done.*

2/22: Nurse documented: "restless with pain." Family wanted hospice back. *Urinalysis still not done.*

2/23: Nurse documented: "generalized edema (swelling due to fluid all over the body) resolved, 300ml dark amber urine." (Note: first reference to the swelling since my assessment on 2/19.) *Urinalysis still not done.*

2/24: Nurse documented "stable" twice, that's it. *Urinalysis still not done.*

2/25: At 5:20 a.m., nurse documented: "No respirations. Cannot obtain blood pressure or pulse." At 7:29 a.m., hospice pronounced death. *Urinalysis never done.*

Human error is inevitable, excusable, and most often reparable. I'd like to say that Oma's suffering and death were simply human error. Some of it was; some of it wasn't. Some of it was (as I've grown to say often) a major lack of give-a-shit. I'll let you decide which was what. The facts are spelled out.

The hospital, in a smaller town, is (in my humble opinion) very nearly a joke. And on 11/25/19, they should have ordered, at minimum, a repeat UA and weekly CBC until Oma could be seen by a nephrologist. Everybody knows you cannot call up a specialist and get in the next week. In my humble opinion, the hospital should have cultured and treated that abnormal urine with the 4+ bacteria with an antibiotic until Oma could be seen by the nephrologist. But that's the hospital's bad.

As for us in long-term care, this is where we fell short:

On 11/29, those responsible for doing so should have reviewed Oma's hospital records close enough to know that she had an abnormal urinalysis, and they should have obtained related orders to protect, and to ensure prudent care for, Oma.

- The doctor (PCP) should not have started the diclofenac on 12/22 with a diagnosis of chronic kidney disease.
- Huge! On 1/15, the nurse failed to obtain the renal ultrasound and the urinalysis, and she failed to discontinue the Vitamin D3, as ordered by the nephrologist (at which point all of this may well have been prevented, or at least managed and minimized). The nurse prevented timely diagnosis and treatment.
- Huge! On 1/16, the nurse failed to report the lab results, with the elevated WBCs and the whacky kidney function levels, to the doctor. She chose instead to fax them (thus, the doctor never saw the results). And the nurse failed to send the lab results to the ordering nephrologist. The nurse prevented diagnosis and treatment.
- Huge! On 1/25, the facility discharged Oma home with elevated WBCs, the UTI never addressed or treated, the urinalysis ordered by the nephrologist never done, the renal ultrasound never done, and with resident still taking Vitamin D3, which had been discontinued by the nephrologist due to acute kidney injury.
- Huge! On 2/18, the aids failed to notice and report, and the nurse failed to notice and address, that Oma had no urine output for—my educated guess is—about eighteen to twenty-four hours, or more.
- Huge! On 2/19, the nurse failed to place a foley catheter immediately upon finding Oma's bladder distended. She went home and left Oma in pain, with backed-up urine and a bulging bladder.
- Huge! On 2/19, the oncoming nurse failed to place a foley catheter immediately upon finding out Oma's bladder was distended, and the nurse whom she had relieved hadn't done anything about it.

- Enormous! On 2/20, the nurse failed to obtain the urine specimen/urinalysis ordered on 2/19 (the UA I told her was "critical;" the UA needed because the UA the nephrologist had ordered over a month prior had never been done; the UA needed because Oma's white blood cell count was rising despite three different IV antibiotics; the UA needed because Oma's kidneys were swollen with urine and her bladder was no longer emptying).
- Purely disgusting! The nurses failed to monitor Oma's urine closely (color, odor, amount, etc.) and failed to obtain that UA from 2/20 through the early morning hours of 2/25, when Oma suffered her last moment and left this world for good.

Johnson James:

The hospital is notorious for discharging on Friday, specifically Friday evenings, just before, during, or after dinner. As a rule, it seemed everybody's status improved sufficiently for discharge on the doctor's Friday morning rounds, and of course, it takes all day to actually get the patient discharged and out the door.

So, the EMT rolled Johnson and his wheelchair in through the front door and up to the nurses' desk right at dinnertime.

Johnson grinned up at me from beneath a noticeably custom brown and beige cap that read, *Jesus Rocks.* He announced in his loud, gravelly voice, "Hi, there. I'm tired, hungry, and grouchy."

"Well, hello, tired, hungry, and grouchy." I headed around the counter, glancing briefly at the dressings covering both of Johnson's legs from ankle to mid-thigh. "I'm tired, hungry, and delightful. Nice to meet you." I grinned, stretching out my hand.

Johnson smirked and said, "Make you a deal, delightful. If you fix the tired and hungry, I'll fix the grouchy. Then we can both be delightful."

"It's a deal!" We shook on it before I took his wheelchair from the EMT and rolled Johnson down the hall to his room, admiring his cap from behind as I pushed his chair.

Two minutes later I handed Johnson the remote control for the television.

"What would you like to drink with dinner, Mr. James? Tea, milk, juice?"

"All three!" He chuckled. "And call me Johnson. No, skip the milk, but double up on the other two. Add thirsty to my list." He grinned.

Ten minutes later I walked back into Johnson's room carrying a tray laden with food, tea, and juice.

Johnson raised wiry brows over honey-gold eyes, which were wide with anticipation. "You kept your end of the bargain, so now I'm gonna keep mine." He laughed.

I set his tray on his overbed table and slid the table in front of him.

"Thanks," he quipped without an upward glance, immediately busying himself unrolling silverware and removing lids and plastic; my presence dismissed entirely.

I watched him, just for a moment, touched by his blatant enthusiasm. *What is that on his cap?* I thought to myself. *I didn't see that before.*

Leaning in to look closer, Johnson still oblivious to my presence, I stared intently at the speck. Out of the corner of my eye, I noticed another, slightly larger, "speck" on Johnson's shoulder. Instinctively stepping back, I noticed tiny "specks" freckling Johnson's khaki shorts and brown t-shirt, and the dressings on his legs and feet.

Oh my God! They're moving! I screamed to myself. *That's bugs!*

Following the direction from which the shoulder bug was crawling, I held my breath and leaned to the side, peering behind Johnson. Reflexively, my hand flew to cover my gaping mouth as I stared wide-eyed at the bugs swarming out of Johnson's wheelchair like ants swarming from a mound that's been poked with a big stick! Alarm blaring in my brain like a train whistle, I glanced at my feet, unable to resist the urge to look closer at the bugs already scattered over the floor, scurrying like tiny roaches running for cover.

My skin crawling, I hurried out on tiptoe, shut the door solidly behind me, and ran for help. Panting, I huddled my co-workers together and, in a frantic but hushed tone, described what I'd just seen.

"Oh *no*," Cynthia, the aid, exclaimed in a loud whisper. "That's bed bugs!"

"*Bed bugs?*" I cried! I'd never seen a bed bug in my life! And I would have happily lived out the remainder of it without having done so.

No more than six or seven minutes after the time I left Johnson's room, Cynthia and I returned, trash bags over our feet and up to our knees.

Johnson, having found a ballgame on television, was still devouring his dinner, and he never even glanced our way.

Bugs dotted the bare blue mattress of the second bed. Cynthia silently pointed at the white trash bag holding Johnson's belongings, which was setting atop the mattress. Like a tiny seething volcano, bugs steadily oozed from the tied top of the bag. Cynthia snapped a picture as we soundlessly backed out of the room, again ensuring the door closed solidly behind us.

Back at the nurses' station, we zoomed in on the picture and counted twenty-three visible bugs. Cynthia quickly googled bed bugs and thrust her phone into my view, a picture of the entire bed bug life cycle displayed on the screen.

"Oh crap!" I whispered. "No doubt about it, that's bed bugs!"

I'd been a nurse for many years and had never, not once, seen a bed bug! Itching all over and scratching madly with one hand, I grabbed the phone with the other and called the director of nursing at home.

"Melanie, they are literally swarming that entire room!" I emphasized.

"The hospital didn't notice? Crap! Have Cynthia take him to the shower immediately, and put all his clothes in a plastic bag. Tie it up tight," Melanie said. I cringed and scratched.

Melanie gave me full instructions and informed me she would be calling Timmy, the administrator, but she was first going to call the hospital. I said I'd call the ambulance company, hopefully before they used that truck to transport anybody else.

"Absolutely! Thanks." Melanie hung up.

"Good grief," the person at the ambulance company spouted. "Y'all didn't tell us he had bed bugs." Disgust oozed through his tone.

"My apologies if I sound rude, as that is not my intention, but I have a situation on my hands, sir. I was simply taking the time, making the effort, to give you the heads up that we didn't have the honor of receiving ourselves." Having reached my limit bugs ago, I continued, "How the man stayed in the hospital for eight days covered with bugs and nobody noticed is beyond me. It took me less than five minutes to spot the problem. But if you truly feel the need to vent your dissatisfaction with your related circumstances, I suggest you call the hospital from which *you* transported the gentleman, and his bugs, to *my* facility. Thank you and goodbye." I hung up the phone, took a deep breath, and scratched.

As per instructions, Cynthia rolled a highly pissed off, grumbling Johnson to the shower and scrubbed him down while I, covered with isolation garb and trash bags, went to his room. I bagged up his few personal items, triple-bagged the white bag holding his belongings, and did my utmost best to bag the wheelchair. Yes, I had been instructed to bag his wheelchair, and let's get real here, all one can do is their very best when pulling bags over a chair. Then, off I went with my bagged feet, pushing a bagged wheelchair, holding bagged belongings as I hurried down the hallway, then out the back door to the rear parking lot. Again, per instructions, I placed the bagged spectacle so that it would get full, direct sunlight all day the following day. Ripping off all my protective garb, I tossed it all atop the spectacle, and stomped like an angry child back across the parking lot and in through the back door.

"Mr. James wants to see you," Cynthia said in passing. "And get ready. He ain't happy. I put him in room two-oh-four this time, like Melanie said, and I posted a do-not-enter sign on the door to his old room."

"Thanks for everything, Cynthia."

Sighing heavily, I knocked on Johnson's door. Thirty-five minutes later, Johnson had calmed down and apologized for chewing me out. However, it wasn't until Cynthia showed him a picture that he believed we had *actually* seen bugs.

"Look, I know you guys are doing what you have to do, but I don't have to like it." He sighed.

"Nope, you don't. We don't like it either, nor do we have to," I replied. "But it has to be done." Shrugging, I asked, "Now, may I rebandage your legs? We need to get you healed up and back home."

Johnson had open wounds covering almost the entire surface area of his legs, stretching from his toes to just above his knees. Apparently, he'd developed cellulitis six months before, and though the cellulitis had been resolved with treatment, the home health nurses hadn't been able to heal the wounds. Ultimately, they became infected, and Johnson ended up in the hospital, then discharged from the hospital to us. In my way of thinking, we may well have stumbled upon the reason behind his wounds not healing; or the reason may have crawled in upon us. In fact, it was highly possible that the cellulitis started with a bug bite.

After finally completing Johnson's time-consuming and tedious wound care, I called Melanie back. "What's the plan? You talk to Timmy?"

"Yes, he was ticked off at the hospital," Melanie replied.

"Well, me, too, but what is he going to do?" I pushed. "Cleaning Johnson up and moving him didn't kill those bugs."

"I know, I know. Timmy is calling our exterminator."

"Okay, good. Yes. That's what I was looking for."

Melanie laughed, thanked me for being so "awesome," and hung up. I didn't feel awesome at all; I felt buggy.

I drove home that night and stripped naked *on my porch*, hoping no neighbors were sitting on theirs, enjoying the night air and my random strip show. Tossing my clothes out in the center of my driveway so the sun and pavement could bake them the next day, I streaked inside! Heading straight to the bathroom, I proceeded to scald myself and scrub my skin raw. While drying my raw skin, I found a classic bite on the front of my right thigh; three in a row, breakfast, lunch and dinner. Shuddering, I took a picture of the bites to send to Melanie and Timmy the next morning.

Exhausted, I fell into bed only for my eyes to pop back open as visions of bed bugs danced through my head. Sleep eluded me entirely as my worries grew legs and multiplied. Over the next few months, the slightest tickle sent covers flying as I shot out of that bed, flipping on every source of light in the room so I could closely inspect every inch of the mattress and linens before wearily climbing back in and trying again. Cynthia said she was having the same trouble.

I left my clothes lying in the center of the driveway for three days before picking them up with a long stick and throwing them into the outside trashcan, sacrificing the many items in my pockets, as there was absolutely no way I was digging in to retrieve them.

On Saturday I arrived at work to find that Johnson had been moved to room 207, per Melanie's instruction. The nurse had seen bed bugs in Johnson's new room, 204, so the process had been repeated. And no exterminator had come. I sent Melanie a text, ensuring she was aware that we still awaited the exterminator. Melanie replied, "I'll text Timmy."

On Sunday I arrived to find that Johnson had been moved to room 304 deep in the night, per Melanie's instruction, due to a bed bug being found in room 207. When I asked, I was told no exterminator had ever come. I shot Melanie a text to let her know, and she replied, "Okay."

On Monday I walked into work just in time to hear Timmy berating the nurses. His face and neck were as red as an apple as he shouted, "I want to know who told Mr. Webster about the bed bugs, and I want to know right now! I'm going to find out, and when I do, it's going to be immediate termination!" He ranted on as we glanced at one another, rolling our eyes, weary of the entire situation but not concerned about his threat of termination.

The man ranted on for fifteen to twenty minutes, spitting out one threat after another, as I sat there and wondered how one could possibly be such a selfish imbecile. The spectacle still sat outside in full view of the smoking area, where Mr. Webster and his daughter spent their entire daily visits, sometimes twice daily. The staff had been instructed to move Johnson from room to room, hall to hall, including the rooms next to and across the hall from Mr. Webster. They had us post "Do Not Enter" signs on the door of every room they'd had us move Johnson out of. And finally, on Monday, they had an exterminator fumigating those very same rooms, and only those rooms. By the way, once the exterminator did finally come, we discovered Johnson was not only infested with bed bugs but also with body lice.

Mr. Webster had poor balance. Mr. Webster had weak lungs and needed to stop chain smoking. But Mr. Webster was not stupid. He was nosy, and he loved to talk. But stupid was simply not something one could rightfully pin on Mr. Webster, aka "Trouble."

For that matter, even Cooper noticed things were amiss. Cooper, who spent most of his time inching himself around in his wheelchair, peering into doorways in an attempt to figure out where he was. Cooper. Even Cooper noticed. "Hey" he pointed at the 'Do Not Enter' sign, "What?" his brow creased, shoulders shrugged.

"No telling" I shrugged in return.

Only an imbecile would think no one would notice.

Per his norm, Mr. Webster showed up at about three forty-five for the four o'clock smoke break. "I'm sorry, Pinecone," he said to me as he stood towering over the counter at the nurses' station. "I didn't mean to cause a ruckus."

"Don't give it another thought, Trouble. You didn't do anything wrong," I reassured him. "And I got your pinecone." I laughed.

Trouble had asked me to put his cigarette butt in the ash tray one day when I had taken the smokers out. I'd taken his butt from him, walked toward the ash tray, then stepped on a pinecone, which rolled beneath my shoe, my balance rolling with it. I didn't just fall; I *fell!* I fell all *over* that sidewalk and in slow motion, bruising things I hadn't even known I had! Ever since that day, Trouble had called me pinecone.

That Friday, when I arrived at work, the director warned me, "The state is here on a complaint about the bed bugs. The complaint is that we didn't address the bugs timely, which placed the residents at risk."

So, the state was in the building, conducting an investigation. Good job, state! Fist bump!

An hour or so later, I was down the hall with my medication cart when a gentleman walked up and stood to the side of my cart. He introduced himself as "Don," informed me he was with the state, and showed me his ID.

"May I have a few minutes of your time to ask a few questions about Johnson James?"

"Absolutely. I welcome the opportunity to answer any related questions you have." I smiled genuinely.

Don then asked me questions regarding the infestation and related details, actions, timelines, and the sequence of events.

I answered all questions honestly and directly. Out of ethical loyalty to my employer, I offered nothing in the way of opinion. However, out of rightful loyalty to my residents, I answered honestly, clearly, and concisely.

In fact, Don ultimately asked, straight up, "Do you think the situation was handled appropriately?"

I replied emphatically and without hesitation, "My opinion doesn't matter. I've told you the facts. Your opinion is the only one relevant to the investigation. Yours is the opinion which will determine the safety, in similar situations, of the residents living here and in other facilities."

Don smiled, shook my hand, thanked me for my time and assistance, and walked away.

Agree or disagree, in my humble opinion, it was fairly simple. Not a lot of "investigation" was even necessary:

Did you have a bed bug infestation issue?

Did you contain it immediately?

Did you take action to resolve it immediately?

Our answers: Yes, we did the best we could, and nope.

Don, I told you we found the bed bugs on Friday and that the exterminator didn't come until the following Monday; this after moving the source to multiple rooms on different halls. What more could you possibly need to know to find the complaint justified? Truly. What, Don?

When I rolled my cart back up to the nurses' station about two hours later, Melanie was grinning like Garfield. "We were cleared on the complaint!" she exclaimed, throwing me a high five.

Slapping her palm, I smiled. "Well, look at you all relieved and excited!" I laughed.

Melanie laughed with me, apparently not one with the ability to read between the lines.

Timmy bounced up like Tigger from 'Winnie the Pooh'. "Cleared!" He threw Melanie a high five. "I was sweating it there for a few hours. I thought he was going to nail us for sure! But it's cleared. I can't believe it!" Glancing at me, he turned and walked away.

"Me neither!" I replied, smiling. "I'm shocked."

To this day, I do not understand how Melanie and Timmy justified their actions, or lack thereof, or how Don justified clearing the complaint.

The man came in literally swarming with bugs on Friday.

He was moved three times in two days due to repeated discovery of more bugs, and each move exposed more of the facility to direct infestation, therefore placing more residents at risk.

They waited until Monday to bring an exterminator in, which allowed more time for the bugs to spread and hide, again placing more residents at risk. Then they treated only the rooms they'd actually had Johnson placed in. Think on that.

Yet the complaint was unfounded? It wasn't valid? I'm betting that if Timmy's or Don's AC went out in August, the AC guy would have been called out on Saturday. I'm betting that had they found bed bugs in *their homes*, an exterminator would have been called out on Saturday.

Johnson James was discharged home once his Medicare days were used up. I mean, that meant he no longer had full funding, and he flat-out refused to pay anything out of pocket. His legs finally healing nicely, he was returning to the same place where it all began, and his home hadn't been fumigated. It was his choice, and he apparently hadn't "ever seen any bugs at home".

But we had. We had seen a host of bugs. And over time we saw more bugs in more rooms on every hall. After each sighting, we moved the resident, or residents, to an empty room while we fumigated their infested room, then moved them back. Timmy unwittingly, but successfully developed an in effective and routine bug management system, if you will.

No point calling state. Right?

Just a bit of selected information that relates specifically to the actions or lack thereof:

Bed bugs are fast! They do not play. Depending on the surface, bed bugs can travel three to four feet per minute. They get from room to room at about the same pace as us, maybe a bit faster.

The common advice regarding bed bug infestation is, if you find a bed bug, stop looking and contact a professional! (we waited until Monday). Live bugs or eggs may drop off while moving things from one place to another – items with bed bugs should be sealed in a bag before moving them (try sealing a wheelchair in a bag!). … warn your friends. Not informing others robs them of the chance to avoid bringing bugs into their homes and businesses." (we not only didn't warn anybody, but were threatened with immediate termination because Timmy merely 'thought' somebody had warned someone; what about Webster's daughter and her family?)

"If bed bugs land in one room of your home, then they will soon spread to all rooms. How fast they spread depends on whether they hitch a lift or go there by their own foot power. I wonder. Did Don have the slightest clue about bed bug infestations? I can say without hesitation or the slightest amount of guilt that Don was wrong to clear that complaint. Moreover, Timmy was wrong to wait until Monday to call in an exterminator. Melanie was wrong to stand by Timmy's decision to wait. Ultimately, the two of them placed every resident and employee, along with everyone's families, at risk so as not to dent the precious budget.

Shindy:

Shindy was the first "little people" person that I'd ever personally met. Her mother must have had a strange sense of humor, as she'd named her tiny baby "Shindy." Shindy Schindler was a whopping eighty-nine pounds, most of which was her adorably large hazel-eyed head, which was topped with thick, light brown curls. She was much like a brunette version of a Shirley Temple doll. Shindy smiled quick, easy, and often, despite the fact that she had absolutely zero use of, or feeling in, her doll-sized body; she felt nothing from the neck down. One might have thought she was doomed from the start, having been born a paralyzed little person, but Shindy had more life in her than twenty people up and running. The facility purchased a special call light that Shindy could use by turning her head to the side and pressing her cheek against it.

Nobody has noticed, but I have stepped back completely from Shindy's case. I still visit her, make her laugh, and change her television channel, but medically speaking, I'm out. I'll tell you why later.

For now, though, Shindy had labs drawn, a CBC and CMP (complete blood count and comprehensive metabolic panel, or chemistry profile) by the mobile lab on March 6. The results either were not received from the lab for some reason or they got lost in the shuffle. Regardless, the records must show timely, prudent care (I roll my eyes). So, later, at some point, the assistant director of nurses was doing her thing, going through an in house system produced report of all recent lab orders. The ADON was reviewing the report and ensuring we had results of all labs drawn in each person's records. She found we had no results for Shindy's March 6 draw, so she logged onto the lab site, printed out results, noted at the bottom that they were received and that the doctor was notified on the date the labs were drawn, and then put them in the to-be-scanned stack. Thus, she lied, and the doctor never saw the results. But the records looked good.

I only know this because I happened to be standing by the printer when the lab results printed, and the ADON stepped up to retrieve them. I watched her note them, then watched her slide them into the stack. Most importantly, while watching her note them, I noticed immediately that Shindy's potassium level was critically low at a potentially heart-stopping 2.8.

The records would look good, though.

The nurses should have been looking for those results, should have seen to it that they received them. Heck, the nurse on duty probably did not even know Shindy had had labs drawn that morning, as very few LTC nurses ever keep up with labs. When I put pending labs on the report, the night nurse dropped it off. With rotating shifts, tons of things are lost in the shuffle.

I quietly assessed Shindy for heart-related issues, obtained an order to repeat the labs, and took it from there.

Watering Red Geranium:

Having forgotten whose PICC line Lois had asked me to pull, I asked her relieving charge nurse, Dana.

"Oh, that's Sophie, but I might need to get a chest x-ray on her. She has a cough. See what you think."

I introduced myself to Sophie and asked her about her cough, which she said was "just an old smoker's cough." I assessed her lung sounds and didn't note anything concerning, so I told her I was going to pull her PICC line (her IV site) and that she'd need to lie down for thirty minutes after it was pulled.

"Well, I've got to pee first." She chuckled. "That's why I took my oxygen off. I was going to pee."

A few minutes later I helped Sophie back into bed and started putting her oxygen tubing back on her, when I noticed that my hand and sleeve were getting soaked as water splattered from the nose piece on the tubing with every bubble of the oxygen concentrator. Glancing behind me at the concentrator, I saw the water container hanging sideways, dangling from the concentrator by the connection tubing, steadily bubbling water into Sophie's nasal cannula tubing. Reaching to right things, I found that the concentrator no longer had the elastic to hold the water container in place. *Okay, I get it; things break. We do what we gotta do. But we do not blow water up people's noses.* I thought to myself

"Ms. Sophie!" I quickly turned the concentrator off. "You can't wear oxygen tubing that's blowing water up your nose."

"Oh, I know it. I take it off every now and then to get a break. It waters me so much I feel like a geranium, a pretty red one." She smirked. "But I have to have my oxygen, so I put it back on and try to swallow the water."

"You can't do that little Red." I couldn't resist chuckling. "You're risking pneumonia." I threw her tubing into the trash. "You have to tell the nurse so she can fix it."

"Oh, honey, I told the nurse my second day here." Sophie looked up at me quite seriously. "It was okay the evening I got here, but the next morning I woke to a puddle on the floor. It was big enough to go swimming in." She snickered. "The nurse had them come in and mop it up. I've told all my nurses, but—"

"Wait!" I held my palm in the air. "It makes a puddle?"

"Oh yes, a big puddle. They mop it up every morning so I don't slip and fall in it. They also change my linens on my bed every morning because my bed gets soaked. They got me a waterproof pillow, too, but I don't like it. It crinkles when I move my head." She shrugged. "But this way they can change the pillowcase, and I have a dry pillow again. I didn't like trying to sleep on the wet one. It made the pillowcase damp even when they changed it. They dry the puddle up with towels from time to time during the afternoon and evening, but in the morning, it needs a mop and bucket."

"No, darlin'! That is unacceptable." I laughed at the lunacy. "I'll be right back."

Fifteen minutes later I had Sophie new tubing and a new water container, which I taped to the concentrator and to the wall, hoping to keep it upright, as I was unable to locate a replacement concentrator. Ensuring the bottle was secure, I told Sophie, "You can't move the concentrator. It's taped to the wall and won't budge, so when you go to the toilet, you'll have to use your tank on your chair, like you do when you go to therapy."

"Thank you, honey. I look forward to a good night's sleep in a nice, dry bed, without water bubblin' up my nose." She laughed, reaching up for a hug.

"So, what do you think?" Dana asked me when I returned a few minutes later. "I need to get a chest x-ray?"

"Well, her lungs don't sound bad, but it's a miracle," I replied wearily. "Her concentrator has been blowing water up her nose since she got here.

She said they've been mopping the puddle up each day, and she's been trying to swallow all the water being blown up her nose. I rigged it so the bottle stands up, and won't bubble water into the tubing anymore; told her to tell you guys if it does. She said she's been telling all her nurses. I'm glad she's going home soon. I think she's safer there."

"Oh," Dana, her nurse, replied.

Breathless

"I can tell you right now that breathing treatments aren't happening tonight. I have had the worst day," Brandi, a nurse, proclaimed as she hurried up the hallway to begin her shift.

I was new at the facility, and they had me "training" on a night shift, on the other unit, so that I would be able to float to other units if needed. I've never understood how one could think one shift prepped one for working the unit, but it is what it is. And that is the extent of "training" in the vast majority of nursing positions anywhere. Chill out nursing supervisors. I said most; I did not say all. But realistically, in long-term care, once you have worked one unit, you can work them all just about as well. You either care to do it right, regardless of how long it takes, or you do not.

So, back to Brandi. Brandi was a PRN nurse, meaning she worked elsewhere and only worked at this facility when she was needed, and when she desired, to fill a spot or cover a shift. Brandi unloaded her backpack and an armload of bags filled with her snacks for the night, then looked at me.

"Hi, I'm new and training on this unit tonight," I quickly explained.

"Okay, well, good. Like I said, it's been a long day." Brandi laughed.

That was just about the summation of my interaction with Brandi for the entirety of that shift. I stopped orienting myself to the unit, instead I began quietly researching who all had breathing treatments that needed to be administered through the night. It turned out that there were a total of fourteen treatments due for a total of nine residents, out of which four currently had pneumonia, and out of those four, one was a quadriplegic with a trach. That meant he breathed through an opening in his throat, with a tube holding it open for air to pass through. In short, his respiratory system was compromised enough already. Add the pneumonia, and come on now, Brandi. How can you live with that?

So I quietly proceeded to administer breathing treatments. As I went along, I'd find I couldn't sign for the administration, as Brandi had already signed that she'd administered. She stayed one step ahead of me through the night and never paid me enough attention to realize that I was administering the treatments. It worked out all right. I admit I was shocked at her lackadaisical attitude. I was new to long-term care, thus naive. I've since learned Brandi's attitude is the norm. Mine is the abnormal.

Danella:

Danella was better known as Ella. Ella fit her better, anyway, as she was one who liked things simple and routine. Ella was somewhat of a contradiction. She was witty, blunt, and outspoken, yet she expressed feelings of complete vulnerability, and I never once saw her out of her room except when on a stretcher en route to the hospital. Ella also appeared fully cognitively functional. After simply visiting with her, one would never recognize her memory deficit. In fact, I wasn't aware of it for several months myself. But little things escaped Ella's memory completely. However, if anything was repetitious, she had a memory like an elephant.

Unfortunately, Ella was medically complicated. In addition to having no use of her legs, she had issues that, if treated optimally, would complicate her other issues. Thus, Ella's healthcare required one to be extremely conscientious, to consider the potential outcome of any and all care, and to take nothing lightly. Yet when one looked at Ella, she appeared to be a fairly healthy, big-boned, mildly obese, middle-aged woman. Ella did not look to be her seventy-seven years. Most fragile for Ella was her respiratory system. For whatever reasons, though she had more potentially fatal diagnoses, her chronic obstructive pulmonary disease caused her the most frequent problems. Thus, Ella was on breathing treatments routinely, had several related oral medications, and she was to wear a BiPap (bilevel positive airway pressure) at night and during naps. This was far from complicated; it simply involved securing the mask over her mouth and nose, ensuring the air hose wasn't kinked or tangled, switching her oxygen source from nasal cannula to the mask, turning the BiPap machine on, and double checking the settings. Time consumed was about three to five minutes max.

Ella's breathing treatment medication had to be stored in the refrigerator. This meant extra steps for the nurse, or, as in my case, the nurse needed to grab it from the fridge before heading down the hallway. On my first day working with Ella, I had to open a new package of the Brovana, a long acting bronchodilator (meaning it facilitates keeping the airway open), so I pulled my sharpie out of my pocket, then initialed and dated the package as is required. Two days later, though Ella got the treatment twice a day and though there were only five doses per package, I failed to notice things weren't right. I'm a nurse, not a detective. Sadly, over time, I realized that I needed to be both in order to even attempt to ensure my patients' wellbeing. After two days off I returned to work on Friday, and when I went to grab Ella's treatment, I noticed my date still on the package in use. I quickly checked the box for another open package but found none.

Even if someone opened another package, possibly not seeing this one , that package wouldn't be used up, I thought, the wheels innately turning. So I asked Ella a short while later.

"You getting your breathing treatments twice a day, Ella?"

"Only when you're here." She replied without hesitation. "I wasn't getting them at all before you came."

"I'll be right back." I assured Ella as I hurried out. I returned to the medication room, checking the date on the box of Brovana. The contents would expire eight days from that day. "Wow." I then got on my computer and ran a quick pharmacy audit on the Brovana. It was last filled eight months prior, and each box contained sixty doses, a thirty-day supply. Ella had been hospitalized three times in the past seven months for acute respiratory failure.

I returned to Ella's room. "Ms. Ella, have you told anyone you don't get your treatments?"

"Yes. I told my son. And he has talked to them up in the office several times. I don't say anything to anybody else because I don't want them mad at me," she said matter-of-factly.

"So, if I hadn't asked, you wouldn't have told me?"

"No, ma'am. But I did tell you." Her expression spoke volumes. "I wouldn't tell anyone else, even if they asked. I'll only tell my son and now you. That's it." She looked me in the eye, clearly communicating the finality of the topic.

"Okay, I get it Ella. I understand," I assured her before pressing in a different direction. "So, your BiPap. They putting it on you at night?"

"Nope. And before you ask, the same thing applies. I told my son, and he has told them in the office." She raised her palms into the air. "But nothing changes. I used to always use my call light and ask for it at bedtime. It scares me when I wake up suffocating. But the aid would answer my light, and the evening nurse would never come. So I gave up. Now, sometimes that night nurse puts it on me if I wake up and push my call light. It depends on which nurse is working. My son knows about all this, and he knows you've been giving me my treatments and putting my BiPap on. I feel so much better since you came to work here. He noticed and asked what had me feeling so good. I told him!"

Ella's words broke my heart, but her expressions caused an irresistible chuckle.

"Ella, I'm glad you feel better, and I'm proud of you for telling your son when things aren't right. However, you need to get on that light every time you don't get what you need. I'm sorry you even have to do that. You shouldn't have to. But do it. You've got to have your treatments and your BiPap, but I know you know that. Okay, let's get this treatment going."

Ironically, the next afternoon I met Darrell, Ella's son, in the hallway, though "whirlwind" would have been a more suitable name for him. Darrell was on it like white on rice.

"You've got to be the one!" he exclaimed as he shifted packages so he could shake my hand. "Mother described you in detail. I was amazed at how much she remembered. You've got a fan there for sure! Mother thinks you should be a doctor. Thank you for taking care of her. She's getting sassy again. That's a good sign that she's finally starting to feel safe here."

I smiled, listening and processing. Just as much can be said without words as with.

In just under five minutes, Darrell had filled me in on Ella's medical history, his attempts to ensure Ella's care in the nursing facility, and the responses he'd received and from whom. He'd ended with, "But the buck stops here, and the shit's about to hit the fan." He grinned as he sailed away into his mother's room.

Dear goodness! My ears are burning, and my head is spinning. I thought as I headed on my way as well.

284

Three days later, I walked into work and was greeted by the Director of Nurses, Danielle.

"I guess you know Darrell called the state on us," she sneered. "Even wrote them a letter in which he mentioned you by name, saying you were the *only* one who gave his mother her breathing treatments or put on her BiPap at night. I guess you are going to tell me you didn't know anything about that." Danielle rolled her eyes.

"No, ma'am. I did not."

"Okay." She smiled sarcastically.

"Well, Ms. Clueless," Danielle continued, "thanks to you, everybody, including you, has to sign off each night, confirming the BiPap is on." Turning to walk away, she added over her shoulder, "So you can thank yourself for that."

"Somehow, the point became the state as opposed to the care." I shook my head in frustration. *We're already signing off for the BiPap on the treatment record.* I thought to myself. *And I didn't know a thing about him calling state.*

Too little too late, I found Ms. Ella, as confused as a goose, her lung sounds crackling when she inhaled and silent as night when she exhaled. Knowing this likely meant the confusion was carbon monoxide buildup, I gave her a breathing treatment to open her airway, then placed her BiPap on her to maximize ventilation. I called her doctor, and Ella was hospitalized for acute respiratory failure again.

Within the week, Ella was back, much to my relief. However, her nebulizer treatments had been changed from Brovana twice a day to Albuterol every four hours. If you think about it, the hospital doctor had every reason to think it needed to be changed. From his perspective, the Brovana obviously wasn't working, or Ella wouldn't have been such a frequent flyer at the hospital with respiratory failure. However, a week or so later, I realized the Albuterol just wasn't going to cut it. Ella was asking for her treatment before it was due. It simply wasn't as effective for her as the Brovana had been. So I called her doctor and he was livid.

"Nobody told me they had discontinued her Brovana!" he shouted into the phone. "In fact, nobody told me she was back from the hospital!" He raved on for what seemed like forever. Then he stopped and sighed. "Okay. Just start her back on the Brovana, right now, and call her pulmonologist in the morning. Make an appointment for tomorrow. I'll call him myself in the morning to make sure she can be seen."

I administered the Brovana, put her BiPap on, and Ella was sleeping peacefully within just a few minutes, her breathing regular, even. I stood for a minute, watching her breathe, and recalled having asthma as a small child. I remembered how terrifying it was to struggle for air.

I knew my Dad would take me to the emergency room if the episode didn't pass. I was confident. Yet it was terrifying, and I had no clue of the potential dangers. Imagine how it must feel to be an adult, wise to all that is and could be, and to be struggling for breath while completely unable to take care of yourself. *Imagine this, while being constantly in the hands of people you don't even trust to call for help, people who have long proven they won't come.* I shuddered to think, as I proceeded to see to all the others.

Helen:

Helen was on hospice. I saw Helen once each evening to administer a breathing treatment, and that was about it. I'd heard Helen could be quite feisty with the aids, but every time I saw her, she was just sleeping.

Helen had pictures of herself and her family on her wall. I've always loved looking at the pictures in the rooms of those lucky enough to have them. I liked seeing the people they still were on the inside, beneath the wrinkled, saggy skin and often-hazy eyes. Helen may not have been considered a beauty, but she looked happy. Even in the snapshots, she was never without a genuine smile. Not one of those "look at me, I'm pretty" smiles, but one of those "life is good" smiles, which spreads to everyone who gazes upon it. So I smiled every time I saw Helen's smile, until that evening.

I walked into Helen's room and immediately noticed she was so pale that she blended in with the white linen on her bed. Her lips were a purply blue. Hurrying over, I saw her fingertips already had a blueish hue to them, as well. There was thick, stringy mucous hanging from the corner of her mouth, clinging to a dry, crusty pile on her pillow. Helen's chest heaved as she unknowingly struggled for air.

Hurriedly, I started her nebulizer treatment to moisten her secretions, then raised the head of her bed to a sitting position. Her hard breathing changed quickly from a quiet, shrill whistle to a coarse bubbling. Helen was still struggling for air. Hurriedly, I began to set up the suction machine so that I could suction her airway clear, removing the excess mucous she wasn't strong enough to get up on her own. Then I realized there was no Yankauer, which is the piece you insert into the mouth to suction with. I had the suction machine and all the tubing, but nothing with which to suction. Running to the supply room, I found none, so I ran to the crash cart and took the Yankauer from it, then ran back to Helen. I suctioned a large, thick wad of mucous that was partially dried to such an extent that it simply clung to the suctioning, as opposed to being sucked into the tubing. Like a vacuum cleaner hose when it encounters an object too large to suck in, it merely picks it up and holds it.

Helen suddenly gasped, taking a few fast, deep breaths. Placing an oxygen mask over her face, I watched the color return to Helen's cheeks, the blue fading to pink on her lips and fingertips. Helen's eyes popped open. She stared at me with wide eyes for a few seconds, then smiled as big as Texas. It was the same smile I had admired in her pictures so many times before. I smiled back, partly because her smile was indeed contagious, partly out of relief. Helen nodded her head ever so slightly, then closed her eyes and appeared to sleep once more.

I sighed, realizing for the first time just how weary I was. After cleaning up my mess, I finished with my round, and then I notified hospice and briefed them on what had happened. I was still horrified at the lack of Yankauers when shift change arrived.

"Who the hell is going to gather everything needed for the suction machine, except for the suction tool itself? What good is the tubing without the Yankauer?" And on and on I went with no one appearing to be paying me any mind. "I haven't eaten today, and I am starving! Do you mind if I run grab something to eat real quick? I'll give you report when I get back." I asked Rora, my oncoming relief nurse.

"No, go ahead. I'm in no hurry. I'll eat my yogurt while you're gone." She smiled.

"Thanks! I'll hurry," I said as I jogged to the break room to clock out.

When I walked back inside after grabbing some food, things were… different. I could feel vibes, but I had no clue what or why. I did notice everyone was quiet, which was unusual and wasn't the case when I left. I shrugged it off.

"Rora, you ready for report?" I asked.

"Sure, if you are." She smiled.

But that smile is different, I thought. *What the heck?* I was baffled but too tired to care.

Then Rora confirmed my suspicions and royally pissed me off. I'm no saint.

I began giving her the details of the incident with Helen.

What is that goofy look about? I wondered as I observed Rora's face, then continued with report.

Rora maintained the goofy expression throughout my entire report as she leaned against the counter, listening, or pretending to listen. I don't really think she heard anything beyond Helen, because as soon as I said, "That about wraps it up," she spoke.

Still with the goofy expression, Rora said nicely, "Why are you so upset about the Yankauer? It's okay. Helen is on hospice."

I stared at her. My brow creased, mouth open, I just stared, waiting for something to make sense, but she said nothing more. She just stared back with that same goofy smile, which by then I fully recognized as patronizing. However, that was far from what pissed me off.

"Okay, maybe I'm missing something here. I am tired, so in all fairness, maybe my brain is fried," I said quietly, struggling to maintain self-control. "Help me. What has hospice got to do with the Yankauer not being at the bedside with the suction machine?"

Rora smiled bigger, her big brown eyes merry with patience for the ignorant. "Well," she started, her brows raised as if I should be catching on by then, "I mean, she's on *hospice.*"

"Yep, she is. And I'm still not following." My eyes then squinted, and my chin ducked as I readied myself for the blow which I felt certain was coming, yet I could not stop hoping I was wrong. I held my breath, realizing for the first time that the others were silent, watching.

As if explaining the facts of life to a child, Rora said, "Well, she's on hospice because she is in the last phase of her life." She looked at me as if I should have been comprehending, then seemed to realize I was still baffled. "Sooo... she is expected to pass. I mean, we know she is going to die."

I stared at her.

She raised her arms in the air and finished, "In other words, there was no need to panic. She's on *hospice.* She is going to die regardless, and nobody would have held it against you if she did. See?"

Rora's sweet face literally radiated, "It's okay, you silly woman! You made a big deal out of nothing. But we understand. We love you, anyway."

"No! I don't *see*, Rora!" I snapped. "What has *hospice* got to do with the lady smothering? *Hospice* is all about comfort and dignity during the last days of life, not struggling for air as you smother to death because some imbecile nurse was too stupid, lazy, or *both* to ensure the proper equipment was available at bedside!"

Rora's eyes widened, and her brows shot up defensively. The room grew noisy as the others decided they no longer wanted any part of the situation.

I turned and glared at each of them in turn, though they had all turned their backs to us.

I was nice! I could have pointed out that I am well aware it's the night shift's job to ensure the equipment is available! I thought to myself.

Rora was gone when I turned back around. Nothing more was said on the matter. Everybody was unusually busy for the remainder of the time I was there.

Get ready.

The next day, upon my arrival at work, Danielle reprimanded me for taking the Yankauer off the crash cart, leaving everyone else at risk of needing one and not having it available. Let us overlook the fact that it was the only one in the building because no one had seen to it that we kept them available in supplies.

I laughed. My mind was spinning too fast for anything else. I just laughed.

"I see how seriously you take patient care." Danielle smirked.

A short while later I submitted my resignation. I simply didn't know anything else to do.

"What's this?" she asked incredulously. "I can't lose you! You're the best nurse I have! What can I do to keep you?" Danielle exclaimed.

I laughed, picked up my resignation, wadded it up, chucked it in Danielle's trash can, and stared her in the eye for about ten seconds before I turned and walked out of her office.

Ina:

Ina had been with us before, so I knew her well. She was a portly, robust, outspoken woman who seemed to think the world was as hard of hearing as she was. Ina didn't say anything; she yelled it. If Ina told a secret, we'd all know at once.

She'd sold her home and had her son put a trailer in his backyard for her to live in. That was where she'd been for the past two years. I clearly recall how perturbed she was that her son had failed to situate the trailer so that the kitchen window was where it ought to be. She'd grumbled, saying, "Boys just don't think."

Oh, but nobody else could say anything negative about her kids! In fact, Ina tried to persuade me to allow her to fix me up with her son. She thought I was "the purtiest and smartest little thing" she had ever seen. "I ain't never met nobody with a heart as good as yers," she added sincerely, and loudly. I was touched beyond words, but I found all kinds of "ethical" reasons to avoid the potential son catastrophe!

However, Ina never forgot. Over two years later I walked into her room just to say hello. I was working extra to cover for the director of nursing so she could take a few days off, yet an RN would still be in the building for the number of hours required by the state. Ina's blood sugar was running high in the evenings, and the nurse practitioner kept raising the evening dose of insulin (which was only going to result in lowering the blood sugar in the middle of the night) instead of raising the morning dose (which would obviously lower the blood sugar in the evening; thus, she would require less insulin at bedtime as opposed to more. You may not be medically educated, but I bet that makes sense to you). So, I was going to try once more to educate Ina on the importance of a high protein bedtime snack. I was really concerned about the risk of her blood sugar bottoming out during the night because of the high doses of evening insulin.

"Come on in!" Ina yelled when I knocked on her door.

"Hey there!" we said in unison, both cracking up in unison, as well.

"Brilliant minds," she chortled. "When you gonna let me introduce you to Billy? He's still single." She grinned like a mischievous child.

"Oh Lawd, Ina." I laughed. "You haven't dropped that idea yet?"

"I didn't drop anything." She looked confused, then took a deep breath. "Did I?" she asked as she struggled to sit up, nearly rolling off the bed.

"Hey, hey, whoa!" I hurried over. "What're you doing, lady? Trying to crack that hard head of yours?" I helped straighten her up, and she immediately leaned back over, looking at the floor. "Ina , look at me!" I half laughed as a niggle started deep in my gut.

"What?" She looked at me. "I'm a'tryin' to see what I dropped."

"You didn't drop anything."

"Well, you said I did!" She giggled, weaving a bit where she sat on the side of her bed.

"No, I said - never mind." I laughed. "You sure seem out of breath since you sat up. You feel okay?"

"Oh, I feel okay. I'm just dizzy." She whirled circles in the air with her finger, then grabbed the edge of the mattress when the small movement caused her to lose her balance. "I told 'em down there in therapy this mornin' that I just couldn't do it today. You know me. I do my therapy." She glanced up to ensure I was readily agreeing. "So, if I say I can't, I can't."

"Okay, that's all right. Just sit still and catch your breath, love. Stop flappin' them lips." I grinned as I tried to count. "Okay, I'm sorry. Stop laughing. I'll hush."

"No, you won't." She continued laughing. "You flap your lips as much as I do."

Twenty-eight. Her respirations were twenty-eight per minute. (Normal is 12-20)

I began speaking in a hushed tone, but still loud enough for her to hear me. "Really, Ina, be quiet for a minute, relax, and breathe. Purse your lips and push the air back out slow and steady for as long as you can."

I stood close and held her steady.

"Girl, I been stumbling around all day," Ina said, breathless. "I done tole that nurse so many times that I give up." She raised her hands in the air and fell forward, her head bumping into my chest, but I stopped her from falling on her face.

"Shhh, breathe." I sat her up straight, pulling my stethoscope off my neck. Using my free hand, I placed it against her back, moving it to assess her lung sounds in each lobe, and found that she had absolutely zero sound on expiration. "Well, my friend, I need you to lie back ."

"Oh good."

I helped her lie back, then raised the head of her bed so she was almost sitting up straight. "Now be still, and purse those flappin' lips, woman."

I tousled her cropped gray hair. "Take short breaths in, then blow out slow and steady for as long as you can. I'll be right back."

Ina was pursing and blowing as I hurried out to find the doctor who just happened to be in the building at just the right time.

"So, I think she's in acute respiratory failure," I quickly finished.

The doctor jumped up and went to assess Ina as soon as I had filled him in. Within minutes, he came hurrying back. "Spot on!" He grinned. "You are spot on! Once again, you amaze me. Send her to ER. We can't do blood gasses here."

Not wanting to step on toes, I told Homer, Ina's nurse, that the doctor wanted Ina sent to ER. I told him why and even offered to do the paperwork for him.

"No, I'll do it myself." He frowned. "But she's just going to be sent right back." He rolled his eyes.

I bit my tongue, and stuck around to make sure he took care of it right away. I listened to him call and report to the nurse in ER.

"Yeah, so, I'm sending over Ina Sanders. She's a little short of breath, but she has COPD, so nothing unusual. I'm sure you'll send her right back, but I was told to send her over, so I'm sending her. Just remember when she gets there that it wasn't me who thought she needed to come."

I listened as Homer said pretty much the same to the other nurses, telling them I got "all worked up". I really didn't care what Homer *said* provided Ina went to the emergency room right quick and in a hurry.

I kept my mouth shut. I continued to keep my mouth shut for the next six days, and I even managed to keep it shut when Ina finally came back on day seven with a diagnosis of acute on chronic respiratory failure. I never said a word about any of it. I didn't want Homer to think I was "all worked up."

Royalty in the making

"Why are you doing this instead of the help?" Ms. Jackson asked as I wiped her behind. "You are the nurse. You have more important things to do. You need to let the help do this kind of thing," she said as she plopped back down on the toilet. "I'll sit right here and wait while you go get the help. I don't mind waiting."

I smiled big on the outside, sighing heavily inside. "Ms. Jackson, I don't see what difference it makes as long as your behind gets cleaned. Stand back up, please, ma'am."

"I don't mind waiting. I'd rather not have my nurse wiping my behind, anyway." She frowned. "Makes me wonder how clean your hands are when you do my eyedrops at bedtime. By the way, they have to be a full five minutes apart, you know," she said as I silently recited the words along with her, having heard them so many times before.

"Ms. Johnson, I fully intend to wash my hands, as always. However, I'm not going to stop wiping your behind and wash my hands simply to go find the aid and have her come do what I could have finished doing myself," I said flatly. "Stand back up, please. You're right about one thing: I do have other things to do. For now, though, I need to get your behind clean, please, ma'am."

She sighed dramatically, stood dramatically, and huffed and puffed dramatically.

After finishing, I washed my hands and started to leave her room, but she asked me to hand her the box of Kleenex setting on the empty bed, which was layered with stuffed animals. I started to point out that the box was two feet away from her and that she could easily roll her chair over and get it, but it was faster, I thought, to simply hand it to her. So I handed her the box. She ignored the box and took out two Kleenexes. I set the box back down and, once again, attempted to leave the room.

"Oh, uh, nurse?"

"Yes, Ms. Jackson?"

"Wait just a minute while I clean my nostrils…so you can throw this Kleenex away."

"No, ma'am, you can handle that yourself." I smiled and walked out, rolling my eyes.

A short while later Ms. Jackson rolled up behind me in her wheel-chair. "I have to have my medicine at four o'clock, and it is now ten minutes past four."

"Yes, ma'am, and I was just about to bring it to you, but here you are." I smiled.

"It's ten minutes after four."

"Yes, ma'am." I reached out my hand to give her the tiny cup holding her stomach pill.

"I have a contract. I am supposed to get my medicine *at* four o'clock."

"I know, Ms. Jackson. You have a contract, but contract or no, I have an hour to legally administer your medications. Actually, I have two hours. An hour before and an hour after the designated time. This allows a nurse to both legally and timely administer more than one person's med-ications at a given hour."

"Well, I have a contract. That rule doesn't apply to *my* medication."

"Do you want the capsule or not, love?" I smiled. "I'm not going to debate the issue. All my patients are important, including you."

"I'll take it this time, but from now on, it would serve you well to bring me my medication on time. I have a contract, you know," she finished as she took the cup.

That night I took Ms. Jackson her eye drops, administered the first one, and said, "I'll be back in five minutes to do the other drops."

"No, you'll stand right there and wait the five minutes to make sure you put them in my eyes in exactly five minutes. You may use that clock." She pointed her stout old finger at the wall.

I turned and walked out, running into the aid on my way.

"Oh, are you with her now?" Kendra asked, hope gleaming in her eyes.

"Yes, but you go ahead. I have eye drops to do in a few minutes; other-wise I'm finished with her."

"Oh. Okay." The hope vanished, and Kendra hurried in, closing the door behind her.

A few minutes later I knocked and entered, eye drops in hand.

"You'll have to wait now," Ms. Jackson drawled. "I'm getting ready for bed. I told you to wait, and you could have finished before we got started," she reminded me smugly.

"Ms. Jackson, it's after seven o'clock, and I have lots of people to see before bedtime. I'll do your drops now or not at all. That's up to you."

"Well, I'm sure Kendra wouldn't appreciate that," she snipped, as if she cared a hoot about Kendra. "She has things to do, too."

Kendra looked up from folding Ms. Jackson's clothing. "I don't mind. You aren't holding me up. I've still got to run the water in the sink for ten minutes so I can wash Ms. Jackson's feet."

I glanced at Kendra. "Ten minutes?"

"That's how long it takes for the water to get warm enough," Ms. Jackson leered. "Girl, you need to fold my socks, too."

"Her name is Kendra, Ms. Jackson. Tilt your head back, please." I administered the drops, handed Ms. Jackson a Kleenex, and hurried out the door.

At eight-forty-five Kendra came stomping up to my cart in the other hall.

"I will not go back into that room! That woman done flipped her fancy wig!" she shouted. "I do not have to stand there and be treated like that!"

"Calm down and tell me what happened." However, I had a pretty good idea it was the same thing that happened with all the aids who were ultimately kicked out of or refused to re-enter *that* room.

"She had me wash her feet, then lotion 'em. *Then*, she gone tell me to wipe the lotion off her toes!" Kendra threw her arms in the air. "She crazy! She look for ways to annoy you. She want things don't nobody want, just to put you in yo place. She has a certain way she wants her bed turned back. The fold in the blanket has to be ten inches wide, no more, no less. She gone pull a ruler out of her drawer to measure it. Then I finally get her in the bed, and she asked me to hand her another Kleenex. I did, and then she tole me to wait while she cleaned her nose so I could throw it away! I ain't touching her boogers! I sits her trash can next to her bed so she could reach it herself. That woman told me to go wash the trashcan, that she ain't gone sleep with no nasty trash can next to her bed.

I tole her it ain't nasty, and she said not to argue with her, just to go wash it. She said 'the niggers' are sposed to be silent, just do as the master of the house tells 'em to do. She say she the 'master.'" Kendra's lip curled. "Now, that's it! Don't she realize she black as I am?" Kendra fumed.

I burst out laughing. "Kendra, don't let that silly old woman upset you. Some people are just mean and ignorant. For some reason she feels the need to belittle others in order to make herself feel important. Maybe she never felt like she mattered to anyone. I don't know. I know it's hard, but just ignore it. Do your thing and get out."

"That's just it! I can't get out! She takes nearly two hours to get changed and in the bed. Anybody else takes fifteen minutes or less! I don't have time for that. She needs one-on-one care if all her little demands are going to be met, but they ain't gone be met by this girl never again." Kendra reached both hands to her head and pulled her own hair in dramatic frustration. "Woman gone make me pull my curls out." She laughed, then shook it off.

So, Ms. Jackson had gone through the last aid on staff, and her call light was blinking. Dreadfully, I headed for her room, hurried in to turn the call light off.

"That girl left before my needs were met." Ms. Jackson snorted, her nose in the air. "I'm about to call my sister and report her. Would you like to wash my trash can before I speak with my sister?"

"That girl's name is Kendra, and she will not be back in your room tonight, nor any other night. You can't call the staff names, Ms. Jackson. I'm surprised at you. Such behavior is beneath you. Regardless, no, ma'am, I don't care to wash your trash can. It's fine. You go ahead and call your sister." I turned to leave.

"I have a contract, you know."

"Yes, ma'am, you've told me that at least three times every day since the first day I met you, so I couldn't forget if I wanted to. But I don't have a thing to do with contracts. *That* is between you and the administrator. Talk with him about it tomorrow. For now, good night. Sleep well."

"I'm going to report you and that girl."

"Yes, ma'am, you should always report your concerns," I replied, silently hoping Kendra and I would be forever banned from her room, like so many others.

A short while later Kendra said, "The master's light is on again."

I trudged wearily back to Ms. Jackson's room.

"I need my light turned out, thank you." Ms. Jackson smiled sweetly, her arms crossed over the ten-inch fold in her blanket, "My sister said I should use my call light to get some help with it."

"Yes, ma'am. Well, you did just as she said, didn't you? I'm sure she'll be proud of you. The string right there"—I pointed— "the one next to the button you pushed to turn your call light on, that string turns your light off, but then you know that." I smiled just as sweetly.

"Oh, my goodness, you're right." Ms. Jackson looked me in the eye as she pulled the string, turning the light off. "Good night now. I'll see you tomorrow," she sang through the darkness.

King Tutt:

"My wife said you have to feed me," George proclaimed as he pushed the button on the remote control, surfing the channels.

"Eat, George." I chuckled. "Your hands work just fine now."

Ten minutes later Mrs. George arrived and began fussing, saying that somebody needed to feed George.

"Ma'am, George is much stronger than he was, and he doesn't need to be fed anymore, unless. of course, you want to continue feeding him once he gets home." I shrugged.

"Well, no, of course not," Mrs. George sputtered. "But while he's here, he should be fed to make sure he eats enough to get stronger."

"Mrs. George." I resisted a sigh as I repeated the daily do-over. "George won't get stronger if he does nothing for himself. And we check everybody's plate and offer health shakes to anybody who doesn't eat adequately. After all, even when we fed George, he only ate what he ate. We can't force food down him."

"George, do you feel strong enough to feed yourself, honey?"

George looked from me to his wife, then back to me, saying nothing.

"Eat, George." I rubbed the top of his head. "I'll check back on you in a little while."

Mrs. George sailed into the dining room just a few minutes later. "George needs to use the bathroom. Come now."

"Ms. George, we're serving dinner to everyone else." I smiled. "You know we can't stop serving dinner to take George to the toilet, but someone will be there shortly," I assured, knowing Mrs. George would time the staff, as always, making notes in her little journal next to George's chair. George always seemed to need to pee during Mrs. George's visits.

"He didn't eat much," she added pointedly before hurrying back out.

After dinner, I asked Keesha to take George to the toilet, during which Mrs. George came to find me to let me know how many minutes George had had to wait.

Later that night, after Mrs. George went home, I asked George if he needed to use the bathroom before going to bed.

"Oh hell, not you, too," he grumbled. "Seems my bladder has become more important than world hunger. Everybody always asking me if I need to pee. My wife asked me right in the middle of dinner! I said no, and she actually said, 'Yes, you do,' like I don't know if I need to pee or not." He shook his balding head. "I guess I better pee, or you're likely to write that in her little book."

A few days later Mrs. George was already there, standing in George's doorway, when I arrived at work. She saw me walk in and began waving for me to come running. Needing to punch in, I stuck my finger up, indicating I'd be there in a minute. That wasn't good enough. Two minutes later she sailed up to the nurses' station, her poofy black hair bouncing with every step.

Uh oh, I thought to myself as I noticed the bounce, *this isn't going to be pretty.*

"How is George supposed to get a nap with the head of his bed up like they had it?" she all but yelled. "And he was wet when I got here. He didn't like lunch, but nobody got him anything else to eat. His water jug is empty. They had that thick blanket on him. I told them he likes the ones I brought from home, and I don't think he got a shower. They say he did, but I don't think so. He says he did, but I still don't think so. I can feel it when George is uncomfortable. I want him showered now, while I'm here, so I can be sure." She finally took a breath.

"Now, that's a lot to take in all at once." I smiled, forcing my sarcasm deep down inside. "Give me just a minute to get report, and I'll be down to George's room so we can talk."

A short while later I stopped, took a deep breathe, and then walked into George's room, where Mrs. George twittered around like a crazed magpie, instructing George on what made him comfortable.

"You don't like that pillow behind your head, George, remember?"

"That was when my blood pressure was high and I had a headache. I don't have a headache anymore."

"Move the pillow, George."

George sat there, noticed I'd entered, grinned at me, and then looked pitiful once more.

Mrs. George hadn't noticed my presence, and she continued rattling. "You don't like tea, George," she said, picking up his nearly empty glass from lunch. "Why are you drinking tea? And tell the nurse when she comes in that you need a shower. I don't care what you say. You haven't had a shower today. You aren't comfortable until you've had your shower."

I cleared my throat.

"Oh, you're here," Mrs. George exclaimed, clapping her hands. "Good. George was just telling me he doesn't like tea, so just bring him juice at dinner, please. And he said he needs a shower. Didn't you, George?" She looked at George.

I looked at George.

George closed his eyes, pretending he had fallen asleep. He let his head lean to the side and began a light, obviously phony snore.

I bit my lip to keep from grinning.

"Well, I guess he's exhausted from sitting up in that chair so long. Can you get them to lay him down? I'll go on home if he's just going to sleep. But make sure he wakes up to eat dinner. I guess he can wait until tomorrow morning for that shower. First thing, though." She held up a finger.

"Yes, ma'am, you go on home now. Get you some rest. I'll see to it that George eats his dinner and then gets right into bed."

Keesha and I went in to help George into bed after dinner, but George had the ballgame on and refused. Mrs. George called to tell George to tell us he needed to pee. George handed his phone to Keesha.

"Umm, hello? This is Keesha, the aid."

"This is George's wife. Tell him he needs to tell you that he needs to pee before he goes to bed."

"Yes, ma'am, I sure will." Mrs. George ended the call, and Keesha looked at George. "You need to tell me that you need to pee before you go to bed."

George rolled his eyes. Keesha looked at me, and we laughed quietly as we walked out, leaving George to his game.

The next day was going about the same. Mrs. George arrived and immediately pushed the call light, standing in George's doorway to make sure we knew she was waiting impatiently.

"I know you all don't have enough help, but George needs someone to come just as soon as his light is on. Don't you, George?"

"Yep." George stared at the television.

"And don't bring him tea for dinner. He doesn't like tea, and it will make him wet himself in the night. Won't it, George? It's okay," she reassured, "tell the nurse you don't like tea."

"Nope."

"And George needs to lie down right after dinner so he gets his rest. Don't you, George?"

"Yep."

"And George needs his shower first thing in the morning, before he gets tired. Don't you, George?"

"Yep."

"And—"

"Whoa!" I laughed. "Mrs. George, you do realize whatever monster you create here will be the monster you take home with you soon, don't you?"

Mrs. George stopped and gazed out the window.

I waited.

George stared at the television.

"George," Mrs. George finally quipped, "stop being so demanding." She snatched up her purse and sailed out of the room.

George looked up in surprise, grinned, and said, "Well, I'll be damned." He laughed so heartily that the pillow slipped from behind his head. "You may be the smartest woman I ever met!" Then, crossing his ankles, he added with a wink, "Bring me some tea with dinner, and grab my pillow before you leave, would you? I'm going to relax a while."

Emerald:

Emerald preferred to spread her pills out on her table, then take them one at a time. Being a hypochondriac, she took a million. Emerald also loved to sleep. Now, that part, I get completely. However, Emerald would sleep through an entire meal and almost through the next one, and then she'd complain because her food was cold. She'd have the staff warm it up for her, then complain that it wasn't any good all "warmed over like that."

Emerald also had a tendency to stretch the truth, meaning she'd lie her socks off, and she created a vast array of new and unexplainable symptoms for which one could never possibly find an answer, but one had to keep looking, as the complaints kept rolling in like waves on a stormy sea.

She frequently had diarrhea, mostly due to her diet, so Emerald would need to poo, almost inevitably, every time I took her medications in. And since she took them one at a time, of course, I'd have to scoop them back up into the cup and come back in a few minutes later to watch her swallow them. Or I'd have to crawl around on her floor, finding the one that rolled away when it "just jumped right off the table" on her. Emerald squealed with delight when you'd found it, while you trudged out to obtain a clean replacement for the runaway. After all, the two-minute rule cannot apply in the "house of germs." Sometimes I wondered if Emerald didn't drop her pills just for the kick of it.

Like a bat, Emerald slept most of the day and woke at night, ready to roam for prey. I always knew Emerald was coming when I heard that rhythmic swishing sound her house-shoes made against the floor as they were dragged along beneath the weight of her enormous legs and backside. And, like a coin, Emerald had two sides: ornery and whiney, or silly and delighted to the point of near elation, much like a school girl who's just been invited to the prom by the boy she'd crushed on since elementary.

Emerald would swish into the lobby, plop her wide load into the chair just across from the nurses' station, and do one of two things: She'd laugh like a hyena about anything she heard, good or bad, or she'd grumble and complain about any little thing she could think of, good or bad. I never was certain which I preferred, the shrill or the shrew. But that was it, one or the other, until the evening we sang. Emerald never forgot that moment. It was that evening that I decided Emerald must have been a looker back in the day, considering the way she pruned and crooned as that song swept her back in time, transforming her into the Emerald of yesteryear, just for a little while. It took her back to days of vigor and vanity. That evening left a mark on Emerald so strong that she tried many times, almost desperately, to recreate the moment. But it had been random, spontaneous; it simply wasn't something one could intentionally *do* and discover the same magic. Or, as much as it surprises even me, I'd have done it for Emerald.

I banged my medication cart into place just outside the door to the dining room on our unit, locking it just as Junius, aka Junebug, slammed his cart against the wall on the opposite side of the door. Both of us immediately and methodically began opening and closing drawers and containers at the speed of light, our hands prepping the remainder of our pre-dinner medications as our minds traveled elsewhere at a matching speed, even as our eyes glanced back to check the records.

"Your cheating hearrrrrrt," I randomly burst into tune, my twang as thick as Hank Williams Sr.'s himself.

Delighted, Junebug joined in the duet, not missing a beat, singing, "Will tell on youuuuuu."

"You'll cry and cryyyyyyy." A deep baritone belted robustly from somewhere in the dining room.

Kindred spirits with twin brains, Junebug and I instinctively leaned in sideways to peer in through the open doorway, just in time to see Ms. Myrtle raise her wispy white head and squawk, in a scratchy soprano, "The whole night throuuuuuuugh."

"You'll walk the flooooor," Clinton howled at the ceiling, concentration pinching his eyes closed.

"The way you doooooo," Grumpy bellowed, ole Jed joining in for the "do," bobbing his knobby little head.

"Your cheating hearrrrrt," we all sang together, blowing the roof off, "will tell on youuuuuuuuuuuu."

That dining room teemed with life as everyone clapped their hands, purely delighted in the moment, laughing and teasing and chattering like woodchucks.

My eyes swept the room, happy tears stinging my eyes as I watched Myrtle, who was grinning like a kid, scoop mashed potatoes onto a spoon and then raise it to her mouth, as if she did so every day, as if she hadn't grown silent, developed a blank stare, and slipped away from us into the maze of her own mind months before.

Jed was glancing about at his table mates, aware of and interested in his surroundings for the very first time in a very long time. His hand was in his plate, of course, but he wasn't just pushing his food around his plate that evening; Jed was busy licking pureed carrots from his fingers, savoring every lick. Jed was eating independently!

Junebug stood next to me, wearing a big, goofy grin.

Suddenly, a high, piercing squeal silenced the room. Emerald, who absolutely never came to the dining room with "all the annoying common people," and who seldom left her bat cave before dark, was standing in the doorway, her face aglow as her eyes flitted about the room. "Let's sing it again!" She shuffled inside.

All eyes on her, Emerald transformed mid-stride, the weight of her huge, fluid-filled legs seeming to dissipate more with each shuffle. Then, stopping mid-shuffle, she leaned her head back, face to the ceiling, and crooned, "Your cheating hearrrrrrt." Releasing her grip from her walker, she spread her arms like glamorous wings, tipped one toe while coyly tilting her knee and winked at Clinton as she ended her solo.

Spurred by flirtation, Clinton picked up where she left off, and the round began once more as Emerald literally pranced about the room. Her house shoes—two inches of purple fluff poofed out around her feet and ankles, as if she'd stepped up onto a purple cloud—sailed to opposite sides of the room as Emerald kicked them off before leaning down to hug ole Jed, who leaned his knobby head back and grinned, oblivious to the food dripping from his chin.

Easily able to visualize pink ballet slippers upon her feet, I watched in amazement as Emerald spun around and sashayed over to Wyverne, who was singing her solo. She met Emerald's entrancing gaze and bopped Myrtle in the face as she, too, spread her wings.

Myrtle, surprised, dropped her spoon, rubbed her nose, and cackled as Emerald popped up behind the ladies, pulling their heads together in a group hug.

"Oh my!" Emerald placed her hands over her heart, shaking her head and swinging her loose brown curls from side to side. "I feel like a girl on a moonlit night, and it feels so goooood!" She giggled wildly, then twirled round the room, giving another round of hugs before prancing back to her walker, grabbing her purple fluffs on her way, and sailing back out the door, her laughter trailing behind her as the room begin to buzz with chatter once again.

When I checked on Emerald later that night, I found her fast asleep. It was the first time I'd ever seen her sleep before the wee hours of morning.

"I feel like a girl on a moonlit night," I heard in my head, "and it feels so goooood!" I smiled, closing her door behind me.

The next night, while sitting at the station and charting, I heard the familiar "Emerald swish" approaching from my right. I waited for her to pass, en route to her seat across from the station. But Emerald's house shoes caught my eye; the inner side of the backs, where her heels had forever squashed the purple fluff, combined with the swishing sound, tugged at my heart with every shuffle.

"I need a snack," Emerald grumbled as she plopped her heavy hips down into the chair. "I guess all you have is pimento cheese or peanut butter." She rolled her eyes, scowling.

"Yes, ma'am. I'm sorry. Which would you like?"

"Well, I don't *like* either one of them. But unless I want to starve to death, I guess I'll take one of both. I'll see which one might be edible," she snapped. "How they manage to screw up peanut butter is beyond me, but they do." She continued grumbling as I stood to unlock the door, getting her a snack.

I walked over and handed Emerald her sandwiches. "The magic is gone." I chuckled to myself.

Emerald snatched the sandwiches from my hand. "I guess you expect a thank you for this garbage," she barked while ripping off plastic wrap.

"Yep, Cinderella has no doubt left the ball." I laughed to myself. "And the wicked stepmother has taken her place."

Ignoring the bark, I walked back to my seat at the station and resumed my paperwork, ignoring Junebug's antagonizing grin as he ducked his head lower behind the counter.

"Well, that was as awful as I thought it'd be," Emerald grumbled as she chewed the last bite of her second sandwich, rolling the plastic into a ball with her palms. "Somebody want to come get this, or do you expect me to eat this garbage, too?"

I spun around to face Junebug. "Don't say it!" I whispered through gritted teeth, knowing I would purely howl with laughter if he did. Junebug froze, mouth open, delight dancing in his black eyes like fire against a night sky.

Infection Control Methods or Myth?

Darcy:

Darcy was determined to get home within the two weeks her doctor had "promised" so she could cook Thanksgiving dinner for her family, just as she always had.

"Douglas will pout like a baby if I don't make my banana pudding, and the kids will never let me live it down if we don't have Darcy's dressing," she explained as I removed the bandage from her hip.

"Darcy's dressing, huh? Sounds like there's a story behind that one." I distracted her while examining her incision site, feeling the redness surrounding the wound for warmth, swabbing the thick, yellow drainage for a culture.

"Oh, yes, ma'am." Darcy frowned. "Douglas's mother, Cora, found a way to have me do any and every little thing that she didn't want to do herself. Douglas and I married in October. October twenty-fifth, nineteen sixty-four. As newlyweds, we lived in a tiny garage apartment, and all our furniture was junk other people didn't need or were planning to throw away. But that didn't stop Cora, not for a minute." Darcy laughed. "Cora dropped in to see Douglas and me just six days before Thanksgiving to tell us she'd borrowed a table or two, and a few chairs, from the church, and Doug senior was bringing them by on Wednesday evening, the day before Thanksgiving.

"Douglas asked her, 'Why are you dropping them off here, Mama?'

"Cora smiled real big; hugged me real tight; put her old, conniving hands on my cheeks; and said, 'Now that she's part of our family, I wanted to let Darcy here have the chance to be the family's official Thanksgiving host! It's a surprise weddin' present to Darcy from her new mama!'" I just about choked, and Douglas just stood there like an idiot, didn't say a word! Cora made a big announcement on Thanksgiving that she was glad Darcy's dressing was edible. She's been at her meanness and tricks ever since!" Darcy squealed with laughter.

"Oy my gosh! So Darcy's dressing was born, and Cora has never let it die!" I laughed. "Well then, let's get you home for Thanksgiving." I pulled Darcy's blanket back up over her hip.

"Does the incision look bad?"

"No, it doesn't look bad. Let's just say it looks like it might be thinking about going bad, but I'm thinking we'll prevent that and keep you right on schedule. The antibiotic the doctor ordered is a good one. It should fix you up. Just to make sure we're on the right track, though, he ordered this culture, which, speaking of, I need to take over to the lab so they can get it going." I smiled and hurried out.

"Hey, Norah, I'll be back in a few. I'm running this wound culture to the lab." I waved my bio bag in the air as I passed the nurses' station.

"You better call Susan about that," Norah hollered at me. "She don't like cultures being done."

I stopped mid-step, backed up, and peered around the counter at Norah. "Huh?"

"Susan don't like us to do cultures." She shrugged.

"Why?"

"I don't know." She laughed. "Ask Susan."

So I did. I called Susan.

"I don't like to do cultures. We know we have bugs. Every place has bugs. People come from the hospital with bugs. When you get into the cultures, you start getting into contact isolation and all kinds of crap, whereas, if you just treat the infection, the patient heals up, and everything keeps rolling without all the added complications," Susan explained. "If one antibiotic doesn't work, you just try another. Besides that, if you start having a bunch of MRSA or something, it looks bad and flags with the state. So it's best to just treat the infection and skip the culture. No culture, no bugs. See?"

I did. I saw crystal clear. That right there was a new broom, a model I had not seen before. Obviously, a model that is highly functional in sweeping dirt under the rug.

Winston:

Winston was an intelligent, educated, well-spoken, and successful retired engineer.

"He expects his wound care to be done every afternoon *at two*. There he is, sitting in his doorway, waiting," Mia whispered. "He'll refuse if it's not done in the next thirty minutes or so. And trust me, he needs it done. He has MRSA in the wound, and he is nasty!"

I headed down the hallway, my lungs involuntarily cutting my breath short as I neared the end, where a thick, revolting odor slammed into my nostrils. Glancing around for what could possibly be the source, I pushed through, making my way to room one-twelve, the stench, and thus my dread, growing stronger as I grew nearer. Turning left, I entered the room, horrified to discover the floor so sticky that it tugged at the soles of my shoes with every step.

Urinals containing varying amounts of urine decorated the quarter bedrail, the windowsill, the bedside table, and even the floor. The second bed was buried beneath…stuff. I can't tell you what, because I tried to get back out of the cloud of acrid stench as fast as I possibly could, before it attached itself to my lungs, nostrils, and clothing. It was unequivocally and indescribably the foulest, thickest odor I'd ever encountered. Raw sewage would have been a blessed relief to my nose. Flies swarmed the urinals and the remnants of food scattered throughout the room.

"Well, hello there." Winston smiled at me, the corners of his sweater-gray eyes crinkling. "What brings you by my way on this spectacular day?"

"I need to change the dressing on your foot, please," I said, immediately panicked, realizing that speaking would make me breathe deeper and more frequently.

Winston raised his legs, propping them on a pillow at the foot of his bed. Gauze, which was stained black from the floor and saturated with drainage, hung loosely from his foot like a decaying mummy in a horror movie. Winston smiled pleasantly, completely oblivious to the odor he'd long since grown accustomed to. In perfectly appropriate medical terminology, he began instructing me on the proper way to perform his wound care.

Concentrating on shallow breathing, I completed the task at hand as efficiently as possible, making no comment. Placing a layer of antimicrobial dressings over the draining areas, I then covered them with thick, absorbent pads, then wrapped his entire foot and lower leg with layers of fresh gauze.

Needing to take a good deep breath, I hurried back out, my shoes sticking to the floor all the way back down the hallway. Making a mental note to wear shoe covers into Winston's room from that day forward, I stopped in the shower room at the entrance to the hallway, washed the soles of my sneakers, and tried to steam my nostrils clear at the sink.

Later in the dining room, as I prepped for dinner, I noticed Winston come through the door, his head held high. He was sitting so tall and straight that I almost didn't notice his wheelchair at all.

"Hello again." I waved from across the room as he approached me, waving back and smiling.

An invisible cloud of stench enveloped me as soon as Winston was within ten feet of me. Eventually, I would come to realize that I always knew when Winston was approaching, as the distinct odor was much like a calling card, announcing his arrival. The odor reached our noses before Winston ever got close enough to speak.

One afternoon, I encountered Winston, en route to the dining room with his foot dripping a trail behind him because he had once again refused to allow his nurse to do his wound care. Not wanting to embarrass him, I quietly explained that he needed to have his wound care done if he wanted to eat with the others in the dining room. It wouldn't be prudent for him to do so with drainage dripping from his foot.

"Well then." Winston raised his chin high. "You may bring my dinner to my room. If she cannot come to do my wound care timely, I shall not allow it to be done."

The following day I was informed that Winston had the right to eat in the dining room, and he had the right to refuse his wound care. All we could do was encourage him not to refuse.

I responded, "Of course he has a right. No question. But he also has MRSA in that wound. The only reason he doesn't require contact isolation strictly within his room is because the site of his MRSA infection can be contained by covering the wound to protect others. Therefore, if the MRSA isn't contained—and it isn't if he's dripping drainage everywhere—he is putting others at risk. So, again, he does have a right to eat in the dining room, but only if the wound is dressed and dry, because the others have a right to be safe."

My words fell on deaf ears. Winston continued eating in the dining room, grabbing snacks from the snack tray and dripping about the facility at will, often coming out of his room in the wee hours to grab another snack before dripping back to his room at the end of the hallway.

To make matters worse, one evening I noticed that the seat of Winston's wheelchair was dripping so heavily that streaming might have been a better word. It, too, left a trail behind him, much like the trail made on the pavement after one has climbed from a swimming pool.

Upon closer inspection, I noticed that Winston was sitting on three full-sized, folded blankets, which were atop the pressure reduction cushion in the seat of his wheelchair.

Well, that's not doing any good whatsoever with blankets stacked on top, but more importantly, what's causing Niagara Falls? I thought as I took a deep breath, then hurried to Winston's side.

Leaning down so no one could hear, I whispered, "What's up with the drip, sir? You're leaving quite a trail behind you." At this point, it was clear that the cushion and blankets were saturated to the point of holding no more; and they were pouring.

"That's urine," Winston snapped blatantly, his head rearing back indignantly. "I have a little problem with urine leakage, and that is something over which I have no control. So I'll just be on my way." He popped his eyes open wide, dipped his chin dramatically in dismissal, and began to roll on toward the dining room.

"Sir." I stopped him, leaning down once more to whisper privately as urine splattered onto my shoes. "You're right; you have no control over the leakage. That is a common problem shared by many later in life. However, you do have control over dripping urine down the hallway. You have control over changing your brief. You—"

"I put a fresh brief on every morning, young lady," Winston interjected, cocking his balding head to the side. "I use a urinal, and occasionally the toilet, so the brief is only for the leakage. It is not my fault that the manufacturer cannot produce a brief that does the job adequately."

"Again, sir, you do have control over changing your brief," I whispered wearily, "and once you do so, and once you change your wet pants, you are more than welcome to join the rest of us in the dining room."

Winston stared up at me, eyes wide, mouth gaping.

"I'd be happy to assist you, as those blankets must go to laundry, and your wheelchair cushion must be washed. And by the way, the cushion does nothing to prevent pressure on your buttocks if you stack blankets on top of it." As an afterthought, I added in desperation, "Winston, you're a delightful, intelligent man. You deserve to be clean. How about I help you get a quick shower before dinner?"

"I get my shower before I go to see my doctor, because he won't see me unless I do so. He doesn't care that the process is tiring for me, and it is quite evident that you also care not," he quipped as he turned his chair.

I stared, speechless, as I watched Winston grab the siderail to expedite his turn, realizing he'd just admitted he only showers before his doctor's appointments, which occurred no more often than every three to six months.

The following Tuesday, when I returned to work, I was counseled once more on Winston's rights. Once again, to no avail, I referenced the rights of all the others, of the staff, to be as germ-free as possible.

Ms. Adams was first. Notorious for removing the dressings on her lower legs, thus touching the wounds with the same hands she used to touch the table she shared with Winston, Ms. Adams developed a MRSA infection in her wounds, as proven by a wound culture.

Next was Johnny, who was a bit OCD and picked up every little thing he saw lying on the floor. Johnny was a quiet guy, didn't say much at all, but when he did, it was inevitably at top volume, as if he were at a concert, trying to be heard over the music and the crowd. Johnny just about caused me to have a heart attack on several occasions, as he would suddenly yell into the back of my head while handing me something he'd found on the floor, as he was doing right then.

"Johnny!" I laughed, spinning around, pointing at the trash can on my cart. "Just throw it away, sweetheart. You don't have to tell me!"

Johnny grinned down at me, exposing all five of his teeth. That's when I noticed the crusty drainage matting his eyelashes, along with the intense redness to the whites of his eyes.

"What's up with your eyes, dude?"

"ITCHY!"

I called his doctor and told him I had cultured the drainage. The doctor started antibiotic eye drops. I called the director and suggested contact isolation, which she felt was an overreaction. She said, "Try keeping Johnny in his room," and laughed. Five days later we received the culture results, and as I'd suspected, it had grown MRSA which required different treatment.

Meanwhile, Corrine continued her habit of repeatedly pushing herself up from her chair unassisted while sitting in the lobby. Corrine was a busy bee and a chatter box wrapped into one adorably challenging package. Over time, Johnny had adopted her. He felt it was his civic duty to jump up and grab her hand, holding her steady as he announced, "FALL," so I could come running. Corrine had allergies, so she rubbed her nose constantly. Quite naturally, though I'd been wiping both her hands and Johnny's with disinfectant wipes habitually since Johnny's eyes had become infected, Corrine developed a nasty cough and ultimately grew MRSA in her sputum culture.

I was directed to stop all cultures.

"Just get an order for an antibiotic," the director barked. "No more cultures."

Within two weeks we had two more respiratory infections being treated. Ms. Dillon was one, and she seemed to be getting worse instead of better as time went on. Ultimately, I collected a sputum sample and sent it for a culture. It grew MRSA, and the doctor had to change to an antibiotic the bug was sensitive to, the first one having been a waste of time. By then Ms. Dillon was severely ill. We started the IV antibiotics, but she got so short of breath in the night that the nurse had to send her to the hospital. Ms. Dillon returned over a week later. I was threatened with a write-up for getting the culture. I'd planned to tell her to save her ink, but she never said another word about it. So all was well there, too. But MRSA lurks.

Popcorn is inevitably a frequent "activity" in long-term care. The activity director at this facility held a popcorn party early Friday afternoon. At dinner that evening, the popcorn still speckled the floor, crunching beneath our shoes as we served dinner. I thought surely the plan was to clean the popcorn up after dinner with the routine cleaning, since it had not already been swept up. It turned out there was no routine cleaning. Sailing through the darkened dining room that night, cutting through to another hall, I felt a crunch beneath my shoe. I stopped, looked around, and shook my head as I saw popcorn still scattered over the now dimly lit floor. Most of it was squashed like bugs, but other kernels were still white and fluffy. When I returned to work on Tuesday, I found the popcorn still there, all squashed except for what was in the corners. Some of the squashed popcorn now speckled the hallways, having hitched a ride on the bottom of shoes or wheelchairs. I asked if they'd had another popcorn party. The activities director responded dryly, "No, we only do popcorn on Fridays." Finally, on Thursday, the popcorn disappeared, and thank goodness there wasn't another popcorn party on that Friday. I felt certain it would have purely exhausted the housekeeping department.

Same facility, same dining room. I was hurrying to get Charles more tea, and a dried spill caught my eye. Laughing, I pointed it out to the residents sitting nearby.

"Look, the Eiffel Tower!"

They laughed.

"It is indeed." Winston grinned. "I observed it as I approached the table. It is certainly no Monet, but the resemblance is uncanny." He chuckled, urine dripping from his chair, drainage dripping from his foot.

Having taken it upon myself to disinfect the floor and table after Winston left the dining room each evening, I almost cleaned up the Eiffel tower but didn't. Instead, I observed. The Eiffel tower remained for more than a week before they started cleaning up, preparing for our "window for state," meaning the time period in which state survey was expected.

"Well," Winston commented at dinner, "I take it the janitor got tired of viewing the Eiffel Tower and mopped it away." He chuckled, his gray eyes sparkling as he dripped.

Before I move on, I must tell this. I want to laugh, but I'm told it's inappropriate in nonfiction. So, just know I'm laughing. I wink.

One harried night, at the end of a particularly difficult shift, I finished administering G-tube medications to a resident and turned to rush back out of a room. Suddenly, a loud splat, from behind me, snagged my attention. Knowing the nurse aid was providing incontinent care to the other occupant of the room, I turned to see if my assistance was needed. Through the gap, between the curtain and the wall, I saw a brief clinging to the wall, just stuck there like home décor.

"No, Ms. Jenkins." I heard the aid instruct wearily. "Don't touch it again."

I observed an old, bony hand reaching for the brief.

"That's nasty." The aid stressed. "And now you done got shit all over the wall."

Calling out to the aid, I asked, "You need some help?"

"Naw. I got it."

Chuckling, I thanked my lucky stars that I was about to be off for a few days. And I headed back up the hallway in hopes of wrapping that day *up*!

Two days later, I return to work, walk in that same room, and there it is. A shit stain as big as a basketball! Grabbing some bleach wipes and gloves, I tried to scrub it off, but it was too set in the paint by that time. But as I was wiping, Ms. Jenkins came unglued.

"You erasin my picture of my mama!" She wailed as I scrubbed. "You can't rase my mama!"

"It won't scrub off." I heard myself say aloud.

"That's cause my mama don't take no shit."

Do NOT say it! I laughed to myself.

Ms. Jenkin's 'mama' was still on the wall when I left nearly a year later.

Again, I could go on forever.

Tricks of the Trade

Sadie:

The first time I met Sadie, I knew she was a heart stealer. She looked up at me with huge, oval-shaped, brown eyes that literally shined from her pale, moon-shaped face. She scratched her little bald head with a plump little hand as she laughed. "Look, honey, I got myself a fairy winkle nurse!"

I laughed, glancing at Paul, her husband, who was staring at me in complete silence as he held Sadie's hand.

"Paulie? You still with me here?" Sadie chuckled.

He shook his head from his apparent daze and laughed with Sadie. "Looks like them hospital nurses are getting all the food before these rehab nurses can get a bite!"

"Actually, I like fairy winkles." I laughed. "Don't tell anyone, but I still have my daughter's fairy winkles in a box."

Sadie's eyes grew even bigger. "I still have my daughter's fairy winkles!"

"Awww, you girls can play fairy winkles together," Paul teased, adjusting Sadie's covers with his free hand.

I glanced at Sadie, noticing her purposeful, rhythmic breathing.

"Sadie, are you hurting?"

Paul looked at me. "She needs a pain pill. I know she didn't ask for one, but that's my Sadie. She never complains."

"I could sure use one, if you have time." Sadie smiled.

Sadie had cancer everywhere, and time proved she would tolerate just about anything with a smile on her face and a witty comment to make you laugh. I finally convinced her to use her call light and get her needs met, but I told her I thought her hair probably fell out simply because her head had gotten so hard. Sadie roared with laughter, saying, "Paulie's gonna love that one!"

Sadie was a fighter. Over time, she and Paul shared her entire story with me. Dear God, how does a person endure such? I found Sadie purely remarkable. Her spirit had not diminished one ounce along the way. Sadie was my hero.

One afternoon the medication aid was administering Sadie's medications when he found one missing. Alex came to ask me about it, telling me there were three tablets remaining the day before, but the entire blister pack was missing. He could not find any in backup supply, either. I stopped what I was doing, explaining that the med was a chemo drug as I walked with Alex back to the nurses' station. Therefore, it wouldn't be in backup.

Ultimately, I found the remaining three tablets in drug destruction. There was an order for the medication to be discontinued. And the diagnosis for the medication had been deleted from Sadie's records altogether, with an appropriate order to do so, of course. So Sadie, who had cancer everywhere, no longer had cancer, according to her records. I was baffled. Even the diagnosis for her pain medication had been changed.

I called my supervisor. In short, the medication was too expensive. When one is "skilled," the facility is required to pay for all medications, procedures, and appointments. Therefore, the medication had been discontinued until Sadie's skilled days were completed. When her days were used up, we could restart the medication, if she still wanted to."

That was supposed to make things okay.

I stood, speechless. If you knew me, you'd understand that speechless is simply not something that happens to me. But I had absolutely no clue what to do, say, or think.

My face scrunched with confusion, and I slowly walked back toward Sadie's room, hesitating at the doorway. Creeping in, I found Sadie sleeping, Paul sitting at her bedside staring at her. Paul glanced up, his thick black brows scrunched together in deep thought.

"What do you see? When you look at her, what do you see?" he asked quietly.

"Paul, I see an amazing spirit with beautiful eyes, an amazing spirit, and an endless smile."

Tears welled in Paul's eyes, rolling down his weary face as he whispered, "I see you."

"I'm sorry. What?"

"I see you." Paul sobbed quietly.

Sadie stirred but didn't wake.

Paul started aggressively pressing buttons on his cell phone, then thrust it at me, tears dripping from his jaw onto the floor.

Taking his phone in my hand, I gazed at a petite version of Sadie with waist-length, shiny, auburn hair flowing on a breeze. Her eyelashes went on for days above big, sparkling, brown eyes, which highlighted the most amazing pink-lipped smile I'd ever seen. She was wearing cutoffs with pink Nike's and a hot pink sweatshirt that read *Choose Happy!* in purple.

Speechless, I handed Paul his phone, touched his shoulder, handed him the box of Kleenex, and walked back out the door. I went down the hall to the bathroom and cried. I'd never have realized that was Sadie.

I called my supervisor on my cell from the bathroom.

"Do they know about this?"

"No. Not yet. Just don't say anything. The social worker is going to talk to them tomorrow. I know this is hard for you, but sometimes hard decisions have to be made."

"Hard for who? Who made the decision?" I insisted.

"I'll talk to you about it tomorrow. I promise."

"You should have talked to me about it today. More importantly, you should have talked to them! I don't need your promise. I don't need your talk."

Paul and Sadie knew nothing about the changes. I called Doc who knew nothing of the medication being discontinued, pulled the medication back out of drug destruction and gave Sadie her pill.

The next day I arrived to find Sadie had been signed up with hospice. Everything was being swept neatly under the rug. Paul and Sadie had no clue the decision had been made without them. They genuinely thought they'd made the decision solely on their own. Sadie's comment was the only thing that kept me from blowing the proverbial fuse.

"You know, Winkle? At first, I was angry! Who are they to tell me it's time for me to die? But they told me the decision was all mine. They were only giving me food for thought because they see me suffering. I realized they were speaking out of love." I winced as she continued. "I feel better than I have in a long time. Relieved, in fact. I wasn't going to win the fight, but I had no idea when to hang it up. Paul needed me to keep fighting. Now he just needs me to love him until the end." She smiled like an angel. "And that is easy."

Meanwhile, corporate demanded staff be cut even more. I was moved to a new hall, meaning I had that entire hall with thirty-two residents, half of the other hall on the same side of the building, and half of my original hall on the opposite side of the building. It was insane. It was *hard*. But more importantly, it was dangerous. The change took us from having three nurses on duty to two, with both nurses having to run all different directions. I spoke up to the director, as my conscious would *not* allow me to stay quiet.

"You know this isn't safe. There is absolutely no way to provide prudent, thorough, proper, timely, effective, or safe care under these conditions. It's dangerous."

The Director of Nursing, Beva, smiled sweetly, cocking her head to the side, "Yes, I know, but you all are still here. None of you have resigned." She shrugged, turned, and walked away. Beva was implying that if we resigned, she would have ground to stand on to convince the corporate office we needed more staff. Otherwise, she was simply going to allow it.One catastrophic evening, I had a resident with chest pain on one hall, a fall with severe bleeding and a protruding bone on the second hall, and a leaking urinary catheter on the third hall. Sadie was the one with the leaking catheter, which resulted in Sadie being soaked in urine. By that point, Sadie was very near the end. Literally running, I quickly removed the leaking catheter, told the aid to change Sadie's linen, and put a brief on her until I could get back to replace the catheter. Having an aid holding pressure on the bleed, I ran back to the first hall to finish dealing with the chest pain.

Ultimately, the chest pain resolved with interventions. I sent the resident who had fallen out to ER. Finally, I headed for Sadie.

Paul was sound asleep in his chair, his head dropped to the side, drool at the lower corner of his mouth, his arms dangling toward the floor. The man was exhausted. I crept around him and froze, mid-step, as my eyes screamed to my weary brain, and my heart ripped right in two. Urine dripped off the mattress onto the floor like a slow-dripping faucet, pooling with the puddle already drying beneath the bed. Sadie had no brief on. The linen was never changed. And Sadie was dead.

My mind whirled!

Sadie! Sweet, precious Sadie took her last breath while lying in a chilly, malodorous lake of urine.

Willing away tears and nausea, I stood in front of Paul, blocking his view of Sadie. Waking him gently, I asked him to step out into the hallway so I could clean Sadie up. I was grateful beyond description that Paul was too groggy to ask any questions or insist on kissing Sadie's cheek before stepping out. He pushed up from the chair and stumbled out to the hallway, where he sat on the floor, leaned against the wall, and immediately fell asleep again.

Tiptoeing past Paul, I found someone to help me with Sadie and someone else to mop the floor. We got everything cleaned up, and Sadie was fresh as a daisy before I woke Paul, as I knew he'd go straight to Sadie's side and grab her hand. I tried to talk to him, but he rushed to Sadie's side, so I held my breath as he leaned down to kiss her cheek, then reached his free hand to her face, felt her cheek, and buckled. I grabbed him from behind and guided his frame down into the chair next to the bed.

Paul looked up at me, his eyes wide, glimmering with tears. His face was twisted with grief.

"I wasn't holding her hand!" he sobbed. "I let her down! I broke my promise!"

"Paul! You didn't! You kept your promise!"

His face to the floor, Paul shook his head violently as tears poured through his fingers and splattered off his boots.

Placing my hand on his shoulder, I shook him. "Paul, listen to me! Hear me! You kept your promise! You were sleeping, but her hand was in yours. She was gone before I woke you. I simply wanted you to get a little more sleep while we got her prettied up for you. I had to keep my promise to her, too. You put her hand in the hand of Jesus, just like you told her you would."

Paul looked up at me with the snotty face of a young boy, eyes begging for my words to be true.

"Paul, have I ever lied to you?" I asked with no conviction whatsoever.

That big man stood up and all but fell against me, sobbing, "Thank you! Oh, dear God, thank you!"

I held him up as long as I possibly could.

"Paul, sit down and hold her hand while I take care of things for you."

Paul sat obediently, gently taking Sadie's hand and kissing it.

By the time I made it back into Sadie's room, Paul had pulled himself together and sat quietly holding Sadie's hand.

Looking up as I walked into the room, he leaned over, and with his free hand he pulled a small wad of paper from Sadie's bag on the floor.

"Just take it. Don't look at it now, please," he whispered, his eyes tearing once more. Then, chuckling, he added, "Good Lord, you girls are goofy, but damned if you aren't the light of our lives!" He laughed softly, wiping his nose on his sleeve, "Thanks, Winkle, for everything."

I took the cue and left them alone. I stuffed the wad into my pocket and thanked God for keeping Paul asleep until I could get Sadie cleaned up. I could *not* imagine the pain with which that man would have had to live had he seen, had he known.

Anger resurfacing, I hunted down the aid who had left Sadie in such a manner.

"It was my break time," she quipped. "I was going to clean her up when I got back from break. But you got it. It's all good."

I wrote her up and sent her home right then.

She signed the write-up with a sarcastic smile, adding, "This don't mean nothin'. I'm glad to go home early. Thank you." Then she sidled out the door.

I reported her the next day.

She still works there today. And the facility saved a lot of money by having Sadie sign up with hospice. Thing is, Paul and Sadie thought Sadie had come for rehab. But the facility, they took Sadie knowing she had cancer and knowing they had absolutely no intention of paying for her treatment. Hospice was the facility's plan from day one.

Poof:

Remember the Prom King? Gilmer? The sweet man with the puppy-dog eyes. The one who unintentionally and much to his dismay made the ladies go wild?

Gilmer's son was concerned about his safety, his sense of wellbeing. Gilmer was confused, sometimes fearful, and his son had noticed the prom queen forever at Gilmer's side. He'd noticed her demanding personality, and he'd seen the fear in his daddy's eyes even before his daddy expressed fear of the prom queen. The family had, in fact, had to request the prom queen leave the room so they could visit with their father and grandfather privately. Ultimately, management had to get involved and insist she leave Gilmer's side so the family could visit him in private. At that point the family requested the prom queen be kept away from Gilmer as much as possible and that they never be allowed to be alone together. Thus, we were instructed to see to it that the two of them were never together out of our sight. This was complicated by the fact that Gilmer was often confused and easily influenced, and he considered the prom queen his friend when she wasn't intimidating him, resulting in his fear of her. He often forgot entirely that he was afraid of her.

"Why?" he asked, completely baffled, and a little aggravated. "She helps me a lot," he said when I encouraged him to keep a distance.

So we, the staff, tried to keep the two of them in line of vision at all times, but the four of us provided all aspects of care for an entire facility, which included numerous individual rooms, two shower rooms, a lobby, a large dining room, and four hallways. Needless to say, one evening, upon looking for Gilmer, who cannot be taken with us into another room while we provide care, I found him missing. Immediately, I called out, and the aid checked Gilmer's room as I ran to the prom queen's room. Finding her door closed, knowing she never closed her door, I knocked and opened it simultaneously, fully expecting to find Gilmer inside.

That said, nothing could have prepared me for what I saw as the door swung open.

There was Gilmer, brown eyes wide with fear as he lay on his back on prom queen's bed, prom queen straddling him, her hands on his cheeks as she tried to kiss him. He peered frantically around prom queen's wrist as the door bumped the wall. Seeing me, his face scrunched in confusion as he raised his palms into the air on each side of prom queen, who pierced me with icy blue eyes.

"Come on with me, Gilmer," I said quietly.

"Why does he have to come with you?" prom queen snipped as Gilmer struggled to get out from beneath her.

"It's best, sweetheart. His family wants him with the staff at all times."
I tried to explain without embarrassing her. "It's better if you just visit
in the lobby. Let him up now, and don't bring him back to your room,
please, ma'am."

I pushed Gilmer down the hallway in his wheelchair as prom queen
followed, by then genuinely lost as to what she had done wrong.

Later I documented the entire incident, leaving out prom queen's name
and all unnecessary details. I called Gilmer's son, as is required with any
incident, but got no answer, so I left a message requesting a return call.
I called prom queen's daughter and informed her of the situation. Then I
called the director of nursing and informed her.

The next afternoon, when I arrived at work, the director called me into
her office. She asked me to rewrite my nurse note and redo my related
incident report on Gilmer. She said, "It doesn't look good. Just leave out
the part where you found them on her bed."

I refused, of course. Nicely. Politely. But my note was appropriate and
accurate; so, I denied the request.

Poof!

The entire two pages on which I'd written my note just disappeared,
along with other pertinent documentation that had been written by
other nurses before and after my note. The entire incident was swept
under the rug. The director told me Gilmer's son had returned my call
that morning, and she'd told him I had called to let him know Gilmer had
fallen again. "But he's okay. No injury, so no harm done," she'd told him.

When First We Practice:

It has always been my practice to write my assessment, related meds,
allergies, etc. on the lab or x-ray results before contacting the doctor and
sending them over. This was intended to expedite effective treatment and
to save the doctor the time of asking for the same information. I also
drew a line beneath the results, indicating I'd reviewed all of them, then
initialed and dated beneath that line. Ultimately, I noted any related new
orders on the results as well to facilitate ease in tracking the issue, patient's
full status, communication with Doc, and orders received for intervention.

I had been doing my norm, as above, at this particular facility for over
seven months before I was asked not to do it anymore. It was explained

to me that it had just "always been their practice to scan in clean copies noted by the nurse, with nothing else on them". This happened after I had made a notation that a patient's lung sounds did not correlate with the chest x-ray results, which is pertinent when you're asking a doctor to treat a respiratory infection the x-ray failed to indicate.

I suppose the ADON was so accustomed to redoing my lab and x-ray results that she didn't realize she didn't need to. One day I was reviewing a patient's records due to an acute illness when I ran across urine culture results that I had handled.

What the heck? I puzzled as I stared at the ADON's initials on the report. *I know I processed, noted, and documented those results. I remember calling the lab to get them faxed over because they hadn't sent them yet. Where are my initials?*

Then I noticed. She had obviously placed a piece of paper over the line I'd drawn across the paper beneath the results (indicating I'd reviewed all), covering my date and initials and assessment data, allergies, etc. However, she had just as obviously failed to keep the piece of paper straight while making her "clean copy," as the last of my line was still visible on the new, clean copy. Further, she'd changed the date to reflect that the results were received and noted by her on the same date the specimen was collected and processed. What she failed to notice in her efforts to cover up something that didn't even need to be covered was that the results were culture results; therefore, it was absolutely impossible to receive, date, and initial the results the same day the specimen was collected. It takes five to seven days to grow a culture.

I pointed this out to the director. Not surprisingly, that new, clean copy was removed, a newer, cleaner copy taking its place in the records, this time with an appropriate, yet false, date of notation. The other, not-so-clean copy joined my original in the abyss of lost truth.

Zero-Deficiency Survey:

What is it?

The state surveys each long-term care facility annually. A zero-deficiency survey means the state found nothing 'significantly wrong with/at the facility'. This meaning, from my humble yet educated perspective, that the state didn't find your stuff. Every time I've experienced a state survey, directly or otherwise, I've wondered how the facility passed at all.

When one gets zero deficiencies, I marvel at just what the heck the state did while in the building. This, I hesitate to say, as we certainly don't need more "state regs." In fact, we need less. What we need is a systems overhaul based on use of good ole not-so-common-at-all common sense.

I digress. So this facility had a running record of zero-deficiency surveys. Corporate had an intricate, motivational reward system for their facilities that promoted census focus and encouraged employees to go the extra mile so that, ultimately, corporate made more money. A zero-deficiency survey was part of the criteria for a facility to win the prestigious corporate award, and of course, the administrator and director of nursing get a nice bonus if they win.

This facility had banners hanging in the back hallway, celebrating so many years of zero-deficiency surveys. They passed out victory t-shirts, which, in effect, advertised the facility when worn in the community. Truth: if you want to see a hopping facility, go visit during survey. You will see faces in the hallways that are otherwise rarely, if ever, seen outside an office. That is the one time of the year that everybody is concerned with and actively involved in patient care.

So, back to my point, this facility had a meeting every weekday morning, and in this meeting they completed a finely tuned, highly intricate process involving multiple checkpoints to ensure documentation was complete. If a nurse failed to document "no adverse reaction to the multivitamin," the system would catch it, and the nurse would be called in to correct the horrific omission. And yet this same facility missed significant care issues. For example, Oma's missed renal ultrasound and urinalysis. Mavis's missed colonoscopy, even though she had a history of cancer, and later had a diagnosis of colon cancer. Where is the finely tuned, intricate system for ensuring patient care? For ensuring quality of life? How do you hold this lengthy meeting every day while your staff literally blows water up a lady's nose for weeks, your housekeeper mops the resulting puddle from the floor, and your aid changes the resulting saturated linen? And it continues day after day while you hold your meetings to ensure a zero-deficiency survey.

This same director was literally perturbed when I stumbled across and addressed an abnormal urine culture from two months prior, which was never treated, and the patient's urine had by then turned deep red with blood. I was at home when she blew my phone up to ensure I was aware that those results had been received, faxed to the doctor, and documented. I wondered if she realized how silly it made her look to point these things out, being unable to also point out where the urinary tract infection had been addressed and treated. After all, her nurses faxed things all the time that should have been called in so treatment would be immediately obtained. Regardless, it is the nurse's responsibility to stay on top of things until an answer is received from the doctor and said answer is documented and carried out. All the director managed to point out was that, yes, indeed, we knew about it, we received it, and we filed it, but we never obtained treatment for it. *That* is what she pointed out. But I let it ride. I was weary of her blowing up my phone. I had work to do in attempt to ensure quality care.

They carried on with their morning meetings, catching that omitted documentation, and chasing that prized zero-deficiency survey, which means nothing except that the state didn't find your dirt. You got dirt. You've all got dirt. I've seen your dirt. Better nail those rugs down. Hopefully, folks are about to come lift 'em.

Word Game

I'm a good nurse. Really. You can ask anyone. Though there are a few who would plead the fifth, not wanting to give me any credit or kudos. But I am no wound care expert. I can allow God to heal a wound via my hands, but it is solely Him who gets the credit. I am simply following His lead and applying common sense, which He gave me, so either way you look at it, the glory is His. That said, He did give me common sense, which I utilize regularly. It was just that which I applied the day I realized, without a doubt, that somebody had been playing the word game. Before that day, I'd had absolutely no clue the game existed. I guess I thought I'd seen them all. But nope. This was a new one for me.

So, our treatment nurse resigned. She was a good employee. She excelled in patient care, or seemed to, and genuinely loved the people. She was kind to them. All in all, I think highly of her, and I don't give credit to anyone who doesn't deserve it. I think if one chooses to go into the people business, one best be ready to take care of the people, like it or not, and realistically, some people are hard to like. Regardless, if you go into the people business, you have got to take care of all the people.

Human error is one thing; lack of give-a-shit is quite another. She did; she cared. But she, too, was sucked in by the corporate game, lulled into deceit in order to excel in management's eye, gain recognition, and be considered valuable to the management team. This chick *needed* to feel important, bless her heart. Ultimately, she had other aspirations and stepped out of the position.

So we got a new treatment nurse. Suddenly, our pressure wounds soared in numbers. Now, this was partly due to the fact that the new treatment nurse didn't move like the old one. The old one moved as fast as the Road Runner for as long as the Energizer Bunny. In fact, if the new and the old started out at opposite ends of the hall, the old one would run the new one over as the new one took her third or fourth step. Just a difference in people. However, the rise in pressure wounds was, by far, more due to the fact that the new nurse did not share the same proficiency in terminology. She just wasn't an experienced player in "the word game." If she saw a pressure injury or wound, she called it just like she saw it: pressure. The old treatment nurse had a host of fancy words, I was told by the new one. Being a fan of the old one, and being a firm believer that one should form one's own opinion of others based on one's own experiences as opposed to the opinions of others, I hesitated to believe such things. In fact, I defended the old treatment nurse, saying, "Hold up, now. Have you witnessed this, or is this simply your conclusion after pondering the rationale behind the increased number of pressure wounds under your care?"

I still don't regret the question; it's a valid question. But I did have the opportunity to witness the word game up close and personal. I stood at the bedside of an extremely large patient while the charge nurse and aid rolled him to his side so the old treatment nurse could look at his backside, as the aid had reported breakdown. I was only there to start an IV for the charge nurse.

Because I was standing on that side, I saw the pressure wound myself. Had this been an admission, it would have been documented as a pressure wound. Naturally, as the hospital would be responsible for it. However, the patient being one of our own, having been in our care during the development of the wound, we would be responsible for it. And, pressure wounds effect the facility numbers, or ratings. However, much to my surprise, the old treatment nurse glanced and said, "Friction wound." Just like that, "friction wound."

I leaned in closer, examining the appearance of the wound. Then, not being a wound care expert, I said, "Wouldn't a 'friction' wound exhibit signs of 'friction'? Wouldn't that look more like an abrasion than a non-blanchable red area?"

"Nope. Friction wound. It's not over the coccyx. A pressure wound is only over a bony prominence," she replied, nodding her head rapidly and smiling like she had won a prize, she knew more than *the RN.*

"Okay" I shrugged. "You the expert, but it sure looks like it's over the sittin' bone."

"The sitting bone?" She laughed as we walked out together and up the hallway.

"Yeah, the two rounded bones at the base of the pelvis that we sit on, the curve of the ischium bones, the sittin' bones. You probably don't know because you don't sit still long enough to feel yours."

"And you probably do know because you're so skinny you feel yours as soon as you sit down, because you don't sit any more than I do." She laughed, but she didn't turn around and reassess, and she didn't change her verdict.

Later that night she had been doing her notes for a little while when I walked out to say good night. She stood, rubbed her butt checks, chuckled, and said, "I know what you mean now. My sittin' bones are aching."

"Yeah, and you rubbing right about where her "pressure wound" is. I mean, her friction wound." I winked.

"Hey, friction doesn't count against us." She smirked, flashed me a thumbs up, and winked back.

Haglund:

Haglund had fallen at home prior to being hospitalized with a urinary tract infection. His right wrist, knee, hip, and ankle were all x-rayed in the hospital due to pain. Some were noted as red and swollen, but no fractures or dislocations were found.

Haglund continued with persistent complaints of right knee pain to the extent that it interfered with his therapy.

I asked the doctor if I could repeat the x-ray, which ultimately indicated no injury same as the hospital's x-rays.

I then told the charge nurse, "Maybe we need a CT scan to see if there's a hairline fracture or some such that the x-ray is missing."

"They're not going to want to pay for a CT scan," she replied. (they being administration because the patient was skilled, meaning the facility pays for everything)

"Well, what if he can't do his therapy?"

"He can take a pain pill and hit it!" She grinned like a champion.

"What if he's walking on a hairline fracture and we make it worse by pushing?"

"They can find it after he goes home." She flashed that champion grin again.

That's why she's in training to become an assistant director of nursing and I resigned from director, I thought to myself. *I'm just not comfortable with the line of thinking corporate nurtures and demands.*

"Okay," I blurted, "What if it were your daddy's knee?"

She cocked her head to the side. "I'd take him home and get his knee scanned."

"Well then?"

Raising her palm, she interrupted, "I don't make the rules."

"Is quietly following them any less wrong, I wonder."

No comment.

The next day I braced myself for termination or, at a minimum, a butt chewing. I went down to see Haglund.

"No, my knee feels better today." He chuckled, mystified. "Thing has been hurting every day for weeks, and then suddenly I wake up this morning, and it feels like a new knee." Haglund shrugged, grinning.

"Thank you, Lord," I whispered as I trekked back up the hallway, no longer needing to take a stand that would likely cost me my job.

P,P, & D:

Per Patient Day (PPD) calculations are determined by the number of residents in a skilled nursing facility (census) and the number of clinical staff caring for them each shift. Notice, all based strictly on numbers. No level of care considered whatsoever.

I counted one day. Large facility with one hundred and ten residents/ patients. I'd just returned to my office after waiting to inform the charge nurse of new orders I'd obtained on one of her residents. While I waited, standing quietly next to her, in a whopping three-minute time span, said charge nurse was "needed" for one reason or another by seven different people. I repeat, in three minutes time.

Having been a charge nurse for many of my twenty-eight years, I knew just how much she had hanging over her head that was yet to be done and how many more needs would arise as she tried to do it. And that is simply the daily do in the nursing world. That morning I'd noticed the pile of fifteen IV bags she had to hang in the same hour, most of which would finish dripping back to back, beepers going off like slot machines in a casino.

Just a few minutes before, I had been hurrying back from another unit when I passed the conference room. It had struck me how many people sat around that table, sitting through those endless and multiple daily meetings, while one nurse on the unit I had just left had sixty individuals in her care. One nurse/sixty patients. And said nurse was to supervise the medication aid and three nurse aids while providing nursing care to those sixty people, all while running to grab ice, juice, coffee, and sandwiches; answering the phone; sending and receiving faxes; reviewing lab results; listening to concerns and complaints; talking to families, doctors, staff, and supervisors; hunting supplies; checking on meds; ordering meds; and documenting, documenting, documenting…

As I turned the corner into my office, I caught a glimpse of several administrative personnel farther down the hallway. They were talking and laughing amongst themselves as they also headed to the afternoon meeting. A thought struck me. I stopped, counted, sat down, counted again, called the charge nurse in, and asked her to count.

"Just real quick. I know you're swamped, but count the heads in the offices." I looked Shanna in the eye.

"Okay." Her gaze shifted to the ceiling as she mentally counted. "Eleven?"

"You're missing some." I laughed. "Name them off as you count."

Shanna began naming and counting on her fingers, her eyes growing wide.

"Twenty!" Shanna exclaimed.

"Yep, twenty heads in the offices. Twenty-one if you count the marketing position."

Shanna stared at me.

"Now count floor staff."

Again, her gaze shifted, but only briefly. "Nine."

"Yep."

"Damn!"

"Yeah, twenty people! Twenty administrative staff handling the "business," and *nine* people on the floor providing the actual back-breaking daily care, nursing and basic. Nine people striving to meet the endless needs of one hundred and ten individuals. Twenty staff to handle the business end of 'caring for people.' Nine staff members to provide the care. Twenty people to push the pencils, and nine to push the meds, carts, shower chairs, beds, and wheelchairs. Oh, and to answer the incessant phone when the twenty are *too busy*." Topper? Census gets what they consider "low"? First thing they do? Every time? Without fail? They make those nine people take longer lunch breaks to help the PPD; in other words, to save corporate money. From my long-educated-in-the-real-world-perspective, that means an additional fifteen minutes of working off the clock, as I have never had time to take the thirty minute lunch break, so how am I going to take a forty-five minute break and meet all the needs? In fact, if it were not for the timer on my cell phone, I would never remember to clock back in, as, without fail, I get busy, too distracted to remember to punch back in without the reminder. Sometimes I'm not able to stop whatever it was I've gotten busy doing to go clock back in when the alarm sounds, so I end up forgetting, anyway.

On the flip side of that nasty coin, let state come in. Ha! Those forty-five-minute breaks come to an instant halt. In fact, no one is allowed to leave the facility for break. They want it to appear as if we always have plenty of staff to meet the needs, so actual breaks are eliminated, and pizza is brought in to make the staff feel better about not getting a real break.

Sadly, everyone is so desensitized to the realities of long-term care life that they don't even stop to consider the irony of it anymore. It's just, "Oh, state is in the building, so it's thirty minutes again? Okay." So they clock out, grab some pizza, scurry back to the floor to break their bodies some more, and then thirty minutes later they run, clock back in, grab another piece of pizza, and scurry right back to the floor.

"That's our biggest expense," the round-faced administrator with the fancy cowboy boots replied when I finally asked one day why staff was always cut when census dropped a little.

In twenty-eight years, I have never *personally* seen a business position cut. Never. Not once.

At night, from ten p.m. to six a.m.—or in other cases, from 6:00 p.m. to 6:00 a.m.—there are seven people to provide care for the one hundred and ten residents and patients. Seven. Ludicrously, it may initially be tempting to think as corporate does, "Well, they're sleeping." Chuckle, smirk, patronize.

But stop. Think. We are talking about *people*. People who have been living their own lives their own way, keeping their own schedules for many years.Remember, Emerald, the lady who only came out of her bat cave at night? Slept all day? Emerald has a multitude of associates.

'Doin.' Love me some Doin! Doin sleeps most of the day and gets up every evening around eight p.m. Often working late, I found this out when he repeatedly popped up outside my office door late in the evening, poking his sleepy eyed face in and asking, "Doin?"

Laughing, I'd respond, "I'm working, dude. What do you think I'm doin'?" Then Doin' would roll off, looking for a snack to snatch.

Mr. Coffee, a chronic, life-long napper, slept for three or four hour stretches throughout the day and night, spending his waking hours in one of three ways: drinking coffee, seeking coffee to drink, or walking off the coffee he already drank.

Bea, over five hundred pounds, could not turn over in bed to save her own life. Her body was just too heavy, bulky, and cumbersome. She was so enormous that once she finally managed to move a leg, it was literally the momentum of the fat itself that propelled Bea forward as she slowly waddled her way from place to place with the aid of her extra wide walker. And yet that lady still managed to "sneak" food. She quietly consumed many employees' lunches, along with many cakes that were tucked away in the break room, awaiting some celebration. And without fail, Bea still slipped away and made her way across the building each evening to eat the remains off the dinner trays sitting on racks outside the kitchen door, awaiting the attention of the dishwasher. Ultimately, Bea's blood sugar would be up requiring insulin and monitoring. Further, when Bea fell, it took time, energy, and all available staff to get her back up off the floor. Bea was too heavy for the mechanical lifts to be utilized to lift her. She had a habit of sitting on the toilet for long periods of time, frequently falling asleep while doing so. I'll never forget the night she fell asleep and slid off the toilet, landing so that her head, shoulders, and one arm were pinned into the small space between the toilet and the wall. I still marvel that we managed to get her up without first removing the toilet. Though I did inspect what doing so might entail during my struggle to think of just how we were going to manage the impossible. How five or six of us were going to fit into that tiny bathroom, with that enormous lady covering most of the floor space, while still finding room to brace ourselves so we could use every muscle we had to lift her massive weight…well, that had me baffled. But though it broke our backs, we managed to do just that. Bea, too, was a night owl.

And of course, as everyone knows in the world of long-term care, as the sun sinks lower in the sky each day, confusion's shadows come out to play. Confusion mutates into fear and suspicion as light changes to night, pulling shades over the windows of reality, obscuring the view, thus changing the valid and logical to strange and bizarre. Very often, this causes even the fully grounded by day to drift afloat by night. Staff are faced with the additional challenges of effectively managing a vast variety of resulting behaviors as darkness plays its tricks on the mind.

Not long ago I stood at the nurses' desk at about nine-thirty p.m., updating the charge nurse on new orders, when I caught a glimpse of a gowned figure entering the dim hallway from one of the rooms on the right. Instinctively straining to see more clearly, I leaned forward as skinny legs stumbled across the hall. The figure stood facing the wall, knobby knees slightly bent, arms up, randomly pressing hands against the wall as if trying to find the spot that opens the magic door.

Squinted eyes locked on the figure, I wondered aloud, "Who the heck is that? And what are they doing?"

The staff immediately turned their heads in the direction of my gaze, and the two aids were already running toward the figure. "That's Mr. Sanders," they yelled over their shoulders. "He wanders at night."

Mr. Sanders? My quiet, soft-spoken, well-mannered book worm? I thought incredulously, my mind instantly shifting into high speed and reverse, ultimately slowing as images of Pam entered my mind. She was a shy, highly intellectual loner who surprised me one night as she exploded from her room, stripping off her clothing as she hurried down the hallway to "hide from the aliens" who had come into her room, taken her gown, and then dressed her so that they could take her to their spaceship.

Night may bring a different movie, but the theater is far from closed.

And bear in mind, most medical emergencies/deaths occur at night as well.

That's the thing about one nurse with thirty to sixty patients/residents and the decreased staff at night. There's never enough care-providing staff at any time, day or night. Staffing ratio decisions are made by people who have never provided any actual care, based on a problem-free scenario, as if *people* are ever problem free.

It speaks volumes that the long-term care industry *exists on the needs of people*; exists on the very fact that *'people' need 'people' to provide 'care' for them*. And yet there are over two times more office/business staff than there are *caregiving staff*. Add to that the fact that, if census drops a bit and staff is cut, it's the *caregiving staff that takes the cut*. One human being can only do so much, can only be in one place at a time. *When you cut the caregiving staff, you cut the care*; and *the care is what you are in business to provide*.

"That's our biggest expense," the administrator had said in reference to the caregiving staff.

"No, sir," I wish I'd said. "That's your tool of the trade. The caregiving staff are what you use to do the job that you're in business to do, to provide the services that you are in business to provide."

That is much like a carpenter deciding to cut the expense of a hammer.

One more thing. It sums up the stark reality of the long-term care industry's true attitude in just a few words.

Our regional director of operations (RDO) came to our facility one day to push, threaten, and talk budget and census. Looking all slick in his Italian leather shoes and his expensive tailored suit, he gazed around at us with his piercing green eyes, and in just a few words, he verbally painted a crystal clear picture of corporate's perspective, attitude, and *feelings* (if you will).

The man actually said, and I quote, "Get heads on those pillows. I don't care whose heads they are. Just get heads on those pillows."

That's what you are, what your loved one is, to corporate: a head on a pillow.

They thought they were just being silly; they didn't realize they were becoming desensitized, becoming corporate-minded. But after the meeting, some of the office staff were laughing because one said, "What are we supposed to do? Go to Walmart and start tripping old people?"

Ms. Teenie:

Something red in the corner of my eye, caught my attention. Looking up, I glanced down the hallway. There she was in her long, red, zip-up robe, hanging limply over her bony shoulders. Her skin was so brown that, from a distance, when she blinked, the fuzzy white tuft of hair topping her tiny little head was the only determining feature. Holding to the siderail, Ms. Teenie tottered doggedly up the hallway.

Knowing, from report, that she was a high fall-risk, I slammed the drawer and hurried her way.

"What are you doing?" I laughed. "Where's your wheelchair?"

Ms. Teenies' huge, chocolate-brown eyes sparkled with mischief as she skillfully batted her eyelids, shimmied her knobby little shoulders, cocked her little nugget head to the side, and flashed me the most beautiful snaggle-toothed smile one could possibly imagine. Ms. Teenie was a practiced expert at winning hearts. The woman had it down!

"Oooh, look at you, Ms. purty thang! I was just going to get out and sees who all I might knows in here, say hello." Her eyes widened innocently, and her slender hand raised, palm up.

"Ms. Teenie, you know you supposed to use your wheelchair, so you don't fall." I slipped my arm under hers, just in case.

"Oh shucks." She dismissed me with a wave of the same hand that had demonstrated such innocence just seconds before. "That's that boy of mine's doin'. He say I'm gone fall, but I been a'walkin' for eighty-fo years now. I think I knows how to do it all right." Her lips pooched into a dramatic pout just as heart-winning as her snaggle-toothed smile.

So, I met Ms. Teenie. She had been admitted to the facility that day due to heart problems causing her blood pressure to suddenly, and without warning, bottom out. This had resulted in multiple recent falls at home. Problem was, there was absolutely nothing more that could be done to resolve the issue. The hope was to strengthen her muscles, steady her gait with therapy, teach her to use an assistive device consistently, and to, of course, keep her off the floor in the meantime. With Ms. Teenie, I could clearly that see the latter two were going to be significant challenges!

Ms. Teenie adored her son, bragged on him constantly, and it appeared to be mutual, as David was there nearly every day. He and his wife brought Ms. Teenie everything imaginable in an attempt to keep her comfortable. David's wife swept Ms. Teenie's room every day to keep Ms. Teenie from fussing about "all that mess on the flo." David tried hard to keep his mama happy, despite her wanting to go home. He wanted what was best for his mama. Ms. Teenie, like the rest of us, wanted what she wanted, regardless. Thus, they were at frequent odds, but they mostly loved and laughed.

David was an intelligent, dignified man. He and his wife were both extremely polite, and David never met a stranger. He and I had many interesting conversations about a wide variety of topics. David was an excellent judge of character. He accurately pegged many people during the time we knew one another; and he knew quickly that I genuinely loved his mama, and that I could be "trusted."

Ms. Teenie's second day proved her to be a social butterfly. She was out and about, and she discovered that she knew several other residents. Over time I'd often run across Ms. Teenie in the rooms of other residents, although she refused to revisit "that mean old bitty" Ms. Viola. Sometimes Ms. Teenie had her wheelchair; other times she didn't. She kept us running for the first several weeks, and we still picked her up off the floor six times the first two weeks. I was starting to think her skinny bones were made of rubber; the little woman looked much like a stick figure with enormous eyes. Gradually, Ms. Teenie began to use her chair, but it took a thousand reminders a day and a diligent watch.

One evening I walked in, and Ms. Teenie was watching television. She looked over at me with a smirk and said, "You know, I's smart. I don't just lays in here doin' nuthin'. I be thinkin'." She tapped her temple with her bony finger, then cocked her head to the side of her pillow, her bottom lip snagging on that top tooth when she smiled. "I saw something on the TV a while ago. It was one of them crafty shows, and they hung they rakes upside down, then used the rakin' part to hang stuff on! You know, for organizin' stuff and all. I'm gone try that in my carport when I gets home," she finished smugly. "Mmmhmm."

"That is a good idea." I leaned over to check her blood pressure. "Ingenious."

"Now, iffen I can only figure out how to keeps these peoples from takin' my stuff at night while I be sleepin', at least till I can gets back home." She scowled. "I mean, they be comin' in here when I be sound sleep, and they go through my stuff, takin' what they be wantin'."

"What are you talking about."

"My hair grease! I keeps it right there in that drawer, where I keeps my sugar!" Her big brown eyes narrowed to slits. "And last night I woked up, and that girl...that sassy, lazy one." She shrugged. "Well, that don't help none, cuz most all of 'em is lazy. Last night I just happen to wake up, and when I did, that sassy one that work at night, she was pullin' my hair grease out my drawer!" She pouted.

"What'd you do? You tell anybody about that?"

"She gone go and ask me after I done woke. She ask can she borrow it. Hmph. I tole her naw! I tole her had she woke me up and ask me, I'd of said yeah. But since she try to sneak it, I'm sayin' naw. She put it up, but they done done that a lot. I jest caught 'em this time. Imma tell my son. I sho am. I done tole him before, but he didn't believe me. Guess he gone know now I was tellin' the truth!"

"I have no clue who you're talking about, but I'll report it to the director."

"That Beva? She ain't gone do nuthin' but stand around bein' bossy, thinkin' she purty, not doin' nuthin'. That one there is a snake in the grass. I bet she don't like you, not one bit." She chuckled, then squealed. "Lord have mercy! I bet she don't! You prolly make her plumb mad cuz you got principles! She only like them other snakes!"

Struggling not to laugh, I exited fast, listening to Teenie chuckle as I headed back up the hallway. *Her grammar may not indicate it, but the woman is sharp as a tack.* I smiled to myself.

The next afternoon I walked in, and Ms. Teenie was perched on the side of her bed, her bony legs crossed at the ankle, the picture of innocence.

"Okay, what's up?"

"Oh, nuthin'." She shrugged just a bit to largely. "I was just sittin' here waitin' on my son." She flashed me that beautiful snaggle-toothed smile, batted her eyes.

"Okay, spit it out. What are you not telling me?" I rolled my eyes. "I know that look."

Ms. Teenie squealed with delight. "Lord hep me, you calls 'em like you sees 'em! I likes that!"

Laughing, in spite of myself, I tried again. "Spit it out."

"Well, you see, I's gonna wash up for dinner, so's I went to the bathroom over there." She pointed her long, skinny finger. "What we havin' for dinner, anyway?"

"Nice try. I don't know. What happened?"

Ms. Teenie fell sideways on her pillow, laughing. When she finally stopped, she replied, "Okay, okay, I fell on the flo, but I got myself up, and I ain't hurt none, so it's all right. There now. I tole ya the truth. What's for dinner?" She batted her eyes again.

"Were you at least using your walker?"

Ms. Teenie just sat there blinking at me.

"Well?"

"I ain't sayin'."

"Nuff said. Use your walker. I prefer your wheelchair, but at least use your walker, please, ma'am."

"So what we havin' for dinner? I want me some greens and cornbread. My son say he gone bring me some. I sho hope he do."

"Me, too, Ms. Teenie. You turn sideways, and I lose sight of you." I chuckled as I checked her for fall-related injuries.

After several weeks Ms. Teenie ran out of skilled days, as is always the case. Medicare only pays for so many days, and then the resident and families have to kick in a certain percent, and eventually they have to pay all or apply for Medicaid. In any case, David told me he didn't think Ms. Teenie needed to go back home and live alone, he wanted her to stay right where she was. He was about to go tell her and I didn't care to stick around for that. To top it all off, I knew well that the facility would charge David for that private room, or they would move Ms. Teenie onto another hall, into a room with a roommate. Another thing Ms. Teenie would blow a fuse about. I left David to talk to his mama, and I left the room-change business for the social worker to handle.

The next day I worked, David approached me, as always, to say hello and to discuss whatever topic came up. But that day he had a specific topic on his mind. David wanted my opinion on his mama being admitted to hospice. Apparently, the social worker had contacted him and suggested he consider admitting Ms. Teenie to hospice. David wanted to know why, as his mama wasn't in any pain. He said, "What are they going to do for her that you all aren't doing? Mama doesn't want hospice. She's said that for years, but that social worker thinks I should meet with them, consider it. What do you think?"

I told David the decision was entirely up to him and his mama, and I wasn't real sure what benefit it would serve other than the extra attention. "But I'm no hospice expert, so it wouldn't hurt to meet with them and see what they have to say in regard to how they might benefit your mama."

The following day the social worker informed me a meeting had been arranged with David and hospice for later that night and that David had requested I attend. The social worker then suggested I use the opportunity to encourage him to admit Ms. Teenie to hospice."

"She already signed a DNR, didn't she?" I was confused.

"Oh yeah, a while ago."

"Then what do we care what they decide about hospice?"

"Oh, you know, it's all about money. Just gently encourage. They trust you." She tossed her mousy brown hair over her shoulder as she walked away.

"No, I don't know. Yes, they do trust me. No, I won't encourage," I said to no one listening.

A while later, after being down the hall for a bit, I returned to the nurses' station only to find a doctor's order laying on my desk. The order was written by Karen, the Assistant Director of Nursing. It was discharging Ms. Teenie from her physician's care and admitting her to hospice, under the care of the hospice physician. I picked it up and stared at it, genuinely shocked.

She expects me to just sign this thing and process it, without Teenie or David having any clue whatsoever, I thought, horrified. *David hasn't even met with hospice yet, hasn't had an opportunity to even think about it, much less make a decision!*

I sighed. It seemed I was always having to create a wrinkle. But I was not signing that order. (Mind you, when a nurse takes an order from a doctor, he or she writes the order, and he or she signs the order. Karen didn't "take" the order from anyone, but she wrote it, then passed it to me to sign and process. As if I'd just slithered out from under the stupid but sneaky rock.)

My mind was racing. Karen must have seen my expression, because she walked over and stood in front of me on the other side of the desk, but continued her conversation with Beva over my head. I acted as if I hadn't seen her or her order, and I stayed busy with other things while I mentally processed the situation. Then I lucked out. Ms. Teenie's doctor walked in and stood just a few feet behind me, looking at a chart. He and I had grown to be good friends over the years. He was an excellent doctor and a good man. He had a sincerely caring heart. I turned around and casually commented, "Hey, Dr. K, I didn't know you didn't want to be Ms. Teenie's doctor anymore. What's up?"

"What?" His eyes were wide. "I didn't say that! I adore that spunky little lady. She's one of my favorite people!" His smile was genuine.

"Oh." I scrunched my brow. "Well, I have this order…"

"What order?" Dr. K stepped forward and snatched the order from my hand. He read it and looked quickly at Karen, who stood with her mouth gaping, her eyes wide. "What's this?" Dr. K snapped. "I never said I wasn't going to be her doctor, and I didn't refer her to hospice. What does she need hospice for? Who referred her? I'm her doctor. I didn't!"

"I'm sorry, Dr. K!" Karen stammered, her cheeks bright red. "There must be a misunderstanding. I'll get it cleared up!" She held out her hand for the order, glancing sideways at me.

I looked innocent and mouthed, "I'm sorry."

The order disappeared.

David and I met with hospice later that night, and the next day David told the social worker that he'd met with hospice and spoken with his mama, and they had decided against it. Ms. Teenie would not be admitted to hospice.

The next afternoon Ms. Teenie was still thinking about the whole thing.

"What I'd like to know is who brought this hospice thang up to begin with!" Her brow creased. "And why? I mean, who down there thinkin' I'm bout ta die, and why ain't they tole me?" Her eyes popped open wide.

Feeling her need to vent, I waited respectfully.

She shook her head, chuckling quietly. "I tell you one thang fo sho, I done got old, but I ain't got nowhere near stupid. Hmph! Somehow, they the ones gone gain from me a'goin' on hospice." Her eyes narrowed to slits. "I don't know how they gone gain, but they is." She slowly nodded her head in thoughtful silence for about two full minutes. Then she shifted her gaze to me, cocking one eyebrow. "Well…" She smirked. "They was! They ain't now!" She cackled, raising both of her little stick arms in the air. Lowering them, she reached out a knobby fist.

I laughed, bumped her fist as I turned to leave, and listened to her contagious cackle as I walked back up the hallway.

After dinner, David walked out of Ms. Teenie's room, shaking his head. "Mama said nobody ever gives her a shower."

The aid on duty overheard this, and before I could respond, she stood up from the chair, which she wasn't supposed to have in the hallway – again - then sauntered into Ms. Teenie's room, telling Ms. Teenie it was shower time and that she was going to warm the shower room.

David smiled. "Now that one's good. She does her job. She knows how to talk to Mama."

I smiled. (Not even an excellent judge of character is infallible.) "One day, when you read my book, remember this moment."

"You need to write that book; get it done." David said as he walked away, going back into Ms. Teenie's room. He and his wife left a few minutes later. "We'll see you tomorrow. Mama's in good hands. She's about to get a shower, so we're going to go on home now."

"Okay, see you tomorrow."

Coming back up the hall a short while later, I passed the aid, who was sitting in her usual spot, her face aglow as she busied herself with her cell phone.

The sun was shining bright the next day. I was in an exceptionally good mood myself. That morning was the morning this book took seed. For the first time in years, I had the hope of making a true difference for everyone in long-term care as opposed to just those in my personal care. Anyway, I had extra pep in my step as I headed down the hall. I walked into Ms. Teenie's room and opened the blinds to let the sunlight in.

"Goodness, it's a beautiful day!"

"Ooooh, just look at that sky!" Ms. Teenie clasped her hands and flashed me her snaggle-toothed smile. "Them clouds looks like cotton balls floating cross that blue sky."

"They are beautiful! So did your shower feel good last night?"

"Hmph. What shower?" Ms. Teenie snipped. "I didn't get no shower."

"But I thought the aid was warming the shower room for you."
I stopped and turned to face Ms. Teenie.

"Aww, she ain't gone do nuthin'! She talk the talk when my son here.
Soon as he gone, she gone, too. I done had me about five showers altogether since the day they rolled me up in here weeks ago," Ms. Teenie
drawled, her lips pooched in disgust. "I likes to be clean, so I don't for-
gets no shower. I ain't had nigh one in least two weeks now."

"Ms. Teenie! You gotta tell me these things. Speak up, woman!"

"Oh hell, I spoked up! I been asking them lazy aids to gimme a
shower, and I tole my son." She shrugged. "That got me nowhere right
quick. But I takes care of it myself."

"You're showering yourself?" I panicked!

"Aww! Naaaw!" she crowed, waved her bony hand in the air. Then
she smirked, shimmied her scrawny shoulders, and flashed me that
bottom-lip-jagging, snaggle-toothed smile. "I been at the sink, givin'
myself a polka-dot bath." She ended with her chin tucked, her lips
pooched, batting her big brown eyes, the very picture of facetiously
sweet innocence.

David:

As I said, David was an excellent judge of character. He was a dignified, intelligent man with integrity. But sadly, the best of the best can
be snowed. I wanted to tell him, but that would have been unethical.
I have wanted to tell many family members through the years. But David
and I talked. We shared our perspectives on a variety of topics. David
and I had become friends. I told David I was going to write this book.
I feel certain he had no doubt that I would do just that, though by now
he's probably decided I was full of hot air after all. I told him I would be
saying something to him when I got it written. So here goes:

> Hey David,
> I know how much you loved your mama. I loved her,
> too. That little woman's very bones were spunky and
> delightful! She was proud of you!

Thing is, that aid—the young cute one who "knew how to talk" to your mama? She is the same aid who was supposed to shower your mama. She is the same aid who stacked layers of folded blankets beneath residents' hips to soak up urine and keep her from having to provide incontinent care as often. She is the same aid who limited available fluids to those she considered "heavy wetters."

She is the same aid who requested to be moved off my hall because I made her work. And they moved her, all right. They didn't ask me a thing. They just met her request and moved her to another hall so she could stack folded blankets beneath others' hips and limit available fluids to other thirsty victims. I don't know, but I'm thinking it must be awfully uncomfortable lying in bed with a stack of blankets under your hips, thirsty because someone doesn't want you to urinate. The stack of blankets has got to be bad for the spine. It must hurt. And goodness knows, fluids are crucial to one's health, not to mention the discomfort of being thirsty.

David, the aid you saw was a completely different aid when you turned your back and walked out the door. Ms. Teenie was telling the gospel truth. That aid just put on a show for you. I tried to tell you with my eyes. Remember when you said, "Now that one's good. She does her job. She knows how to talk to Mama?" I tried to tell you indirectly when I immediately replied, "One day, when you read my book, remember this moment."

I love you, David. You are a good man. I loved and wholly adored your mama. She didn't suffer. You, your sweet wife, and I saw to that, so don't get upset. Let's just get busy. We need to work together and make changes.

Thing is, folks, David represents all the families. Now, don't misunderstand. There are some dynamite aids out there, some dynamite nurses. But many do not need to be doing what they do, and all of them—every single one of them—are overloaded.

I think what bothers me the very most is that all these nurses in administrative positions know. They know. They've been there. Nothing in this book will come as a genuine surprise to them, though they will certainly deny such. They know. "It's just how it is," they say. They'll shrug as they continue trying to "fix" things so they can obtain that prized but meaningless zero-deficiency survey.

Speaking of the state, I applied for a position with the state as a long-term care surveyor. I did. I thought that might be a way to help induce changes in both systems, thus making a difference for our elderly everywhere. I was called for an interview. The lady who contacted me initially—the one who had read my letter of interest and had seen my credentials—seemed genuinely interested in our elderly and eager to have me on the team. She "loved my passion for our elderly, my passionate desire to improve their lives in long-term care".

However, she was not the individual with whom I was to interview. I interviewed with two women. One conducted the interview while the other sat listening, saying absolutely nothing, not one word the entire interview. The conductor was very fashion-minded and apparently favored turquoise, as her skirt was turquoise. She also wore a few turquoise bracelets, a turquoise necklace, turquoise rings, and turquoise earrings. She sported a turquoise hair clip, and she wore turquoise framed glasses on her face, on which she had attached a turquoise lanyard. I know this is irrelevant. I just found it distracting, possibly entertaining, as she asked her questions, to which I responded as genuinely as I had been in my letter of interest.

Ultimately, I was asked if I had any questions of my own. By that point, I was far from impressed and was thinking my prior opinion of the state system, though not at all pretty, was likely too generous. Thus, I asked one question, thinking that if the answer was appropriate, I might be wrong in the opinion of which I was fast growing more convinced.

"What do you look for in a candidate for a long-term care surveyor position?" I asked.

- I can think of multiple appropriate responses that would be undeniably indicative of a focused intent to ensure the safety and well-being of our elderly, a true intent to provide genuine quality of life for our elderly.

• I did not receive such response.

Without hesitation, Turquoise responded, "We look for a candidate who will get along well with the group. We spend a lot of time together, we travel together and share the ride to save expenses, so it's important to choose an applicant who will get along well with the group." She smiled and pushed her turquoise glasses a bit higher on her nose, saying, "I'm thinking that's probably the most important thing to look for in a candidate."

I stood and stretched out my hand.

"Thank you for your time." I smiled. "I'm thinking I'm likely not a good candidate for the position, after all. Would you be so kind as to withdraw my application? Thank you, and I can show myself out."

I don't have a thing in turquoise, I chuckled to myself as I exited. *And I now understand how these facilities get zero-deficiency surveys, despite the fact, that so much is so horribly wrong. Maybe the great state needs to hire a few people that don't fit so well with "the group".*

Afterword

Knowing that I could go on forever, yet resisting the burning desire to do so, I am stopping here. I can only hope the things I needed to say have been said, that they aren't buried in this enormous stack of papers, scribbled notes, and notepads filled from first page to last next to my chair. Sadly, this is not even all of them. I never even opened the second box filled with more of the same. However, time is of the essence.

Fully cognizant that some hearts will be touched and that some will not, it is time I sent this ship out to sea. I've been asking myself, "What is it that I need to tell people that will strike the chord that moves them? Which picture can I paint that will touch hearts, making people want to love one another?" Frustratingly, as purely mind boggling as it is, I have seen hearts untouched as they lived and created these very same stories. Of course, some, if not many, who read them will not be touched, will not feel a thing. But that, my friends, is what it is, and it is a large part of the problem with the world today.

However, touched or not touched, the thing I would encourage all to remember is that you are no doubt up next. This *is* where you are headed. Now would be the time to make changes. You can carry right on avoiding seeing for yourself. You can deny things are as they are. You can keep stepping as if your steps lead elsewhere. Those are your choices. But your steps are very likely leading you into a star role in a story very similar to the ones you've just read, or worse.

The people within these pages are real people, with real hearts and real spirits. Real people who, just yesterday, beat a path very similar to the one you beat today. These are real people who traveled the same roads, thinking that where they are now was just as far away, even impossible, as you are thinking it is. Truth? It's right around the corner, waiting for you. Waiting to stash your pain and misery, maybe even your untimely, unnecessary death, on the dusty shelves of the societal closet.

Thing is, if you were to go around asking many of these system-saturated elderly people—the vulnerable as well as the not so vulnerable—they would give you different answers on different days. I know because I've done it. I've asked them if they are happy, if they feel safe and respected, if life is good, and if they ever look forward to tomorrow.

Sadly, and generally speaking, once they acclimate, the system becomes a way of life. They, themselves, literally fade from their own minds and become distant but fond memories. Gradually, without even realizing it, they give up anticipation, sacrifice hope for acceptance, and quiet their thoughts so that acceptance will come easier. They simply become the victims of the corporations. They breathe through the motions while they unconsciously wait for the breathing to stop. Many refer to it as the individuals' "adjustment". I rather see it as their surrender. In fact, as said in Elderly Elementary, for many, once they walk in that front door, their light starts dimming, their spirit, their very essence begins to fade away, and they become like prisoners whose only crime was growing old.

I'm not certain what hurts my heart most: our elderly's quiet surrender, or those moments when they realize the horror of what they've unconsciously allowed by succumbing to mere existence. My heart aches as I watch the thunderstorm of emotions surge through them as they scramble to hear their own voice and remain strong, alive, while resignation already threatens to cover them like an old blanket.

I've heard it thousands of times: "People come here to die."

I've responded a thousand times: "So, live. Live until you die."

I've been asked a thousand times: "How? How can I *live* here?"

To top it all off, we take them from their homes, even from the streets, and stick them into a place in which they can be cared for, be safe from harm. And then we fax critical lab values, instead of calling the doctor, as we would do for ourselves. We risk their sight and just keep on administering ultimately toxic eye drops because we are too lackadaisical to stop and think, too lackadaisical to do for them as we would do for ourselves. Simply put, many simply don't care, others do, but due to the realities of the nursing world, near all ultimately give up. We skip pertinent medications and treatments because, by dang, we are getting off on time. After all, we have lives to live, families to care for, things to do. We leave helpless human beings soiled by feces, soaked in urine, miserable and malodorous because there is more work than one person can possibly do, so we do just enough to get by, get off and go home. We control their meals and snacks, literally lock away whatever we determine their only option will be, as if we ourselves want someone telling us what we can have, how much, when, or if we can have anything at all. On that note, I have always marveled at the snack trays. I have wondered who it is that has mistaken nurses for Jesus, thinking nurses, also, can feed the masses with just two fish. I ultimately started keeping a supply of individually wrapped snacks in my car, and I've bought snacks from many a vending machine, solely because my heart cannot bear hearing a nurse, or nurse aid, tell a hungry person, "We're out. We don't have anymore". We lose sight of important tests and procedures in the shuffle, which ultimately costs the lives of those we forced to rely on us to provide care and keep them safe. We ignore significant issues because we don't have time to address them, so that 'person' pays the end price, the person we assured we'd take good care of. We do not, in any way, do unto others as we would have them do unto us.

It has always turned my stomach to watch the masked faces of most, not all, administrative personnel as they listen to the concerns of the residents/patients, responding as if they, too, are concerned, and then disregarding the individual just as soon as the individual walks or rolls away, sometimes laughing at them, stripping them further of their dignity. Their only true concern is preventing the individual from calling in a complaint to the state.

Every single administrator and every single director of nursing *knows* their facilities are understaffed, even when *fully* staffed. They keep quiet, pretending otherwise, just to keep their jobs, just to keep from making the effort to seek change, just to keep from having to be the one to 'stand up and speak truth'.

Corporations insist on staffing as if they are providing a service to healthy, robust individuals who simply need someone to give them their medication, check their blood sugar, wipe their behinds, give them a shower, and provide three meals a day. Done, son. This is far from the reality of the population they serve. The level of care needed by those in long-term care is even far greater than what it used to be. The level of nursing care provided on "skilled" units is identical to the level of care needed and provided on med/surge units in hospitals, where the nurse to patient ratio is 1:6. However, in LTC the nurse to patient ratio is sometimes around 1:15, but is most often 1:30, and occasionally it is around 1:60, which is insanely unsafe. For that matter, it is inhumane for both the ones needing care, as well as the ones struggling to provide it.

There is a balance, people. We need to find it.

We keep trekking through and adding to a system we all know is broken. We exert great effort to hide, cover, fix, and deceive instead of using that effort to stand up, speak out, and seek change.

We move our elderly people around like checkers on a board. John didn't know he had shoes for over two years, but the facility had successfully moved him from his room to another, emptying that hall he had been on, so they could cut staff, save corporate's bottom line, and make sure those at corporate still got their bonuses. They got their bonus, but John had no *shoes*. Can you imagine how different the world would be if people extended even half the time and effort walking a solid path as they extend scrambling to cover their tracks through the mud?

Think about it: We created the system. We work the system. We ignore the outcome of the system while we feed the system. We are the system. We are all guilty. The negligent way we, as a society, handle the lives of our elderly is a crime that we are all committing, even those of you who commit by proxy.

If we don't buck up, buttercup? We, too, will be sentenced *there*, sentenced to life in the system.

You are up next. This *is* where *you* are headed. *This* is *there*. We need change. We are an intelligent people. Change is possible. All we need is the heart to make it. Without a doubt, our elderly people are suffering, and it's past time we stepped up and put a stop to it.

State regulatory bureaucracies? *Sit* down! Work on your own system. It too, is broken. Many of you match, or exceed, your benefit with your harm. And yet you push on, going through the motions to draw a check while knowing full well your system is not working. This makes you just as guilty as anyone else, more guilty than some.

We are all human. We all fall short. What makes the difference between right and wrong is what you do about it when you fall short.

I truly have no desire to cause anyone any grief. I have every desire to help our elderly. I have told you nothing short of truth. I can tell these stories, and many more, because my conscious is clear, my pillow is soft. If yours' is not, if reading this made you angry, or defensive, I encourage you to ask yourself why, and make some changes.

The sequel, the why, is coming. You now have a fairly good idea of *how* it is *there*. Now you need to know the *why*.

One last thing: Love one another.

Conclusion

My hope is that you now see where our elderly are now, which is where *we* are headed, some sooner than others. My hope is that you, too, now desire change. My hope is that you now see how badly change is needed and how long over-due it is.

Developing and implementing more state regulations is not the answer. Not only is it *not* the answer, but it is a large part of the problem. There are already regulations to regulate the system, and then there are regulations to regulate the regulating regulations.

We are talking about the lives, happiness, and well-being of human beings, of individuals. State bureaucracies know absolutely nothing about individualization. They not only lack the ability to think outside of the box, but in many cases, they construct the box and then nail it shut.

What our elderly need is genuine love and respect which is nothing short of what they deserve. Our elderly *need* for us to step up and resolve the problems related to their care, or lack thereof.

There are solutions. One must first want to find them. However, one must first open one's eyes to see the problem before one can seek the solution.

I am just me. I am nothing special, no hero, no genius, and far from a saint. And yet I have worthy suggestions, and I am more than willing to stand. In fact, I am determined to stand. And if need be, I'll start kicking and screaming.

Why?

I care, plain and simple. That's why.

Do you?

You might want to think on that one.

Remember, and I repeat:

One undeniable fact is that if God doesn't grant you or me an early departure, if we don't have a ton of money to hire private caregivers to provide for us at home, and/or if we don't literally luck out in being one of those very rare souls who maintains good health, functional ability, mental clarity, and financial security until the day we die... we're up next! No doubt about it.

You *are* very likely headed *there*; without changes, you are *not* going to like it. Take it from one who is already there:

Every single time I arrived at work, and many times when I'd come from down the hallway, I would find Gilmer glancing about, searching for something that made sense. His eyes wide with fearful confusion, relief then flooding his face when he'd see me coming, as if life hadn't lost all semblance of order or hope, after all.

Folks, there are few feelings in this world that are half as good, or as significant, as knowing that someone who is lost, vulnerable, confused, and/or scared finds comfort in your presence, because one knows you genuinely care, one believes you can right one's world. Folks, there are few feelings in this world that are half as overwhelming, scary, or heart wrenching, as knowing that someone who is lost, vulnerable, confused, and/or scared finds comfort in your presence, because one knows you genuinely care, one believes you can right one's world. Yet you do genuinely care, and *you* know, that your being able to right one's world is as far from reality as is the voicemail that you will hear when you call that facility.

I stood from doing paperwork one evening and noticed Gilmer sitting in his wheelchair straight across from the desk, his eyes searching, his facial expression alternating between suspicion and baffled devastation, like switching channels back and forth between Sherlock Holmes and Armageddon.

Seeing me, he raised his chin. His bushy brows shot up, and his mouth flew open as he motioned me over, almost frantically.

I hurried to his side.

"What's up, my friend?"

As always, Gilmer asked, "What am I supposed to do?" his leathered palms raised midair.

Having been a busy, productive, successful, and highly active man, Gilmer simply could not understand what he was supposed to be doing there. Doing nothing was literally distressing the man; nothing was simply not something he'd ever dreamed, in his wildest imagination, that *he* would be doing.

Gilmer's grandson once told me, "Pappa Gil never could just sit and relax. He always told us that if we were sitting idle, something wasn't getting done." He chuckled. "Mamaw said she used to ask him to help her do things in the kitchen just to slow him down long enough to spend a little time with her."

Normally, when Gilmer asked what he was supposed to do, he would look up and gaze into my eyes while waiting for my reply. But that evening, before I could reply, Gilmer lowered his hands and continued in complete sincerity, his sad brown eyes scanning the lobby, saying, "You know? I never imagined life could get this bad. This is the worst life has ever been." He slowly shook his head. His bushy brow shot up, and his gaze lifted to mine. "Well, boot camp. I guess boot camp was this bad. But I knew if I hung in there, life would get better." He gazed around again, then looked back into my eyes. "I don't think this is ever going to get any better."

Because I value and respect my elders, because I genuinely love those in my care, and because I see the 'shadows in the twilight', I spoke the truth.

Pulling a chair up beside Gilmer, I sat down so we would be eye to eye.

"I don't know, Gilmer. I hope so. I hope it gets better. I know it's bad, and it's far, far less than you deserve. I can promise you two things." I smiled sincerely.

Gilmer locked his big brown eyes on mine and listened intently. "God is still on His thrown. He sees, He cares, and He is working in His way, in His time. He never leaves us, and He knows and cares about the desires of our hearts. Jesus even made certain to take care of His mother, Mary, as he hung, suffering and dying, on the cross."

Gilmer nodded his head, his expression reflecting deep thought.

"I feel certain He expects us to take care of our parents just as He took care of His. He'll move the right hearts. Hang in there. Secondly, my dear friend, I promise you that I will do anything and everything I can to make life better for you. I do care. And I cannot be the only one who does. Somebody will listen and help us make it better someday."

Gilmer smiled, wiped the moisture from his eyes, and mumbled, "Dear Lord, I sure hope so."

Thank you, Gilmer, for being you, for sharing *you* with me, and for sharing your heart in such a way that I grew even more determined to seek better. For you, my sweet, genuine friend, I will never stop trying.

Most importantly, a huge shout out to all the elderly people whom I have loved and who have loved me right back, no questions asked! I dedicate this book to those who have shared their hearts, their joy, and their pain. To those who have shared their spirits and their wisdom. And to you, my precious friends, who shared with me your last days and minutes on this earth. I am honored, and it is in your honor that I write this book. You are more than worthy, and you are far—so very far—from useless.

Lastly, thank you to all of you who read to this end. In doing so, you have already taken the first step toward a brighter future and a better life for our elderly, for yourself, for your loved ones, for your children, and even for me. You have taken the first step toward changing where our loved ones are and where we are headed.

Blessings!

We all travel *life's* highway which takes us from here to there, from start to finish. Regardless of the specific twists and turns our personal highways may take… ultimately, we all arrive...